The Regulation of Assisted Reproductive Technologies in Europe

This book explores the social, ethical and legal implications of assisted reproductive technologies (ART). Providing a comparative analysis of several European countries, the authors evaluate the varied approaches to the application of ART throughout Europe.

From a global perspective, countries take very different approaches to the regulation of ART. Countries apply restrictions to the access criteria for these treatments and/or direct restrictions to the practice of the techniques themselves. To understand these varied approaches to ART practice and regulation, it is necessary to understand the societal and political background from which they emerged. This book therefore consists of case studies from eight European countries which provide insights into the status and development of the regulation of ART in the last 40 years. The country cases from all over Europe and the three comparative chapters provide insights into the diversity of current ART regulation across the continent as well as into similarities, differences and trends in this regulatory area.

This book will be of interest to practitioners of ART who are interested in understanding the differences in regulation of ART in Europe, as well as long-term trends in this respect. Given the ethical and legal implications the book explores, it will also be of interest to students or researchers in the fields of social sciences, humanities and law.

Erich Griessler is a sociologist and head of the research group "Science, Technology and Social Transformation" at the Institute for Advanced Studies (IHS), Vienna, Austria. His research interests focus on the social, ethical and legal aspects of life sciences, including genetic testing, assisted reproductive technologies and xenotransplantation as well as responsibility and participation in research and innovation.

Lenka Slepičková is a sociologist working at the Olomouc University Social Health Institute, Moravia, Czech Republic. Her research interests focus on the fields of health, illness and medicine in connection with reproduction and family, inclusion, marginalization and stigmatization.

Heleen Weyers is a researcher at the Department of Transboundary Legal Studies of the Faculty of Law, University of Groningen, the Netherlands. Her research is focused on the coming into being of law (politics), its effects (sociology of law) and the relation between the two.

Florian Winkler is a junior researcher in the research group "Science, Technology and Social Transformation" at the Institute for Advanced Studies, Vienna, Austria. His research is mainly focused on controversial technologies (such as solar geoengineering, surrogacy or DNA-phenotyping) and the societal processes around them.

Nicolle Zeegers is Assistant Professor in Political Science at the Department of Transboundary Legal Studies, Faculty of Law, University of Groningen, the Netherlands. Her research interests include prostitution, assisted reproductive technology and other morality issues in a comparative law and governance perspective.

Routledge Studies in the Sociology of Health and Illness

For more information about this series, please visit: www.routledge.com/Routledge-Studies-in-the-Sociology-of-Health-and-Illness/book-series/RSSHI

The Regulation of Assisted Reproductive Technologies in Europe

Variation, Convergence and Trends

Edited by Erich Griessler,
Lenka Slepičková, Heleen Weyers,
Florian Winkler and Nicolle Zeegers

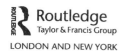

Routledge
Taylor & Francis Group

LONDON AND NEW YORK

First published 2022
by Routledge
4 Park Square, Milton Park, Abingdon, Oxon OX14 4RN

and by Routledge
605 Third Avenue, New York, NY 10158

Routledge is an imprint of the Taylor & Francis Group, an informa business

British Library Cataloguing-in-Publication Data
A catalogue record for this book is available from the British Library

Library of Congress Cataloging-in-Publication Data
A catalog record for this book has been requested

ISBN: 978-1-032-12240-3 (hbk)
ISBN: 978-1-032-26259-8 (pbk)
ISBN: 978-1-003-22372-6 (ebk)

DOI: 10.4324/9781003223726

Typeset in Goudy
by Apex CoVantage, LLC

Contents

Figures

Tables

Contributors

Ines Corti is Associate Professor of Private Law at the University of Macerata, Italy

Sven Geyken is a lawyer with the Georg-August-Universität Göttingen in Germany

Erich Griessler is a sociologist and head of the research group "Science, Technology and Social Transformation", Institute for Advanced Studies, Austria

Anna Krawczak is a researcher on the Interdisciplinary Team for Childhood Research, University of Warsaw, Poland

Magdalena Radkowska-Walkowicz is an associate professor, Institute of Ethnology and Cultural Anthropology at the University of Warsaw, Poland

Janne Rothmar Herrmann is a professor of law at the University of Copenhagen, Denmark

Anna Singer is a professor of private law at the University of Uppsala, Sweden

Lenka Slepičková is a researcher at Palacký University, Czech Republic

Heleen Weyers is an assistant professor of theory of law at the University of Groningen, the Netherlands

Florian Winkler is an STS-researcher at the Institute for Advanced Studies, Austria

Nicolle Zeegers is an assistant professor of political science, University of Groningen, the Netherlands

1 Introduction[1]

Erich Griessler and Lenka Slepičková

Assisted reproductive technologies: from experiment to normalization, sophistication and broadening the range of recipients

Today infertility is an "ongoing global reproductive health problem" (Inhorn & Patrizio, 2015, p. 411) for millions. In the late 1970s, assisted reproductive technologies (ART), including the most well-known technique, in-vitro fertilization (IVF), began as a set of experimental methods designed to overcome female infertility – tubal factor (Calhaz-Jorge et al., 2020). Using the term "artificial" pointed out that human reproduction was not achieved, as usual, via sexual intercourse but in vitro – in other words "artificially". This designation, however, also permitted associations with potential monstrosities which ART could give rise to (Herrmann, 2022; Krawczak & Radkowska-Walkowicz, 2022). For example, during parliamentary proceedings in the United Kingdom, the British Human Fertilization and Embryology Act was called the "Frankenstein report" (Fenton, 2006).

Despite such early reservations, ART in recent decades has become part of mainstream reproductive care. Today, ART is an option taken by many people who suffer from infertility for different reasons. These days, ART is presented and perceived as a conventional medical option that supports reproductive processes, as expressed in the name "assisted reproductive technology", a term which is now generally used.

Thus, ART made its way from an experimental therapeutic procedure to a standard medical intervention in less than 45 years. In 2016, the latest year for which comprehensive numbers are available, 40 countries in Europe reported 918,159 treatment cycles. Over the last few years, the number of cycles performed in many developed countries increased by 5–10% per year (ESHRE, 2020). It is estimated that worldwide, each year, around 2.4 million registered and unregistered ART cycles are performed, with about 500,000 babies born (Gallagher, 2012). In addition to growing numbers of treatments, the range of indications for ART – including male infertility – broadened, and the therapeutic effectiveness of ART increased. Most importantly, ART is no longer only employed for medical reasons in cases of impaired procreation but is also used to help single women and same-sex couples to have children.

DOI: 10.4324/9781003223726-1

The WHO, listing the wide variety of people who may require infertility management and fertility care services, explicitly broadens the group of persons using fertility services to include those whose fertility is not impaired in terms of physical inabilities to conceive but whose "infertility" is related to their sexual orientation, age or partnership status (World Health Organization, 2020). Thus, the definition of infertility moved from strictly medical causes towards a concept of "social infertility", a term that includes many life circumstances that render people unable to conceive or carry a child without medical intervention.[2] In other words, the close connection of ART to physical infertility has weakened in recent decades. In addition, because of the rapidly developing technologies of ART, new actors entered the scene of human reproduction, for example, donors of gametes or embryos, surrogate mothers and brokers of fertility services.

The need for (continuous) regulation

As already mentioned, ART has challenged the boundaries of what is perceived as ethical, desirable, moral, natural and normal since its beginning. As such, it clashes with societal contexts in which it is situated in terms of broad social relations, cultural norms and knowledge systems (Webster, 2002). Such conflicts often give rise to calls for legal regulation. Therefore, from the very inception of the field, rules have been debated, set and reformulated all over the globe that should regulate ART. Many times, national and international regulatory bodies faced and are continuing to face calls from different stakeholders to decide what ART procedures should be permitted or prohibited, which patients should be entitled to or excluded from treatment and who should carry the financial costs. These controversies transcend by far simple debates about the permissiveness of a medical intervention and its cost coverage. In many countries, ART was and continues to be a central arena of political battle (Gal & Kligman, 2000) in which actors such as physicians, different groups of patients and their advocates, NGOs, policy makers, jurists, private and public health insurance companies, political advisory bodies and churches struggle over social, legal, ethical and religious norms in human procreation and biomedicine.

Norms that regulate the use of ART operate on different levels. Legislative gatekeeping determines which medical procedures are permissible and for whom. Legal bans prohibit certain medical procedures (e.g., gamete donation) or exclude certain patient groups (e.g., single women, same-sex couples) and thus regulate availability and access. In addition to that, there is economic gatekeeping. ART is an expensive procedure, which – if not covered by public health insurance – only few can afford. Another type of barrier are the formal and informal organizational policies of clinics that provide treatment. Medical facilities have formal access rules, for example, age of patients; partnership; causes of infertility; and physical, mental and even social conditions. But they also have informal rules; health professionals can give or inhibit access, for example, by not starting, choosing to continue or stop treatment and offering or withholding certain procedures or options of treatment. In addition, legal regulation and organizational policies are not necessarily identical. What is legally permitted is not always done in clinical practice, and clinical practice might circumvent legal regulations.

Today, the majority of the 43 countries in Europe that perform ART have legislation in place that governs ART (Calhaz-Jorge et al., 2020)[3] and that has been introduced and repeatedly modified in the last four decades (ESHRE, 2017). However, despite several commonalities[4] and regardless of their geographical or cultural proximity, European countries surprisingly differ from one another in how they regulate access to and practice of ART, such as in terms of eligibility for treatment (age limits, partnership status, sexual orientation), permissibility of embryo selection, egg and/or sperm donation, donor anonymity, surrogacy or reimbursement and waiting time (Calhaz-Jorge et al., 2020). In summary, ART regulation in Europe, the main topic of this book, ranges from permissive to restrictive, with intermediate regulations in between (Busardò et al., 2014; Engeli & Rothmay Allison, 2016; European Society of Human Reproduction and Embryology, 2017).

The regulatory diversity across Europe raises questions such as what types of procedures and regulations exist and how they affect different patient groups.[5] Comparison shows that discourses on and regulation of ART – a set of medical technologies that are only value free on the surface – are deeply embedded in very specific national, political, social, historical and religious contexts. They exist, develop and change in relation to specific sets of values about, for example, parenthood, family, kinship, sexual orientation, medicine, religion and the availability of human life in principle. Studying these values in their national settings uncovers their diversity and variability but also how they are sustained, rationalized and legitimized.

Country sample composition, guiding questions and methods

This volume assembles case studies from several European countries: Austria, Czech Republic, Denmark, Germany, Italy, Netherlands, Poland and Sweden. Their ART policies range from permissive (Denmark, Netherlands, Sweden) through intermediate (Austria, Czech Republic) to restrictive (Germany, Italy, Poland).[6] Thus, this volume can provide a comprehensive overview on the variation of ART policies in Europe. Also, these countries have been selected to show the variety of political and cultural traditions in Europe and ART and to include nations that are often omitted from international comparison of ART policies. In terms of size, the country sample covers large, medium, and small states; in terms of geographical distribution, it includes two Nordic, a Western European, two Central European, one Southern European and two Central and Eastern European countries. All of them are Member States of the European Union (EU). However, they entered the EU at different moments in its history and with different political traditions. Germany, Italy, and the Netherlands are founding Members; Denmark, a northern country, joined in 1973, Austria and Sweden, two neutral countries which remained apart from the EU for many years, in 1995; the Czech Republic and Poland, two post-communist countries, became Member States only in 2004.

The country cases follow a common theme by addressing several shared questions: What is the legal regulation of ART within a specific country? How and why did this regulation come about? What is the infrastructure of ART services in a country and how is it used? However, the country cases also differ from one another. They analyze the development of ART regulations from the perspective of different disciplines, including history, law, political science and sociology. They also differ with regard to the explanatory angle the authors take, depending on what they regard from their disciplinary background as most relevant topics and/ or moments of national debate to explain ART regulation. Finally, the country cases use different sources such as legal texts, policy documents, records of parliamentary debate, media articles and qualitative and quantitative research on ART.

Individual country cases and comparative chapters

The contributions in this book can be read as individual chapters; however, as a whole, they provide a systematic overview on similarities and differences in the development of ART regulation in eight European countries.

In their chapter "Emerging from Standstill: Austria's Transition from Restrictive to Intermediate ART Policies", Erich Griessler and Florian Winkler analyze a radical regulatory change in 2015 which brought a policy shift in Austria from a restrictive toward an intermediate regulatory regime. The authors put this policy change in the context of a more general change of values and the broad transformation of post-World War II political culture in Austria (Griessler & Winkler, 2022).

Lenka Slepičková provides an overview of assisted reproduction in the Czech Republic. The country is an example of the co-existence of permissive and restrictive elements in ART policies. On the one hand, many ART techniques are permitted that are prohibited in other European countries. As a consequence, the Czech Republic is an important destination country for cross-border reproductive services. Yet, on the other hand, Czech ART policies have restrictive elements such as limiting services to heterosexual couples within a certain age range and excluding same-sex couples and single women because of conservative family values. As Slepičková shows, health care providers, however, find ways to creatively circumvent such restrictions (Slepičková, 2022).

Likewise, Danish ART regulation has permissive and restrictive elements, and Denmark is also a center for cross-border reproductive care. Janne Rothmar Herrmann explains in her chapter, "Taming Technology: Assisted Reproduction in Denmark", how this regulatory combination came about and how ART policies started from a restrictive approach that tried to control ART and developed over time into a more permissive regime (Herrmann, 2022).

In his chapter, Sven Geyken leads us into the German "Regulatory Jungle" of ART, where it has been hotly debated in the country since the 1990s, but policy makers never succeeded in regulating it with a single piece of legislation. The subsequent piecemeal legislation has led to uncertainties that prompt many German couples and single women to seek treatment abroad. Currently, ART regulation is again under discussion in Germany (Geyken, 2022).

Ines Corti's chapter on assisted procreation in Italy shows how decisions of the Italian Constitutional Court completely rewrite a very restrictive law issued by Parliament. The chapter underlines the important role courts can play – not only in Italy but across Europe – in ART policies as well as the strong role the Catholic Church plays in this field, in Italy but also in other countries as well (Corti, 2022).

In their chapter, "Avoiding Ideological Debate. Assisted Reproduction Regulation in the Netherlands", Heleen Weyers and Nicolle Zeegers characterize Dutch ART regulations as permissive in terms of access and moderately restrictive in terms of methods permitted and human-rights orientation. They describe the development of Dutch ART policies from the 1960s onward as a slow and objective discussion which was oriented toward pragmatism and self-governance of the medical profession as well as consensus seeking (Weyers & Zeegers, 2022).

In contrast, the debate on ART in Poland is highly politically charged, and ART legislation is very restrictive, even though it has been practiced in this country for more than 30 years. Poland is another example of a country in which the Catholic Church plays a key role in the public debate on reproductive biomedicine. Anna Krawczak and Magdalena Radkowska-Walkowicz's chapter, "IVF in Poland: From Political Debates to Biomedical Practices", analyzes two important and conflicting myths, that ART is a neutral medical technology and that it would create "baby monsters" (Krawczak & Radkowska-Walkowicz, 2022).

Sweden, in contrast, is an example for slow policy development based on thorough investigation of possible risks and consequences for the child. ART policies developed over decades and without much public controversy and criticism. Anne Singer explains in her chapter, "From Safeguarding the Best Interest of the Child to Equal Treatment. Legislating Assisted Reproductive Techniques in Sweden", how Sweden moved over time from a very cautious view on ART toward allowing new methods and opening toward new family forms. Definitions of what is in the best interest of the child changed; however, the right to know one's genetic origin prevailed (Singer, 2022).

The country cases are followed by three comparative chapters. In her chapter, "Expectations Regarding the Convergence of Domestic Laws on ART", Heleen Weyers addresses the question of whether we can expect convergence of formal domestic laws regarding two topics of ART regulation – non-anonymous donation and access for lesbian couples – in the countries described in previous chapters (and in the European Union in general). To answer the question, she discusses the role of the European Court of Human Rights (ECtHR) as well as value changes as a driving force for convergence (Weyers, 2022).

In her comparative chapter "What Drives the Politicization of ART in Western and Northern European Countries?", Nicolle Zeegers examines whether the "two worlds of morality politics theory" (TWMP) applies to Austria, the Netherlands and Sweden. Comparison between the processes of politicization of ART in Austria and the Netherlands leads to identifying shortcomings in the TWMP theory that seem to be solvable by supplementing it with insights into wedge issue politics (Zeegers, 2022).

Erich Griessler, in his chapter, "Regulating Change in Human Procreation. Value Changes and Imaginaries of Assisted Reproductive Technologies in Eight European Countries", explores the country cases for different meanings of ART. He focuses on similarities and differences between countries in this respect and how they affect ART regulation. He applies the concept of "sociotechnical imaginaries" developed by Jasanoff and Kim (2009) and claims that the development of ART is guided by four contesting imaginaries: unavailability, cure, equality and optimization (Griessler, 2022).

The country cases and comparative chapters of this book show the rich variety and changeability of regulation of ART in Europe: they show the practice and regulation of ART as contextual and historical social phenomena that are strongly interrelated to certain values, themselves rich in variety and change over time. This book clearly shows that ART has slowly changed human reproduction over the last 40 years and that it is interrelated in a seamless web with changing values about sexual orientation, self-determination, family, kinship, biological citizenship, the commodification of the body, commercialization and globalization of healthcare, power and inequality.

With this book, we hope to contribute in a readable and thought-provoking way to situating a particular technology within networks of power/knowledge and values and to "unpack the multifaceted repercussions and cultural transformations currently being induced by ARTs around the world" (Inhorn & Birenbaum-Carmeli, 2008, p. 178).

Notes

1 We want to thank Shauna Stack for language editing.
2 Proponents of a movement in the United States, for example, centered around the idea of fertility equality, claim that one's ability to build a family should not be determined by wealth, sexuality, gender or biology (Kaufman, 2020). It demands cost coverage for reproductive procedures, such as sperm retrieval, egg donation and embryo creation, for all prospective parents in the United States. These claims met with criticism, mainly from feminist activists, especially regarding surrogacy, inevitably involved in the realization of the reproduction intentions of gay men and some straight individuals as well. Paid surrogacy is often connected with the exploitation of surrogate mothers and the commodification of female bodies and children (Kaufman, 2020).
3 Albania, Bosnia and Herzegovina (Federation), Ireland, Romania and Ukraine don't have ART legislation (Calhaz-Jorge et al., 2020).
4 Current laws on embryo protection commonly prohibit the creation of clones, hybrids and chimeras. In some countries, such as Germany, practicing ART is forbidden in facilities that are not legally established.
5 In a situation of European regulatory variety, thousands of couples and individuals engage every year in cross-border reproductive care – travelling abroad to undergo infertility treatment to evade regulations they consider limiting in their countries. Patients and couples are free to make use of regulatory differences and travel across boundaries for treatment, even if cross-border reproductive care creates situations that violate domestic legislation (European Society of Human Reproduction and Embryology, 2017).
6 See Griessler in this volume.

References

Busardò, F. P., Gulino, M., Napoletano, S., Zaami, S., & Frati, P. (2014). The evolution of legislation in the field of medically assisted reproduction and embryo stem cell research in European Union members. *BioMed Research International*. https://doi.org/10.1155/2014/307160

Calhaz-Jorge, C., De Geyter, C. H., Kupka, M. S., Wyns, C., Mocanu, E., Motrenko, T., . . . Goossens, V. (2020). Survey on ART and IUI: Legislation, regulation, funding and registries in European countries: The European IVF-monitoring consortium (EIM) for the European society of human reproduction and embryology (ESHRE). *Human Reproduction Open, 1*, hoz044.

Corti, I. (2022). Assisted procreation in Italy: A long and winding road. In *This book*.

Engeli, I., & Rothmayr Allison, C. (2016). Governing new reproductive technologies across Western Europe: The gender dimension. In M. Lie & N. Lykke (Hrsg.), *Assisted reproduction across borders: Feminist perspectives on normalizations, disruptions and transmissions* (1st ed., pp. 87–99). Routledge.

European Society of Human Reproduction and Embryology. (2017). *Regulation and legislation in assisted reproduction*. www.eshre.eu/-/media/sitecore-files/Press-room/Resources/2-Regulation.pdf?la=en&hash=62013D3DEB410113819200F708DBBB9EF53F2278

European Society of Human Reproduction and Embryology. (2020). *ART fact sheet*. www.eshre.eu/-/media/sitecore-files/Press-room/ART-fact-sheet-2020-data 2016.pdf?la=en&hash=AB68A67B4FEA7723F2125B02BCB93FB837139CD4

Fenton, R. A. (2006). Catholic doctrine versus women's rights: The new Italian law on assisted reproduction. *Medical Law Review, 14*(1), 73–107. https://doi.org/10.1093/medlaw/fwi041

Gal, S., & Kligman, G. (2000). *The politics of gender after socialism*. Princeton University Press. https://press.princeton.edu/books/paperback/9780691048949/the-politics-of-gender-after-socialism

Gallagher, J. (2012, July 2). Five millionth 'test tube baby'. *BBC News*. www.bbc.com/news/health-18649582

Geyken, S. (2022). A regulatory jungle: The law on assisted reproduction in Germany. In *This book*.

Griessler, E. (2022). Regulating change in human procreation. Value changes and imaginaries of assisted reproductive technologies in eight European countries. In *This book*.

Griessler, E., & Winkler, F. (2022). Emerging from standstill: Austria's transition from restrictive to intermediate ART policies. In *This book*.

Herrmann, J. R. (2022). Taming technology: Assisted reproduction in Denmark. In *This book*.

Inhorn, M. C., & Birenbaum-Carmeli, D. (2008). Assisted reproductive technologies and culture change. *Annual Review of Anthropology, 37*, 177–196. https://doi.org/10.1146/annurev.anthro.37.081407.085230

Inhorn, M. C., & Patrizio, P. (2015). Infertility around the globe: New thinking on gender, reproductive technologies and global movements in the 21st century. *Human Reproduction Update, 21*(4), 411–426. https://doi.org/10.1093/humupd/dmv016

Jasanoff, S., & Kim, S.-H. (2009). Containing the atom: Sociotechnical imaginaries and nuclear power in the United States and South Korea. *Minerva, 47*, 119–146. https://doi.org/10.1007/s11024-009-9124-4

Kaufman, D. (2020, July 22). The fight for fertility equality. *The New York Times*. www.nytimes.com/2020/07/22/style/lgbtq-fertility-surrogacy-coverage.html

Krawczak, A., & Radkowska-Walkowicz, M. (2022). IVF in Poland: From political debates to biomedical practices. In *This book*.

Singer, A. (2022). From safeguarding the best interest of the child to equal treatment. Legislating assisted reproductive techniques in Sweden. In *This book*.

Slepičková, L. (2022). Assisted reproduction in the Czech Republic. In *This book*.

Webster, A. (2002). Innovative health technologies and the social: Redefining health, medicine and the body. *Current Sociology*, 50(3), 443–457. https://doi.org/10.1177/0011392102050003009

Weyers, H. (2022). Expectations regarding the convergence of domestic laws on ART. In *This book*.

Weyers, H., & Zeegers, N. (2022). Avoiding ideological debate. Assisted reproduction regulation in Netherlands. In *This book*.

World Health Organization. (2020). *Infertility*. www.who.int/news-room/fact-sheets/detail/infertility

Zeegers, N. (2022). What drives the politicization of ART in West European countries? In *This book*.

2 Emerging from standstill

Austria's transition from restrictive to intermediate ART policies

Erich Griessler and Florian Winkler

Introduction

In 2015, Austria witnessed a change from a restrictive towards a more permissive regulatory regime of assisted reproductive technologies (ARTs). In 1992, Austrian policy makers dealt very restrictively with two of the most fundamental policy problems posed by ART – which technically feasible options should be permitted and who should get access – (Engeli & Rothmayr Allison, 2016, p. 88). The Reproductive Medicine Law of 1992 (Fortpflanzungsmedizingesetz, in the following FMedG 1992) permitted ART only for fertility treatment as last medical resort and banned egg, embryo, and heterologous sperm donation[1] as well as surrogacy and preimplantation genetic diagnostics (PGD). The law excluded single women and lesbian couples from treatment.

The change of the Reproductive Medicine Law in 2015 (Fortpflanzungsmedizinänderungsgesetz, in the following FMedRÄG 2015) was characterized by considerable liberalization. Now egg donation, heterologous sperm donation, and PGD were allowed, and ART treatment was opened to lesbian couples. Nevertheless, some restrictive elements were retained: Austrian law still prohibits embryo donation and the commercialization and advertising of egg and sperm donation as well as surrogacy; PGD is limited to a defined number of indications; ART treatments remain as last resort for infertility treatment, and single women continue to be excluded.

This chapter portrays the change of the Austrian ART regime after a standstill of more than two decades. It (1) describes the regulations of 1992 and 2015 as well as their rationale; (2) embeds the transition in the broader context of change of Austrian political structure and culture; (3) contextualizes the reform with changes in values towards family, same-sex relationships, religion, and individual autonomy. In order to give the reader an impression of how a particular ART is discussed, a special section is dedicated (4) to portraying the discourse on surrogacy in Austria.

For this chapter, we studied policy papers, which includes an analysis of stakeholder comments on the draft FMedRÄG 2015 during the official evaluation procedure preceding the parliamentary debate as well as responses of the Ministry of Health to parliamentary questions. To describe the use of ART in Austria, we used

DOI: 10.4324/9781003223726-2

statistics of in-vitro fertilization (IVF) funds. In order to portray the discourse of surrogacy in Austria, we did a media analysis. We searched Austrian newspapers via the WISO portal[2] for relevant articles between 1.1.2000 and 5.1.2018 with the search string "Leihmutterschaft" AND "Österreich" ("Surrogacy" AND "Austria"). We retrieved a total of 328 articles and categorized them according to their depiction of surrogacy (positive/negative/neutral). Furthermore, we analyzed grey and peer-reviewed literature on ART in Austria and international comparisons of ART, its regulation, and its use, as well as literature on Austrian political culture. Finally, this chapter is based on previous work of one of its authors on patterns of Austrian policy making in biomedicine (Griessler, 2004, 2010), the Austrian debate on prenatal diagnostics, and PGD and egg donation (Griessler, 2012), as well as the development of the Austrian Reproductive Medicine Law (Griessler & Hager, 2016).

This chapter starts by portraying the use of ART in Austria, the public IVF fund that covers part of treatment costs, and the criteria it applies for cost coverage, as well as the ART infrastructure in Austria. The second part describes the restrictive FMedG 1992, which regulated ART, and its more permissive reform in 2015. The following parts sketch the Austrian discourse on surrogacy and report available indications about the effectiveness of the FMedG 1992. The next section describes the manifold changes in Austrian society which enabled the significant policy change from a restrictive towards a more permissive law. In the conclusion, we argue that Austria, with this reform, has changed its position from restrictive to intermediate patterns of ART policies.

Use, funding, and infrastructure of ART in Austria

With a population of 8.7 million (Statistik Austria, 2020), Austria in 2010 was among the European countries – together with Germany, Ukraine, Ireland, and Albania – with the fewest ART treatment cycles per million women between the age 15 and 45 (Präg & Mills, 2017, p. 5). Austria currently has 31 accredited ART centers that provide treatment (Kern, 2021). The Austrian IVF-Register provides detailed numbers on treatment cycles carried out in Austrian IVF clinics (Kern, 2021).

As Table 2.1 indicates, the numbers of treatment cycles increased in Austria from 2012 to 2020 from 7,196 to 10,515. In total, the Austrian IVF-Fund, which covers part of the treatment cost under certain conditions (see subsequently), supported, from 2010 to 2020, 97,931 IVF cycles, which led in total to 29,088 pregnancies (Kern, 2021, p. 30). These numbers do not include IVF treatment that was not covered by the IVF-Fund for not fulfilling one or another of its funding conditions. Yet it seems plausible to assume that the numbers of the IVF-Register provide a rather complete picture of the Austrian situation. Using a survey method with a respondent rate of 27 of 28 IVF clinics, the European IVF-Monitoring Consortium (EIM) et al. (2017, p. 1959) arrived at 7,173 cycles for the year 2013. Given that one IVF clinic did not respond, the numbers essentially accord with those of the IVF-Register.

Table 2.1 Number of IVF cycles in Austria, 2012–2020.

	2012	2013	2014	2015	2016	2017	2018	2019	2020
Number of cycles	7,196	7,478	7,649	9,101	10,097	10,216	10,828	11,028	10,515
Pregnancy ratio	31,6	33,8	31,6	31,7	30,4	29,8	29,0	29,0	28,4
Baby take-home rate per transfer	28,4	30,5	30,9	30,7	30,0	29,7	28,5	28,4	n.a.

Source: (Kern, 2021, p. 30)

Table 2.2 Application of sperm donation and egg donation in 2020.

IVF center	Sperm donation			Egg donation	
	IVF	ICSI	Cryo	Full attempt	Cryo-attempt
Total public centers	8	12	5	-	2
Total private centers	184	45	41	14	20
2018 IVF-Fund	192	57	46	14	22

Source: (Kern, 2021, p. 21)

Table 2.3 IVF spending 2015 to 2020 in Euro.

	2015	2016	2017	2018	2019	2020
IVF-Fund spending	15,710,718	17,134,393	17,186,085	18,353,727	18,238,459	16,823,209
IVF-Fund spending per cycle	1,726	1,697	1,682	1,695	1,654	1,600

Source: (Kern, 2021, p. 30)

Table 2.2 shows the number of egg and sperm donations carried out in Austria in 2020. There were only a few egg donations reported to the IVF register, most of them in private centers. The number of sperm donations was considerably higher than that of egg donations; again, most of them were carried out in private centers.

Table 2.3 provides an overview of the spending of the IVF-Fund since 2015. However, those numbers can only provide a rough picture of the magnitude of the Austrian ART market. The numbers of the IVF-Register only include those IVF cycles covered under the terms of the IVF-Fund but not those for which coverage by the IVF-Fund has not been requested for whatever reasons (e.g., exceeding age limits, covered maximum treatment cycles, or lesbian couples without medical indication).

Since 2000, under certain conditions, the public IVF-Fund covers 70% of the expenses for IVF treatment. Patients and their partners must pay the remaining 30% (Kern, 2021). Cost coverage of IVF treatment by the IVF-Fund is subject to certain provisions the patient and partner as well as the IVF clinics have to fulfill. For patients and their partners, these preconditions include a medical condition, meeting certain age limits, and legal provisions given by the FMedRÄG, as well as a maximum number of cycles. According to the FMedG, ART is only permitted if a medical indication exists, that is, female infertility because of polycystic ovary syndrome, endometriosis, or male sterility. At the beginning of treatment, the woman who wants to carry the child to term must not be older than 40 years, and her husband or her (male or female) legal or life partner must not be older than 50 years. Each couple is entitled to cost coverage of up to four successive treatment cycles. This right is renewed if a pregnancy has been accomplished (Parlament, 1999). The treatment cycles must be carried out by a center which is accredited by and has a contract with the IVF-Fund. In addition, a signed treatment contract between couple and center is mandatory. To receive accreditation, IVF centers must carry out a minimum number of 50 treatment cycles per year and prove a pregnancy rate of 18% per follicular puncture.

The IVF-Fund is administered by the Federal Ministry for Social Affairs, Health, Care and Consumer protection, but the principal funders are the Umbrella Organization of Austrian Social Security Associations (Dachverband) and the Family Burden Equalization Fund (FLAF) (Kern, 2021, p. 31). The FLAF finances family benefits, such as maternity allowance, family allowance, and childcare benefits. It is mainly financed by contributions of employers and is administered within the Ministry of Finance. In 2020, the Dachverband covered approximately 48% of the costs of the IVF-Fund, whereas the FLAF covered 50% (Kern, 2021, p. 31). The remaining 2% is mainly covered by social insurance institutions for civil servants and private insurance.

Regulation of ART in FMedG 1992 and FMedRÄG 2015

The debate over FMedG 1992, which developed over a decade in several stages, was dominated by two questions: what available technology should be permitted and who should get access to ART (Hadolt, 2007)? The FMedG 1992 expressed conservative attitudes towards family, sexuality, and the moral status of the embryo by limiting ART treatment to traditional families and consequently rejecting the creation of new family forms and discriminating against same-sex couples. It prohibited egg donation and indirectly surrogacy to protect women from exploitation. The law permitted ART within strict limits: (1) ART was only allowed as last resort in infertility treatment, that is, if pregnancy by sexual intercourse is impossible because the woman and/or her partner had a medical condition; (2) only married or co-habiting heterosexual couples were entitled to treatment; (3) sperm donation was prohibited in general except for heterologous insemination, that is, insemination with donor sperm if the husband or established partner was infertile; (4) donation of eggs and embryos and surrogacy were not allowed; (5) PGD was not explicitly regulated, but the law permitted genetic analysis only if it was necessary to accomplish pregnancy. Therefore, analysis of the fertilized egg (blastocyst) was illegal, but polar body diagnostics was not covered by the law and therefore not forbidden (Austrian Bioethics Commission, 2012). Polar body analysis provides similar information to PGD but is based on analysis of the polar body instead of the fertilized egg.

The FMedG 1992 was a compromise between restrictive and permissive coalition partners in Austrian government. For the conservative Austrian Peoples Party (ÖVP), strongly binding collective core values within the political debate about ART were the protection of the human embryo, traditional family values, non-commercialization of ART, and the intrinsic dignity of humans and the human body; for the Social Democrats (SPÖ), the protection of women from exploitation by ART and the self-determination of women were central (Hadolt, 2007). The FMedG 1992, however, neglected the needs of many people seeking ART treatment and created several inequalities for different groups looking for ART. Consequently, some Austrian patients bypassed the law and – with the help of Austrian ART physicians who supported cross-border medical care – looked for ART treatment abroad (Hadolt, 2007).

The FMedRÄG 2015, after many years of legal inactivity, brought about several changes in Austrian ART regulation (see Table 2.4).

First, the new regulation provides access to ART to married heterosexual couples, cohabiting couples, and lesbian couples (§ 2 [1]). However, it still permits ART only as last resort in infertility treatment.

Second, the law permits heterologous sperm donation for IVF and intracytoplasmatic sperm injection (§3[2]). Donors must be at least 18 years of age (§ 13 [1]). Sperm must be tested for fertility and be free of any medical threats to the woman and the child (§ 12). To prevent commercialization, donors are entitled to receive limited compensation (in the form of allowances) (§ 16 [1]). A maximum

Table 2.4 Comparison of FMedG 1992 and FMedRÄG 2015.

	FMedG 1992	FMedRÄG 2015
Medical ultima ratio	Yes	Yes (exception: lesbian couples)
Access for lesbian couples	No	Yes
Access for single women	No	No
Surrogacy	No	No
Egg donation	No	Yes (no advertising, no commercialization)
Heterologous sperm donation	No[3]	Yes
Embryo donation	No	No
PGD	No	Yes (for limited indications)

Source: (Griessler & Hager, 2016)

of three donations is permitted per donor (§ 14 [2]). Hospital records must be kept on the donor and the use of the donation (§ 15) to safeguard the fundamental right of children to find out the identity of their biological father at the age of 14 (§ 20 [2]).

The FMedRÄG 2015 also permits egg donation but inflicts age limits for donors (18 to 30 years of age; § 2b [2]), and for recipients (maximum age, 45 years; § 3 [3]). Commercialization and advertisement of egg donations is prohibited (§ 16). To avoid commercialization, donors receive only limited compensation (e.g. in the form of allowances or reimbursement of travel and hotel expense; the law does not define an exact amount) (§ 16 [1]). The child is entitled to learn the name of the egg donor at the age of 14 (§ 20 [2]).

Third, the law permits PGD in specific cases (§2a [1]), that is, after three or more unsuccessful IVF cycles, after three miscarriages, or when there is an increased risk of a miscarriage or genetic disease due to the genetic predisposition of a parent. PGD for genetic screening remains prohibited. In 2016, three institutes received accreditation to carry out PGD (Oberhauser, 2016); indications for which PGD might be used are listed in the gene-analysis register (Bundesministerium für Gesundheit und Frauen, 2017).

Austrian discourse on surrogacy

Surrogacy is illegal in Austria, although it is not explicitly addressed in the FMedG. Two paragraphs are important in this regard: FMedG § 3. [1] states that the use of a donated egg is only allowed for women who are infertile. In reverse conclusion, egg donation into fertile women is banned, which excludes potential surrogate mothers. Furthermore, the use of ART is limited to married or co-habiting couples only (§ 2. [1]) (*Aktion Leben*, n.d.; Barth & Erlebach, 2015)).

In the parliamentary debate on the FMedRÄG 2015, surrogacy was hardly mentioned at all and only as an example of practices of ART that should remain forbidden (Parlament, 2015, pp. 74, 91, 102). In general, Austrian actors seem to reject surrogacy. In September 2017, Aktion Leben, a moderate pro-life organization and lobbying group, asked all Austrian parliamentary parties for a written statement about their position on an international ban of surrogacy.[4] In their responses, all parties unanimously stated their fundamental rejection of surrogacy. SPÖ, ÖVP, and the Green Party did not take a clear stance towards an international ban. The Austrian Freedom Party (FPÖ) clearly approved such initiatives, and the liberal party The New Austria (NEOS) advocated taking the discussion to an international level (Aktion Leben, 2017). It is because of this strong rejection that a change of the legal situation of surrogacy was not considered in the reform of FMedG in 2015.

Austrian newspapers parallel this strong rejection of surrogacy. Most articles studied in our media analysis take a critical stance towards surrogacy; none of them advocate a permissive legalization of surrogacy in Austria. The articles focus primarily on surrogacy cases from abroad (Hammerl, 2016; Kummer, 2016), particularly on celebrities who hire a surrogate mother (Kurier, 2011; Strozzi, 2017).

In 2015, a representative of the Austrian Association for Gynecology and Obstetrics (OEGGG) considered it very likely that surrogacy will remain banned in Austria for a long time, as there are many ethical and medical concerns involved in surrogacy (Steurer & Aberle, 2015). This assessment seems plausible, considering the way that surrogacy was brought up in the parliamentary debate about the FMedRÄG in 2015 (Parlament, 2015, p. 65). The aforementioned responses of Austrian parties to the inquiry of Aktion Leben two years later continue to show a clear of rejection surrogacy from Austrian parties.

Effectiveness

There is only scarce official information about the impact and effectiveness of the law. Besides the already mentioned numbers of the IVF-Fund, no evaluation of the law exists. In 2016, the Ministry for Health and Women responded to a parliamentary question that no violation of the ban on commercialization and mediation of egg and sperm donation (§ 16 FMedG) or inadmissible advertising had come to their attention (Oberhauser, 2016). It seems that the ban of surrogacy in Austria is respected, and there are no cases of illegal surrogacy arrangements known. However, there are a few media reports (Angermann & Trescher, 2014; Steurer & Aberle, 2015; Tempfer, 2017). Austrian physicians seem to collaborate in reproductive tourism as "fertility brokers" (Van Beers, 2014, p. 113) and recommend agencies that provide surrogacies abroad to their patients (Eidlhuber, 2015; Özkan, 2014). How many such arrangements are being made is hard to tell, since no statistics exist. Tempfer (2017) quotes a leading Austrian ART physician who acts about five times a year as a go-between with U.S. agencies. The cost of such professional arrangements is about 75,500 Euro; the surrogate mother would receive approximately half of this amount. As the legal regulations are restrictive, there is no infrastructure for surrogacy in Austria. The only organization that might resemble an infrastructure for this purpose are fertility clinics recommending surrogacy services abroad (Özkan, 2014).

Transition from restrictive to intermediate policies

The following section portrays the parliamentary debate of FMedRÄG 2015 and analyzes why, after years of standstill, sudden change in the FMedG occurred.

The parliamentary debate on FMedRÄG 2015[5]

The arguments used in the parliamentary debate mirror the arguments which have been brought forward in the statements of stakeholders in the official parliamentary evaluation procedure (Griessler & Hager, 2016).

In the parliamentary debate, deputies discussed some practices of ART more frequently and controversially than others (Parlament, 2015, p. 65). Egg donation and PGD were raised several times, both by politicians who approved and rejected the respective changes to the FMedG. Surrogacy and sperm donation, in contrast, were only rarely mentioned and did not evoke much debate. Embryo research and donation where not mentioned at all (ibid., 74, 80, 91, 102, 105).

Politicians from the conservative Austrian Peoples Party, the Social Democrats, and the liberal NEOS who argued in favor of egg donation stated that preserving the ban would lead to reproductive tourism to countries where quality standards cannot be guaranteed, such as the right of the child to find out about its genetic origin (ibid. 106). They also argued that appropriate regulation could prevent commercialization of egg donation (ibid. 75, 89, 106). In contrast, representatives of the right-wing Freedom Party and the small conservative party Team Stronach heavily criticized permitting egg donation. They referred to risks of egg donation for women's health (ibid. 66, 72, 84), casualties because of ovarian hyperstimulation syndrome (ibid. 72), and currently unknown long-term consequences of egg donation (ibid. 67). Furthermore, opponents of egg donation from FPÖ and Team Stronach argued that the introduction of egg donation would favor exploitation and commercialization of (especially poor) women (ibid. 69, 72).

Supporters of the legalization of PGD framed it as a way to avoid severe hereditary diseases (ibid. 75, 95, 101) and suffering (ibid. 97, 104) through miscarriage and stillbirth (ibid. 91, 95, 101). Moreover, they argued that carriers of a genetic disease who want to avoid passing the condition on to a child would currently be forced into a kind of "pregnancy on trial" because the existing law only allows prenatal testing to ascertain hereditary diseases (ibid. 68, 86). This would mean that a child would have to be conceived and tested by prenatal diagnostics, and, if positive, the woman would have to have an abortion. The strain that such "pregnancy on trial" puts on the woman and the couple was deemed unacceptable. Opponents of PGD from ÖVP, FPÖ, and Team Stronach argued that PGD would imply discrimination on the basis on physical and mental disabilities and hereditary diseases (ibid. 71, 85, 103), involve the destruction of fertilized egg cells (ibid. 68), and select between worthy and unworthy, respectively perfect and imperfect, life (ibid. 71, 103).

The connection of PGD and prenatal testing is an example of how existing and permitted medical practices are used to justify new practices of ART. Another example of this way of justifying new ART treatments concerns egg donation; some politicians argued that men and women would be treated unequally if sperm donation were permitted but egg donation prohibited (ibid. 99, 102). Therefore, it would be unreasonable to allow sperm donation and ban egg donation at the same time (ibid. 86). Besides showing that gender equality was also drawn on as an argumentative resource, this way of arguing suggests that the already existing legal framework played an important role in determining which new aspects of ART should be legalized in Austria.

The new law was accepted in 2015 with a great majority of 113 pros and 48 cons. With some exceptions, the majority of deputies from SPÖ, ÖVP, the Green Party, and NEOS were in favor of the FMedRÄG, while the majority of deputies from FPÖ and Team Stronach voted against the new law.

Gradual change of political culture

In order to understand the more than 20-year-long inactivity in Austrian ART regulation, we have to consider the basic make up of Austrian post-war political culture and one of its basic principles, that is, "the avoidance of conflict" (Steiner, 1972, p. 424; as cited in Pelinka, 2006, p. 231). For more than 20 years, ART threatened this basic axiom because of its connection with a primordial conflict of Austrian ART policy making, the unusually intense dispute on abortion regulations in the early 1970s between the Social Democrats on one side and the conservative Austrian Peoples Party and the Catholic Church on the other (Griessler, 2010). After this heavy controversy, which divided Austrian society and ended in an undeclared and fragile armistice between the two opponents that combined liberal law and insufficient and patchy implementation, political actors avoided entering into another similar hot debate and shied away from the discussion of issues that would force them to discuss the ontological status of the embryo and related touchy ethical questions and would threaten the hard-won truce (Griessler, 2010, p. 2, 2012; Metzler & Pichelstorfer, 2020). So, why did change happen nevertheless?

Sketch of Austrian post-war political culture

We have argued elsewhere that the transition from restrictive to more permissive ART regulation is connected to overall changes in patterns of Austrian policy making in general and in biomedicine in particular (Griessler, 2010) and a combination of interlinked changes in the Austrian political system and society (Griessler & Hager, 2016).

As many authors analyzing the Austrian political system have pointed out, Austria is characterized by a number of important cleavages, for example, between conservative/social democratic, capital/labor, religious/secular,[6] and urban/rural. To cope with these many conflict lines, Austria since World War II has developed into a textbook example of a "consociational democracy" (Steiner, 1972, p. 424; as cited in Pelinka, 2006, p. 231). Because of several specific historical experiences, Austrian political culture (Gerlich & Pfefferle, 2006; Pelinka, 2006) after World War II was primarily consensus oriented and paternalistic. As concerns paternalism, Austrian political culture can build on the longstanding legacy and tradition of enlightened absolutism which has characterized Austria since the 18th century and deprives civil society of an active role (Degelsegger & Torgersen, 2011; Gerlich & Pfefferle, 2006; Hanisch, 2005). As concerns consensus orientation, it was the lesson learned from the irreconcilable confrontation between Austrian conservatives and social democrats in the interwar years, an ensuing civil war in 1933, and a totalitarian conservative regime between 1933 and 1938 which was replaced – welcomed by the majority of Austrians – by National Socialism that led to the establishment of a stable system of organized balance between the former enemies, the conservative Peoples' Party and the Social Democrats. Thus, after World War II, the country's politics and political discourse were dominated by a closed circle of a small number of elite actors, mainly from the ÖVP and the SPÖ, as well as social partners representing capital (Chamber of Commerce and Federation of Austrian Industries) and labor (Chamber of Labor, Trade Unions) (Glynn et al., 2003, p. 28). In this time, the SPÖ and ÖVP were able to rely on the support of stable electorates and the allegiance of their voters (Ulram, 2006), which were integrated into the neo-corporatist political system by compulsory memberships in their respective chambers as well as in a plethora of different organizations close to the parties (Pelinka, 2006; Tálos & Kittel, 2001).

Other important political actors in ART regulation are experts and the Catholic Church. Experts, in particular physicians, played an important role in ART politics as advisors (Gottweis, 1988; Griessler, 2010; Hadolt, 2007). ART politics is made "by a fairly regular 'cast' of experts, stakeholders, bureaucrats, and representatives of interest groups" (Metzler & Pichelstorfer, 2020, p. 75). The FMedG 1992 was developed and precooked by a small, close circle of civil servants, parliamentarians and other politicians, medical and legal experts, theologians, philosophers, and natural scientists. It was little changed after it entered the public realm (Hadolt, 2007).

Despite the important role of experts, policy makers and the rules of the political process clearly maintain primacy in policy making The Austrian Bioethics Committee (ABC) is a relevant and telling example. Established to advise the federal chancellor in bioethics in medicine, policy makers do not necessarily follow their advice. In 2002, for example, the minister of research decided to follow the minority position of the ABC and took a restrictive position towards research on human embryonic stem cells; in 2012, a call by the ABC for permissive reform of the FMedG remained without regulatory activity for many years because policy makers could not agree on a reform (Metzler & Pichelstorfer, 2020). Policy makers became active only under pressure by Decisions of the ECtHR and the Austrian Constitutional Court (Leibetseder & Griffin, 2019). One reason for the ABC's lack of influence on policy making is its status within the policy process and its composition. The appointment of its members is decided by the federal chancellor and depends on his/her interest in bioethics, political strategy, and worldview. Since politics and worldviews play a role in the composition and appointment of the ABC and its members, it is not a "depoliticized" space, and when it comes to decisions in the area of ART, it is regularly "divided along religious lines" (Griessler, 2004; Metzler & Pichelstorfer, 2020, p. 88).

The Catholic Church, another significant political actor, takes a restrictive position towards ART, PGD, and same-sex unions/marriages. The Catholic Church has been able to wield a strong influence on Austrian politics because of its close connection with the conservative ÖVP and the settlement of its historical conflict with the SPÖ from the interwar years (Knill et al., 2014; Metzler & Pichelstorfer, 2020; Potz, 2005; Prainsack, 2006). Until 2015, the Catholic Church was able to delay permissive reforms for a long time and impede and "silence" public debate so that topics related to ART hardly made it to the public agenda (Metzler & Pichelstorfer, 2020). The Catholic Church's influence on Austrian society, however, was and is strongest when it is invisible because public attitudes towards family concur with Catholic viewpoints and appear as "cultural or even natural ones" (Metzler & Pichelstorfer, 2020, p. 91). And the Catholic Church is influential, because it is perceived as a strong player by other actors, who avoid topics which might get them into conflict with the Church.

In contrast to politicians, civil servants, experts, and the Catholic Church, the public was little involved in the ART debate and took little notice of policy development of Austrian ART regulation because the debate did not occur in an observable "front stage", but "back stage . . . in working groups, meetings of parties, in intergovernmental committees, or in expert hearings" (Metzler & Pichelstorfer, 2020, pp. 74, 85). The public was little involved but confronted with the solution developed by elite actors.

For a long time, the structure of the Austrian post-war political system was able to generate consensus and allowed political elites to monopolize political debate and decision making. In this way, the Austrian political elites, in contrast to the conflictual interwar period, were successful to "channel conflicts to roundtables, thus producing silence on the streets" (Metzler & Pichelstorfer, 2020, p. 78). But this system also generated immobility and at times petrification, excluded unprivileged actors from political discourse and decision making, and increasingly lost its ability to solve societal problems.

Changes in party system

Since the mid-1980s, Austria has experienced a slow but continuous departure from this traditional political system. The stable two-party system ceased to exist, more parties entered the political arena, and ÖVP and SPÖ continuously and dramatically lost voters, so the political system became more volatile and competition oriented. Since 1986, the populist Freedom Party has vehemently and successfully challenged the basic arrangement of consociational democracy. Pillarization is losing importance; political parties are no longer able to sufficiently distribute benefits to their electorate to secure their support. Today they continuously must secure support by listening to an electorate that is highly mobile. New parties appear and disappear on the political scene (Pelinka, 2006)

Growing importance of dissatisfied citizens and courts

Another important driver for change is the growing importance of courts in Austrian politics. Individual citizens and citizen's movements who are dissatisfied with solutions provided by the political system and therefore fight for their rights in court have emerged as additional unpredictable and at times influential political actors. This has been particularly important in widening access to ART, equality politics for same-sex couples, and, most recently, the reform of assisted suicide (Knill et al., 2014; Leibetseder & Griffin, 2019; Van Beers, 2014; Verfassungsgerichtshof, 2020). Decisions of the ECtHR and the Austrian Constitutional Court "forced" the government to act on the one hand but also provided an undisputable and "depoliticized common ground" which gave the government the justification to work out a new compromise after decades of standstill (Griessler & Hager, 2016; Metzler & Pichelstorfer, 2020, p. 89). Now government had to do as it is told by indisputable court decisions.

Weakening position of the Catholic Church

Other important developments in the context of ART are the weakening role of the Catholic Church in Austrian society not only because of a loss of registered believers[7] but also because it lost influence with the conservative ÖVP, which, with new party leadership, became more liberal on ART questions.

Growing public acceptance of same-sex relationships and new family forms

In recent decades, lesbian and gay couples have become much more accepted in Austria (Griessler & Hager, 2016; Leibetseder & Griffin, 2019). Registered partnership for same-sex couples was introduced in 2010 (Waaldijk, 2017). In December 2017, the Constitutional Court ruled in favor of a formal complaint from a lesbian couple that marriage for same-sex couples was not allowed (Die Presse, 2017), and same-sex marriage became legal in 2019 (Leibetseder & Griffin, 2019). Joint adoption and second-parent adoption have been possible in Austria since 2013 and 2015, respectively.

ART physicians demand permissive regulation

Physicians are "pivotal actors in the reproductive field, enjoying social prestige and professional authority" (Engeli & Rothmayr Allison, 2016, p. 92). Although ART physicians are powerful actors, their impact on regulation might be moderated, and they might be "obliged (in public controversy) to compromise with competing powerful actors in the field such as women's organizations and pro-life movements" (Engeli & Rothmayr Allison, 2016, p. 92). This accurately portrays the Austrian situation: ART physicians are powerful actors in the politics of biomedicine (Griessler, 2010). However, because of the strong opposition of the restrictive ÖVP and the Catholic Church, as well as feminists in the 1990s, they had to make concessions (Hadolt, 2007). Although the reform of 2015 was in line with many demands of ART physicians, they continue to advocate more permissive regulations. The statement of the Austrian Society of Reproductive Medicine and Endocrinology and the Austrian IVF Society during the official evaluation process of the FMedRÄG is an example for this. The statement is signed by the members of both boards. It argues that the law does not do justice to "the current sociopolitical reality and scientific progress" and explains that

> for more than 30 years we can observe a change in the traditional family image "father, mother, child". Our society is increasingly confronted with single mothers (and fathers as well), so-called "patchwork-families" and with significant changes of the role of the women ("self-determination [sic],

fulfillment in the job, changed attitudes towards family planning: decision to childlessness, late pregnancies and birth), split of genetic and social parenthood and the phenomenon of cross border reproductive tourism.

(Urdl, 2014)

They demand access for single women to ART up to an age limit of 50 years because single mothers are a reality in today's society. Single women would seek cross-border treatment. Moreover, they demand "social egg freezing" for non-medical reasons, because they consider banning it paternalistic and violating the right to self-determination of individual life planning by the legislature. Otherwise women would seek trans-border treatment (reproductive tourism). As concerns egg donation, they want to raise the limit from 45 to 50 for the recipient. Again, they warn about reproductive tourism.[8] Moreover, they criticize the law because of a lack of anonymity for the donor, the prohibition on mediation of donators, and the limitation on compensation for expenses. They argue for compensation which covers the real total expenditures of the donor, including damages for pain and suffering. Moreover, they demand egg and embryo sharing using spare eggs and embryos from routine treatment cycles. Donators should be free to stay anonymous or not (Urdl, 2014). Only a few months after the FMedRÄG 2015 came into force, some physicians started to criticize the new law as too restrictive because it prohibits commercialization and brokering of donor eggs and sperm (Der Standard, 2015). ART physicians are not only campaigning for permissive regulations of ART through public statements. Acting as fertility brokers for trans-border surrogacy is an example of how ART physicians are pushing for permissive regulation by providing services to their patients.

Women's organizations are split

Engeli and Rothmayr Allison (2016) argue that women's organizations that are split in their positions and have weak links to other important social actors are unable to push through their positions in the regulation of ART. In the Austrian context, women's organizations are divided into permissive and restrictive camps as well, the first focusing on the right to abortion and reproductive autonomy, the latter on protecting women from exploitation. Whereas in the 1990s the dominant discourse for social-democratic women was on protecting women from exploitation, the discourse switched to self-determination and reproductive autonomy (Griessler & Hager, 2016). This is well captured in the statement of an Austrian policy maker who said in an interview: "Anyone who wants children should have them" (Griessler, 2012, p. 54).

Conclusion

Engeli and Rothmayr Allison (2016) distinguish between permissive and restrictive ART policies and suggest a third category: intermediate policies. An intermediate policy combines "characteristics of the restrictive and permissive dimensions".

Criteria for categorization are "(1) the autonomy granted to the medical community to practice ARTs; (2) the constraints imposed upon access to treatment; and (3) the availability of healthcare coverage for fertility-related treatment" (Engeli & Rothmayr Allison, 2016, p. 89). Engeli and Rothmayr Allison classify Austria as a restrictive country. In line with Leibetseder and Griffin (2019), we argue that Austria has combined restrictive and permissive elements since the FMedRÄG in 2015. It is more liberal towards same-sex relations, egg and sperm donation, and PGD limited to certain severe conditions but continues to adhere to the family model of two parents, a ban on surrogacy, and commercialization of donation, as well as lower age limits for cost coverage by IVF funds and donation. The change cannot be understood only as Austrian policy makers and society becoming more permissive but as a comprehensive change of Austrian political culture and structure.

Acknowledgments

This work was supported by the Austrian Research Promotion Agency and conducted within the project "Genetic Testing and Changing Images of Human Life". It was funded by the Austrian Genome Research Program (GEN-AU), as well as from internal funds of Institute for Advanced Studies. Florian Winkler contributed the section on surrogacy and the Parliamentary debate on the FMedRÄG in 2015. Erich Griessler conceptualized the chapter and wrote the remaining sections. We want to thank Heleen Weyers, Nicolle Zeegers, and Lenka Slepičková for valuable comments and Shauna Stack for language editing.

Notes

1 Insemination with donor sperm was permitted.
2 The Austrian newspapers covered in the WISO Portal were *Der Standard, Die Presse, Falter, FORMAT, Kleine Zeitung, Kronen Zeitung, Kurier, Neue Kärntner Tageszeitung, Neue Vorarlberger Tageszeitung, Neues Volksblatt, NEWS – Nachrichtenmagazin, Oberösterreichische Nachrichten, Profil, Salzburger Nachrichten, Tiroler Tageszeitung, Vorarlberger Nachrichten, Wiener Zeitung.*
3 The 1992 FMedG permits heterologous insemination in case of infertility of the heterosexual husband or partner [FMedG 1992 §3 (2)].
4 Aktion Leben calls for a restrictive regulation of surrogacy and advocates an international ban of surrogacy. The organization set up a homepage which describes surrogacy as both harmful for the surrogate mothers and the children born within such arrangements (www.leihmutterschaft.at/).
5 All quotes in this section refer to the stenographic protocol of the preliminary debate of FMedRÄG 2015 (Parlament, 2015).
6 Because of its historic dominant position in Austria and its high impact on Austrian society and politics, which is strong both in international comparison and in comparison to other confessions, the cleavage is more precisely not religious/secular but actually Catholic/secular.
7 In 2001, 75% of the Austrian population were members of the Catholic Church; with 12%, the unaffiliated, the second strongest group; next were Protestants with 5%. After 2001, only estimates are available since official statistics ceased to collect data on religious affiliation. Goujon et al. (2018, p. 18) estimate that share of Catholic believers in

2018 in Austrian population decreased to 63%; in the same time span, the share of unaffiliated increased to 18%, and the share of Protestants remained the same. The share of Muslims doubled between 2001 and 2018, from 4% to 8%; Muslims have the second-highest share of believers in the Austrian population.

8 It is interesting to note that the reproduction physicians' statement describes circumventive tourism as a negative development and as an argument for permissive regulation of ART. However, it is ART physicians who act in some cases as reproductive brokers and recommend their patients to U.S. clinics, in this way contributing to the development they are claiming they want to prevent.

References

Aktion Leben. (n.d.). Retrieved 30 November 2017, from www.leihmutterschaft.at/pages/leihmutterschaft/mehrinfos/article/451.html

Aktion Leben. (2017). *Parteien positionieren sich zu Lebensschutzfragen*. www.aktionleben.at/site/presse/article/545.html

Angermann, V., & Trescher, T. (2014). Ein neues Leben. *Datum. Seiten Der Zeit.*, *12*, 14–23.

Austrian Bioethics Commission. (2012). *Reform of the Reproductive Medicine Act. Opinion of the Austrian Bioethics Commission* [Statement]. www.bundeskanzleramt.gv.at/themen/bioethikkommission/publikationen-bioethik.html

Barth, P., & Erlebach, M. (2015). *Handbuch des neuen Fortpflanzungsmedizinrechts*. Linde.

Bundesministerium für Gesundheit und Frauen. (2017). *Genanalyse-Register gemäß § 79 Abs. 1 Z 1 GTG*. Bundesministerium für Gesundheit und Frauen.

Degelsegger, A., & Torgersen, H. (2011). Participatory paternalism: Citizens' conferences in Austrian technology governance. *Science and Public Policy*, 38(5), 391–402. https://doi.org/10.3152/030234211X12924093660679

Der Standard. (2015, June 11). Eizellenspende fördert 'gesundheits-tourismus'. *Der Standard*. http://derstandard.at/2000017313805/Eizellenspende-kurbelt-Gesundheits-Tourismus-an

Die Presse. (2017, December 5). Ehe für Homosexuelle kommt 2019. *Die Presse*. https://diepresse.com/home/innenpolitik/5333225/Ehe-fuer-Homosexuelle-kommt-2019

Eidlhuber, M. (2015, August 25). Retortenbaby: Ihr Kinderlein kommet. *Der Standard*. https://derstandard.at/2000020734784/Retortenbaby-Ihr-Kinderlein-kommet

Engeli, I., & Rothmayr Allison, C. (2016). Governing new reproductive technologies across Western Europe: The gender dimension. In M. Lie & N. Lykke (Eds.), *Assisted reproduction across borders: Feminist perspectives on normalizations, disruptions and transmissions* (1st ed., pp. 87–99). Routledge.

European IVF-monitoring Consortium (EIM), European Society of Human Reproduction and Embryology (ESHRE), Calhaz-Jorge, C., De Geyter, C., Kupka, M. S., de Mouzon, J., Erb, K., Mocanu, E., Motrenko, T., Scaravelli, G., Wyns, C., & Goossens, V. (2017). Assisted reproductive technology in Europe, 2013: Results generated from European registers by ESHRE. *Human Reproduction*, 32(10), 1957–1973. https://doi.org/10.1093/humrep/dex264

Gerlich, P., & Pfefferle, R. (2006). Tradition und wandel. In H. Dachs, P. Gerlich, H. Gottweis, H. Kramer, V. Lauber, W. C. Müller, & E. Tálos (Eds.), *Politik in Österreich. Das Handbuch* (pp. 501–511). Manz.

Glynn, S. M., Cunningham, P. N., & Flanagan, K. (2003). *Typifying scientific advisory structures and scientific advice production methodologies (TSAS)*. PREST, University of Manchester.

Gottweis, H. (1988). *Die Welt der Gesetzgebung. Rechtsalltag in Österreich*. Böhlau.

Goujon, A., Reiter, C., & Potančoková, M. (2018). *Vienna Institute of Demography working papers 13/2018. Religious affiliations in Austria at the provincial level: Estimates for Vorarlberg, 2001–2018*. https://doi.org/10.13140/RG.2.2.14612.55688

Griessler, E. (2004). The Austrian Bioethics Commission: Claims, legitimacy and practices. *Journal of Medicine, Life and Ethics, Society, 3*, 1–9.

Griessler, E. (2010). 'Weil das so ein heißes Eisen ist, rühren wir das besser nicht an' Zur Regulierung kontroverser medizinischer Forschung in Österreich. In P. Biegelbauer (Ed.), *Steuerung von Wissenschaft? Die Governance des österreichischen Innovationssystems* (pp. 143–186). StudienVerlag.

Griessler, E. (2012). *'Selbstbestimmung' versus 'Kind als Schaden' und 'Familie': Die politische Debatte um Pränataldiagnostik und Eizellspende in Österreich anhand der Beispiele des Entwurfs zum Schadenersatzänderungsgesetz und des Urteils des Europäischen Gerichtshofs für Menschenrechte* (Sociological Series). IHS. https://irihs.ihs.ac.at/id/eprint/2123/

Griessler, E., & Hager, M. (2016). Changing direction: The struggle of regulating assisted reproductive technology in Austria. *Reproductive Biomedicine & Society Online, 3*, 68–76. https://doi.org/10.1016/j.rbms.2016.12.005

Hadolt, B. (2007). Die Genese der Reproduktionstechnologiepolitik in Österreich: Überlegungen zum Politiklernen in neuen Politikfeldern. *Österreichische Zeitschrift für Politikwissenschaft, 36*(3), 285–302.

Hammerl, E. (2016, March 19). Uterus-Leasing. *Profil*. www.profil.at/meinung/elfriede-hammerl-uterus-leasing-6276542

Hanisch, E. (2005). Der lange Schatten des Staates. Österreichische Gesellschaftsgeschichte im 20. Jahrhundert. In H. Wolfram (Ed.), *Österreichische Geschichte 1890–1990*. Ueberreuter.

Kern, R. (2021). *IVF-Register Jahresbericht 2020*. Gesundheit Österreich GmbH. www.sozialministerium.at/Themen/Gesundheit/Eltern-und-Kind/IVF-Fonds.html

Knill, C., Nebel, K., & Preidel, C. (2014). Die katholische Kirche und Moralpolitik in Österreich: Reformdynamiken in der Regulierung von Schwangerschaftsabbrüchen und der Anerkennung gleichgeschlechtlicher Partnerschaften. *Österreichische Zeitschrift für Politikwissenschaft, 43*(3), 275–292. https://doi.org/10.15203/ozp.193.vol43iss3

Kummer, S. (2016, January 2). Leihmütter als Maschinen. *Die Presse*. https://diepresse.com/home/meinung/gastkommentar/4916756/Leihmuetter-als-Maschinen

Kurier. (2011, January 19). Hollywood im Leihmutter-Boom. *Kurier*.

Leibetseder, D., & Griffin, G. (2019). States of reproduction: The co-production of queer and trans parenthood in three European countries. *Journal of Gender Studies, 29*(3), 310–324. https://doi.org/10.1080/09589236.2019.1636773

Metzler, I., & Pichelstorfer, A. (2020). Embryonic silences: Human life between biomedicine, religion, and state authorities in Austria. In M. Weiberg-Salzmann & U. Willems (Eds.), *Religion and biopolitics* (pp. 73–96). Springer International Publishing. https://doi.org/10.1007/978-3-030-14580-4_4

Oberhauser, S. (2016). *8341/AB vom 17.05.2016 zu 8716/J (XXV.GP)*. www.parlament.gv.at/PAKT/VHG/XXV/AB/AB_08341/imfname_532079.pdf

Özkan, D. (2014, August 9). Leihmutterschaft: Die Mütter anderer Kinder. *Die Presse*. https://diepresse.com/home/leben/mensch/3852455/Leihmutterschaft_Die-Muetter-anderer-Kinder

Parlament. (1999). *Bundesgesetz, mit dem ein Fonds zur Finanzierung der In-vitro-Fertilisation eingerichtet wird (IVF-Fonds-Gesetz) (4.1.2013)*.

Parlament. (2015). *Stenographisches Protokoll der 59. Sitzung des Nationalrates am 21. Jänner 2015*. www.parlament.gv.at/PAKT/VHG/XXV/NRSITZ/NRSITZ_00059/fname_419 486.pdf

Pelinka, A. (2006). Die Politik der politischen Kultur. *Österreichische Zeitschrift für Politikwissenschaft, 35*(3), 225–235.

Potz, R. (2005). Staat und Kirche in Österreich. In G. Robbers (Ed.), *Staat und Kirche in der Europäischen Union* (pp. 425–454). Nomos.

Präg, P., & Mills, M. C. (2017). Assisted reproductive technology in Europe: Usage and regulation in the context of cross-border reproductive care. In M. Kreyenfeld & D. Konietzka (Eds.), *Childlessness in Europe: Contexts, causes, and consequences* (pp. 289–309). Springer International Publishing. https://doi.org/10.1007/978-3-319-44667-7_14

Prainsack, B. (2006). Religion und politik. In H. Dachs, P. Gerlich, H. Gottweis, H. Kramer, V. Lauber, W. C. Müller, & E. Tálos (Eds.), *Politik in Österreich. Das Handbuch* (pp. 538–549). Manz. http://ub-madoc.bib.uni-mannheim.de/21077

Statistik Austria. (2020). *Bevölkerung*. www.statistik.at/web_de/statistiken/menschen_und_gesellschaft/bevoelkerung/index.html

Steiner, K. (1972). *Politics in Austria*. Little Brown and Company.

Steurer, P., & Aberle, S. (2015, July 29). Ihr Kinderlein kommet. *News*.

Strozzi, N. (2017, June 25). Baby auf Bestellung. *Tiroler Tageszeitung*.

Tálos, E., & Kittel, B. (2001). *Gesetzgebung in Österreich: Netzwerke, Akteure und Interaktionen in politischen Entscheidungsprozessen*. Facultas.

Tempfer, P. (2017). Leihmütter. Mutterleib auf Miete. *Wiener Zeitung*. www.wienerzeitung.at/nachrichten/oesterreich/politik/867598_Mutterleib-auf-Miete.html

Ulram, P. (2006). Politische Kultur der Bevölkerung. In H. Dachs, P. Gerlich, H. Gottweis, H. Kramer, V. Lauber, W. C. Müller, & E. Tálos (Eds.), *Politik in Österreich. Das Handbuch* (pp. 512–524). Manz. http://ub-madoc.bib.uni-mannheim.de/21077

Urdl, W. (2014). *Stellungnahme zu Entwurf* (Statement 12/SN-78/ME XXV. GP). Österreichische Gesellschaft für Reproduktionsmedizin und Endokrinologie. www.parlament.gv.at/PAKT/VHG/XXV/SNME/SNME_02390/imfname_376183.pdf

Van Beers, B. C. (2014). Is Europe 'giving in to baby markets?' Reproductive tourism in Europe and the gradual erosion of existing legal limits to reproductive markets. *Medical Law Review, 23*(1), 103–134. https://doi.org/10.1093/medlaw/fwu016

Verfassungsgerichtshof. (2020, December 11). *Erkenntnis 139/2019-71*. www.vfgh.gv.at/downloads/VfGH-Erkenntnis_G_139_2019_vom_11.12.2020.pdf

Waaldijk, K. (2017). *More and more together: Legal family formats for same-sex and different-sex couples in European countries. Comparative analysis of data in the laws and families database* (No. 75; Familes and Societies Working Paper Series). https://archined.ined.fr/view/AWRHxjC8gpz89Adag4VF

3 Assisted reproduction in the Czech Republic

Lenka Slepičková

Introduction

The regulation of assisted reproduction in the Czech Republic is relatively liberal regarding techniques available: unlike in other European countries, all assisted reproduction technology (ART) techniques are allowed, publicly accepted and widely used, including in vitro fertilization (IVF); intracytoplasmic sperm injection (ICSI); assisted hatching; preimplantation genetic diagnosis (PGD); donation of sperm, eggs or embryos – within particular age limits and with the guarantee of donor anonymity. The Czech Republic represents a country with a long tradition and high quality of infertility treatment and favorable legislation, attracting a substantial number of foreign patients every year, coming mostly for treatment with donor eggs, which is anonymous, relatively cheap and highly efficient. However, access to ART is limited, and attempts to open assisted reproduction to women without a male partner or outside the age limit (set at 39 for treatment partially covered by health insurance and 49 for treatment paid by the patient) have not been successful, mainly due to criticism from conservative and Catholic politicians. In this aspect, we can observe tension between conservative policy and liberal attitudes of physicians and the general population.

This chapter will examine the trends in providing assisted reproduction in the Czech Republic and the reasons for the immense popularity of reproductive technologies in this country. The current legal regulations and their development will be elaborated upon, along with recent attempts to change the legislation: to change the age limit for women using assisted reproduction and allow access to ART for single women in 2011 and to introduce non-anonymous donation of gametes for in vitro fertilization and allow access to ART for single women again in 2017. The chapter will also focus on the opinion of the general public and physicians concerning assisted reproduction and the potential changes in its legal regulation and will cite qualitative research on infertile couples that reveals how such regulation affects their experience with infertility treatment.

Infertility treatment in the Czech Republic

Infertility treatment using ART has a long tradition in the Czech Republic – the first "test-tube baby" in the Czech Republic and Central and Eastern Europe was

DOI: 10.4324/9781003223726-3

born in an IVF center in Brno, the capital of Moravia, in 1982, utilizing the gamete intra-fallopian transfer (GIFT) method. In 1984, at the same clinic, the first baby conceived through IVF in the former Czechoslovakia was born. Since then, this branch of medicine has rapidly developed. Nowadays, more than 40 specialized clinics, both private and public, offer their services to the 10 million inhabitants of the Czech Republic),[1] and the number of assisted reproduction cycles provided every year is growing (see Figure 3.1).

Almost all regions in the Czech Republic are covered by clinics and hospitals offering infertility treatment; however, they are primarily concentrated in large cities such as Prague, Brno and Ostrava (Institute of Health Information and Statistics of the Czech Republic, 2019).

High-quality treatment; a wide range of procedures offered, including those prohibited in other countries; and affordable costs, together with various opportunities for travel and sightseeing, attract many foreign patients to Czech infertility clinics, mostly from the United States, Germany, Italy and Israel (Whittaker & Speier, 2010). In an annotation of her book *Fertility Holiday*, which focuses on the journeys of North Americans to the Czech Republic for IVF, Amy Speier (2016) claims:

> As the lower middle classes of the United States have been priced out of an expensive privatized "baby business" the Czech Republic has emerged as a central hub of fertility tourism, offering a plentitude of blonde-haired, blue-eyed egg donors at a fraction of the price.

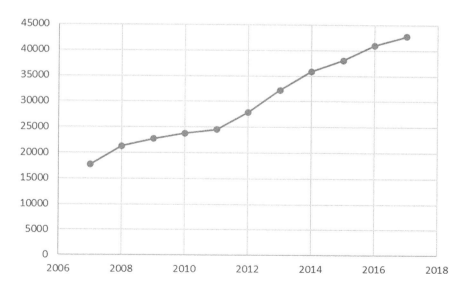

Figure 3.1 Number of cycles of assisted reproduction (2007–2017).

Source: Institute of Health Information and Statistics of the Czech Republic (2019)

One reason underlying this type of travel, in her account, is the quest for empathetic physicians the American patients are finding in the Czech health care system.

An advertisement for infertility treatment in the Czech Republic lists more reasons to come and even promises results:

> Thanks to a broad spectrum of methods, adherence to strict criteria important for successful treatment, and long-term experience, Czech IVF (in-vitro fertilization) teams are among the best in the world, and success rates are also very high: 70% in cases involving donated eggs. Czech comprehensive IVF centres can help up to 90% of couples, often even those whose situation seems to be hopeless.
>
> (CzechTourism, 2021)

The share of foreign patients is increasing in Czech fertility clinics: while in 2007, the share of ART cycles provided to foreign patients was 13.5%, in 2011, it was 26.4%, and in 2013, the share was 34.5% (Institute of Health Information and Statistics of the Czech Republic, 2015). Foreign couples are seeking mostly procedures using egg donors: in 2016, a cycle using donor oocytes in the Czech Republic was provided to 783 Czech patients and to 5,774 foreign patients – the share of foreign patients was 88.1% (Institute of Health Information and Statistics of the Czech Republic, 2019).

Some clinics explicitly focus on foreign clients. However, because donors are anonymous, unlike in other countries, it is not possible to offer a "catalogue" of donors with their current or childhood pictures and detailed descriptions of their personalities, education and hobbies. The match between donor and patient is made on the basis of several criteria, including blood type, hair and eye color and height.

Legal regulation of assisted reproduction in the Czech Republic

First provisions

The first expert discussions over paternity proceedings in the case of conception due to assisted reproduction already occurred in Czechoslovakia during the creation of the Act on the Family in 1963. In the end, it was claimed that no legal regulation was needed, given the state of development in methods of infertility treatment (Thalerová, 2016).

The first legal provisions on ART were passed in 1982. The amendment of the Act on the Family (132/1982), in reaction to the first successful artificial fertilization in Czechoslovakia, stated that paternity of a child born between 180 and 300 days after artificial fertilization provided with the consent of the husband of the mother could not be revoked, except for cases in which there was evidence that the pregnancy occurred by other means (Thalerová, 2016).

However, access to assisted reproduction, as well as the other conditions for providing assisted reproduction, were not regulated by law but only by guidelines from the Ministry of Health (from 1982, 1997 and 2001), which stated that assisted reproduction could be provided only in qualified institutions providing health services, and only for medical reasons, through a written request from both members of a marital couple. The married woman undergoing assisted reproduction could not be older than 35. Donors were to be anonymous, and their age was regulated (Thalerová, 2016). Access to treatment for non-married couples was enabled in 2006 by an amendment to the Act on Public Health (227/2006).

Current regulations

The legal regulation of ART has remained fragmentary. Some general laws dealing with health or family are also applied to the field of assisted reproduction, but complex legal regulation of ART practice does not exist. The first act regulating ART in the Czech Republic was introduced in 2006 (Act No. 227/2006 on research using human embryonic stem cells and related activities and an amendment to some related acts). Until 2006, the Ministry of Health had regulated ART through its guidelines.

Nowadays, the most important legal provisions in the field of assisted reproduction are Acts No. 227/2006, which regulate embryo cell research and assisted reproduction, and No. 373/2011, on specific medical services, which includes several chapters focused on assisted reproduction. Articles 11–14 of the Convention on Human Rights and Biomedicine (that was ratified in 2001) also relate to assisted reproduction. The Convention bans sex selection (except in cases involving the risk of transmitting a serious sex-linked disease). The Convention on Human Rights and Biomedicine also regulates PGD, which can be provided only for medical reasons or research.

Procedures

Unlike other European countries, many ART techniques are allowed and practiced in the Czech Republic – IVF; ICSI; assisted hatching; selective reduction of embryos; PGD; cryopreservation of oocytes and embryos; and donation of sperm, eggs or embryos (within particular age limits and with the guarantee of donor anonymity). The only exception is surrogate motherhood, which is not allowed because Czech law considers only the woman who gave birth to the child its mother.

Access with regard to type of relationship

Legally, assisted reproduction is available only to stable heterosexual couples in the Czech Republic (it is not necessary to be married to undergo ART). The prospective father must sign a form stating that he accepts the treatment and that the child born after the treatment will be legally his child, regardless of whose biological material is used. However, the doctors providing infertility treatment are not

Table 3.1 Overview of the Czech legal regulation of assisted reproduction.

Age limit	Women under 49 (39 = health insurance limit)
Access with regard to type of relationship	Marriage or stable heterosexual relationship (often circumvented by "fake partners")
Coverage	Three or four cycles (with the provision of single embryo transfer in the first two cycles) partly covered by obligatory health insurance for women between 22 and 39
Cryopreservation of oocytes	Allowed
Cryopreservation of embryos	Allowed
Sperm donation	Allowed (age of donors 18–40; anonymity guaranteed; no charge is possible, only reimbursement of direct, reasonable and proven costs)
Oocyte donation	Allowed (age of donors 18–35; anonymity guaranteed; no charge is possible, only reimbursement of direct, reasonable and proven costs)
Embryo donation	Allowed (anonymity guaranteed)
ICSI	Allowed
Assisted hatching	Allowed
Oocyte maturation	Allowed
Selective reduction	Allowed
PGD	Allowed
Surrogacy	Not allowed, not prohibited, practiced unofficially

obliged to investigate the type of relationship. The law excludes only such types of relatedness between partners undergoing assisted reproduction that would prohibit them from marrying. After treatment, who appears as the father on the birth certificate is not checked. Therefore, some single (or lesbian) women are coming to clinics with "fake" partners who sign the necessary forms to obtain treatment.

Hašková and Sloboda (2018) analyze the ways in which access to ART for non-heterosexuals is negotiated in the Czech Republic. They claim that, in practice, the parental rights and obligations of the man who acted as a partner at the infertility clinic may be enforced, which may represent a source of concern for the parental couple. For single men and gay couples, it is impossible to benefit from ART in the Czech Republic either through a fake partner or through a surrogate mother. Some are thus fulfilling their desire to become parents through using surrogate mothers abroad (Hašková & Sloboda, 2018).

Health insurance coverage

Besides the restrictions related to the status of the couple and the age of the woman, the other factor limiting the availability of infertility treatment is its cost.

In the Czech Republic, the system of partial coverage for ART by the general obligatory health insurance is applied. The general health insurance covers three or four[2] cycles of IVF for women under 39. Any additional drugs and procedures (ICSI, assisted hatching, donation, PGD, etc.) are paid by the patients, as only the cheapest drugs and basic procedures are covered. Similarly, any additional cycles after the initial three or for women older than 39 are fully paid by the patients. This stands in contrast to the fact that patient payments for healthcare are not common in the Czech system, with the exception of aesthetic plastic surgery or higher-quality materials in stomatology.

The system of health insurance coverage neglects the fact that half of couples seek infertility treatment due to male infertility. The treatment is covered only from a woman's health insurance, no matter whose physical impairment is the cause of the infertility, and the number of covered cycles is limited to only three or four cycles for women. Men, in contrast, can undergo an unlimited number of cycles a life with their female partners covered by health insurance. The current system of coverage also does not reflect the trends in the type of preferred treatment; nowadays, it is primarily the ICSI procedure[3] that is used in assisted reproduction, but this is the procedure that is not covered by health insurance (as only "basic" IVF is covered).

Surrogate motherhood

Surrogate motherhood has been practiced illegally in the Czech Republic since 1993 as a series of legal and medical steps. Clinics offically claim that patients for surrogate motherhood can be accepted only for severe medical reasons, such as the absence of a uterus.[4] Prospective parents must locate a surrogate mother, as clinics do not enter the process until the IVF cycle is realized. The surrogate mother is preferably single or divorced; if she is married, she must obtain approval from her husband, as he must agree to refrain from asserting fatherhood. The surrogate mother undergoes "infertility" treatment involving the donor sperm of the prospective father, whom she names as the biological father after giving birth. The child is then adopted by the prospective mother. These individual arrangements involve not only informal financial compensation but also much uncertainty and risk, as the rights and obligations of all parties are not legally enforceable. Moreover, the principle of anonymity between donors and infertile couples in assisted reproduction (Act 373/2011) is violated. The number of babies born to surrogate mothers in the Czech Republic is estimated at 50 per year.

The Civil Code mentions surrogate motherhood only once, claiming that adoption is prohibited among relatives, with the exception of surrogate motherhood (§ 804). An explanatory memorandum defines surrogate motherhood as a situation in which a child is born to a woman who is not the biological mother. However, the principle that the mother of a child is the woman who gave birth remains valid. The relationship between a biological mother and a child born to a surrogate mother can be regulated only through the process of adoption. An explanatory memorandum to §775 of the Civil Code clearly states, "The claim of the woman who was the genetic donor against the woman who gave birth cannot be approved".

Surrogate motherhood abroad and the parental rights of gay couples

Gay couples in the Czech Republic cannot marry and cannot share parental rights or adopt a child as a couple. The institution of a "Registered Partnership" was introduced in 2006 by Act 115/2006. It regulates the matters of a partnership and introduces advocating, heritage and maintenance obligations between same-sex couples. Registered partners cannot jointly adopt a child and cannot have access to assisted reproduction.

As explained previously, for gay couples, it is not possible to use surrogate motherhood in the Czech Republic; consequently, some are traveling abroad to realize their parental intentions with the help of a surrogate mother. However, when coming back to the Czech Republic, they cannot be approved as a parental couple. At the moment they cross the border, the parental relationship of one of them formally ceases to exist.

In May 2018, a landmark case was decided in the Czech Republic when two gay men, the parents of a child conceived through surrogate motherhood in California, were approved as parents by the Constitutional Court. Originally, only one of them was approved as the father. But, according to the judges of the Constitutional Court, the best interest of a child should be more important than abstract principles, and both partners are part of a legally approved family protected by the Charter of Fundamental Rights. But, at the same time, the Constitutional Court emphasized that this situation was exceptional, as it was related to a parental relationship that originated in a foreign country.

The Czech general population is quite supportive regarding the right of same-sex couples to adopt a child: 60% of respondents in a survey conducted by the Public Opinion Research Centre[5] agreed with the right of homosexuals to adopt the child of their partner, 47% supported the right to marry and 47% agreed with the right of same-sex couples to adopt a child from institutional care. The support of the rights of homosexuals is stronger among women, younger people (15–44), respondents who assess their standard of living as good, respondents with higher levels of life satisfaction and voters of the right-wing or center parties (Public Opinion Research Centre, 2019).

Surplus embryos

According to Act 373/2011 on specific medical services (Article 9), if there are surplus embryos created during infertility treatment, it is possible to conserve them and use them for another cycle of IVF for the same couple unless the couple expresses in writing their intention to donate them to another infertile couple, to use them for research or to destroy them. If there is no written approval for another use or destruction of the embryos, the provider can, after 10 years of preservation, call upon the couple to express their will regarding the preserved embryos. If there is no response, the provider may destroy the embryos.

Research on human embryonic stem cells

Act 227/2006 (Article 3) states that research on human embryonic stem cells can be carried out only after authorization from the Ministry of Education, Youth, and Sport only in qualified institutions providing health services on imported lines, provided that they were obtained from human embryos in such a way that does not go against Czech legislation or the legislation of the country of origin; their import is allowed only for research purposes, which cannot lead to the creation of a new human being.

Political discussions on ART regulation

2008: Discussing the access of single women to infertility treatment and setting age limit

An effort to redefine the boundaries determined by the legislation governing assisted reproduction occurred in the Czech Republic between 2008 and 2011. This effort was part of the so-called reformation package, which also included the Act on Specific Medical Services. The Act regulates the conditions under which assisted reproduction is available.

There are two issues that have turned out to be controversial in the Czech Republic: access to the treatment for single women and age limits for women receiving assisted reproduction. Age barriers had not previously been clearly defined in the legislation.

The topic of assisted reproduction for single women has provoked much debate in Czech media (Slepičková, 2015). In the end, under pressure from the Christian-Democratic Party and certain church institutions, this proposal was eliminated from the law.

In Czech society, with its significantly low level of religiosity, it is not very common to see the Church intervene in public debates. The Czech Bishops' Conference (2008) declared in a statement: "Permitting this, the father is eliminated from fatherhood. And it is not in accordance with our efforts to support complete families. The ideal type of family for children is a life with biological parents".

It is surprising that in the Czech Republic, one of the most secular countries in the world, the Catholic Church has such political power. The authors of a book on the political discussions concerning early childhood care in the Czech Republic (Hašková et al., 2012) provide several explanations for this paradoxical influence of the Catholic Church on family policy. One concerns the multi-party electoral system in the Czech Republic, which enables small political parties such as the Catholic one (the Christian and Democratic Union – the Czechoslovak People's

Party) to become part of the coalition in almost every government. The other important fact is that family policy is one of the most important issues for this party. The members of this party have always been able to achieve some kind of influence on the Ministry of Labor and Social Affairs – not directly in the position of minister but at least in the position of a deputy.

The second point, concerning the age limit for women seeking assisted reproduction, was widely debated within consultations with professionals and stakeholders during preparation of the bill as well as in Parliament and finally; it was set at 49. The discussion in Parliament was highly paternalistic and male dominated (corresponding to the fact that the representation of women in Czech political institutions is extremely low) (Slepičková, 2015). Women were described as passive objects of medical intervention: the debate was framed by the question "Until what age can a woman be fertilized?" Further, the ridiculing figure of a mother-granny was invoked to depict those that intended to conceive at an "inappropriate age". In contrast to similar debates in other countries (Fenton, 2006), the figure of the "mad scientist", whose actions should be limited by law was replaced with the figure of a money-grubbing doctor.[6] Those who objected to higher age limits argued that doctors working in the field of assisted reproduction also violate the "laws of nature". Arguments concerning the right of a woman to decide about her own motherhood were rarely invoked (Slepičková, 2015).

2017: Single women on the scene again and an attempt to introduce non-anonymous donation of gametes for IVF

In April 2017, the Czech Parliament debated an amendment to the Act on Specific Medical Services that included access to ART for single women. The debate was described as "emotional" (Kopecký, 2017), provoking "heated discussion" and "sharp statements" (Skoupá et al., 2017). František Adámek from the Czech Social Democracy party, who proposed the bill, described the then-valid legislation on assisted reproduction as "hypocritical"; after all, single women were commonly undergoing infertility treatment, obtaining written consent from their "fake" partners, namely friends. The bill was also strongly supported by the minister of labor and social affairs (from the Social Democratic Party), Michaela Marksová, who argued that many single women are intelligent working professionals who really want children and who will care for them very well; accordingly, the state should support their efforts as they would with any child. She referred to the low fertility rate in the Czech Republic as one of the main arguments. She also mentioned that it is common to circumvent the current law using "fake partners". What is more, around 50% of children are born outside of marriage, and the divorce rate in the Czech Republic is also around 50%.

The proposed change to the law, allowing single women to undergo infertility treatment officially, was also supported by medical professionals working in infertility clinics, who referred to the current legal restrictions as "non-functional, useless and humiliating". They are, of course, and it is implicitly mentioned several times in the discussion, suspected to have vested interests in the matter, because a change in the law would bring them more clients. Their argumentation is described in the debate as solely purpose built.

In contrast, the minister of health was against the change, claiming that the topic is a sensitive one and any changes have to be publicly debated before their introduction. Assisted reproduction, in his opinion, should always treat an infertile couple, and the state has to prefer complete families (Skoupá et al., 2017).

The other objectors – mainly from conservative right-wing parties – stated that the right to a child is not a human right. The Christian-Democratic Party, which emphasized its long-standing support for traditional families based on one mother and one father, was against the change as well. The members of the Christian-Democratic Party even stated that if access of single women to the infertility treatment were to be approved, it would block the approval of the entire bill. In the end, this part of the amendment was not approved by Parliament (with only 40 deputies voting for it and 153 against).

The other changes debated included, for example, the introduction of non-anonymous donations of gametes for in vitro fertilization. The group of Members of Parliament, who proposed this change, argued for the right of children to know their origin. This change was not approved, which was expected, even by the deputies who proposed it. The opponents argued that the bill involved neither the rights of the parents (the infertile couple who underwent assisted reproduction) nor the rights of donors to be protected from violating their privacy. The bill even did not include the obligation of parents to tell the child about assisted reproduction. Before rejection of the bill, some physicians working in the field of assisted reproduction publicly expressed their concern about the radical decrease of available donors because of the introduction of non-anonymous donation.[7]

Other rejected changes concerned a change in the age limit for women undergoing assisted reproduction from 49 to 45 when using donor eggs and an explicit ban on surrogate motherhood.

The introduction of an Expert Committee on Family Policy and its unheeded suggestions for changes in the legal regulation of assisted reproduction

In 2015, two years before the debate in Parliament over changes in the access to ART, the Czech minister of labor and social affairs (Czech Social Democratic Party), Michaela Marksová, nominated an Expert Committee for Family Policy for a two-year term in order to discuss and propose actions for supporting families. The members of the committee included a demographer, a sociologist, an economist, a representative of the Czech statistical office and a member of a research institute within the Ministry of Labor and Social Affairs (Czech Social Democratic Party). The resulting policy paper, "Family Policy Plan", published in September 2017 (five months after the last debate in Parliament), includes a section on "What Do Families Need?" in the chapter "Available Assisted Reproduction" (Ministry of Labor and Social Affairs, 2017). The results and recommendations in this policy paper are in sharp contrast with the previous decisions of Parliament, as they suggest a more permissive policy advocating the rights of citizens who cannot conceive naturally and want to use ART in the context of the very low fertility rates in the last decades in the Czech Republic.

The policy paper notes the increasing number of assisted reproduction cycles in the Czech Republic, along with the increasing proportion of children born through assisted reproduction (almost 4%), connecting it to the trend of post-poning parenthood. The paper further covers three issues in the field of assisted reproduction: 1) its availability (costliness and the age limit); 2) the necessity to have written consent from the male partner for a woman to obtain access to treatment; and 3) the fact that treatment is covered by the woman's health insurance, regardless of the medical cause of the infertility.

According to the policy paper, the costliness of treatment represents an important obstacle to the use of assisted reproduction, especially for women who exceed the age limit (39) for coverage by health insurance. This age group of women is, compared to other countries, underrepresented in the group of patients undergoing infertility treatment in the Czech Republic. The paper states, "The health status of women differs and the final assessment of the ability to undergo assisted reproduction should be within the purview of a medical professional instead of being strictly limited by age" (Ministry of Labor and Social Affairs, 2017, p. 52).

The paper also highlights the fact that the written approval from a male partner necessary for a woman to be treated leads to a situation in which many women obtain consent only formally, from men who are not their partners. Some other women without a partner, according to the paper, choose "unsafe and undignified ways" to become pregnant (Ministry of Labor and Social Affairs, 2017, p. 53). By allowing access to assisted reproduction for women without the permission of a male partner, the Czech Republic would become a member of the group of countries that have opened this possibility, such as the United Kingdom, Belgium, Denmark and Spain. This change would be a positive signal for the support of fertility, the paper claims.

Furthermore, it is not logical, the paper argues, that the system of health insurance coverage does not take into consideration the medical causes of infertility; the process is covered entirely by the health insurance of the woman. The fact that Czech families mostly want two children is not taken into account either. The infertile couple is infertile when partners cannot conceive, even if the couple or one of the partners already has a child/children.

The committee recommends that future governments establish an inter-ministerial group led by the minister of health, which would engage in legal regulation of assisted reproduction in the Czech Republic. This group should consider undertaking the following actions (Ministry of Labor and Social Affairs, 2017, p. 53):

- increasing the age limit for assisted reproduction covered by health insurance[8]
- a re-definition of the "cycles covered by health insurance", from coverage of "four cycles for a woman" to coverage of "four cycles to conceive a child", which would increase the number of cycles covered by health insurance

- coverage for complete infertility treatment (including medication and donor gametes) by health insurance
- eliminating the necessity for a male partner's approval for a woman's infertility treatment
- starting a discussion of the role of men in the treatment of infertility and considering coverage for assisted reproduction by the male partner's insurance

Following the recommendation of the Expert Committee on Family Policy, the Committee for Reproductive Medicine was nominated in 2017 by the Ministry of Health in order to "discuss the key issues in the field of reproductive medicine in accordance with the national health policy" (Ministry of Health, 2020). The committee has had only two meetings as of October 2021. In the notes from the meeting, the committee states that the members, mostly physicians, did not support increasing the age limit for women undergoing IVF covered by health insurance to 43 (from 39), and they did not support access to IVF for single women or complete coverage of treatment by health insurance. On the other hand, increasing the number of cycles covered by health insurance from "four cycles for a woman" to "four cycles to conceive a child" was supported. However, as of October 2021, no changes in the Czech law regarding assisted reproduction have been enacted. Minister Marksová ended her work in the government in December 2017 after parliamentary elections.

The Ministry of Health and its attitude toward potential changes in the law regarding assisted reproduction

Just one month after the debate in Parliament, in May 2017, the Ministry of Health (Miloslav Ludvík, Czech Social Democratic Party) released a statement from its ethical committee concerning particular aspects of assisted reproduction (Ministry of Health, 2017) and supporting a rather restrictive position towards access to ART. This statement expressed a moral concern over the current proposals being debated, such as raising the age of mothers or opening access to assisted reproduction for single women: "The natural right to conceive and raise children, grounded in our legislation, does not mean that medical services are obliged to enable every woman to become a mother" (Ministry of Health, 2017). The statement emphasizes "the best interest of the child" as the leading principle in discussions concerning parenthood and assisted reproduction.

The statement is based on a document from the association Adam. Adam is an association founded by the psychologist Hana Konečná focused on the "psychosocial aspects" of infertility treatment. It operates on a voluntary basis. It provides information for infertile couples in the Czech Republic and releases statements on current trends in infertility treatment. It used to be a member of Fertility Europe group, an international patients' organization, but ceased its membership in 2018 because of a disagreement with providing assisted reproduction "outside biological limits" (single persons, homosexuals, persons outside age limits), trends that Fertility Europe supports.

This document is described as "highly qualified opinion based on relevant data" by the ministerial ethical committee. However, the document was created with obvious intention: do not support proposed changes,[9] and its arguments cannot be viewed as the results of the objective analysis. For example, the cited research on adolescents about how old their mother ideally should be (with the strong preference of adolescents to have a younger mother) is not representative of the population of Czech adolescents, and its relevance to the legislative limits of infertility treatment is disputable. Like the final statement of the ethical committee, the document is based on general concepts such as "a mature enough maternal bond", "the quality of the marital relationship", "the maturity of parents", "the ability of parents to carry the burden of parenthood" and so on.

The document published by the Ministry of Health further claims that the proposed changes in the legal regulation of assisted reproduction are not morally acceptable (Ministry of Health, 2017). It also presents changes that would create new barriers in access to assisted reproduction, such as setting the age limit for women using donor eggs to 40, implicitly to "educate" women: by introducing this limit, "the natural loss of fertility would remain the important factor in the decision making over motherhood". The statement also warns against the commercialization of assisted reproduction and calls for open public debate over this problem. According to the statement, access for single women to assisted reproduction is undesirable because the state cannot replace the "missing" parental figure. No adjustments to the system of health insurance coverage for assisted reproduction are needed, according to the statement, in terms of extending the coverage to a (frequently infertile) male partner, but an increase in the covered cycles from four to six is acceptable (Ministry of Health, 2017).

Attitudes of Czech men and women towards infertility treatment

As was stated previously, assisted reproduction is a common popular way of solving infertility in the Czech Republic.

The attitudes of the general population towards adoption as a way of solving infertility are also rather positive, as is shown in Figure 3.2, based on survey data. The sample is representative of the overall Czech population.

Data suggest that infertility is perceived in the Czech Republic primarily as a medical problem requiring a high-technology treatment. We can potentially associate this finding with the very low levels of religiosity in the Czech Republic; religious concerns regarding the ethics of assisted reproduction are frequently cited in other countries.

Czech men and women also hold very positive attitudes towards adoption, which is the second most often considered solution in the hypothetical situation of infertility. However, ART techniques using donors have a relatively low popularity within the Czech population; they would only be chosen by approximately one-third of respondents.

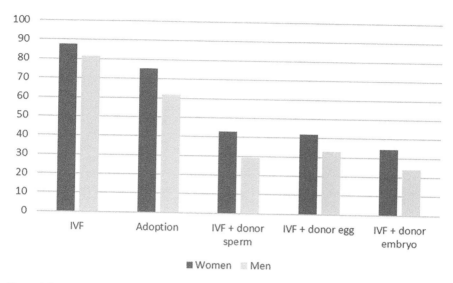

Figure 3.2 Would you consider this solution in the case of infertility? (% answering "YES").
Source: Slepičková (2007)

In comparison, the data from qualitative research conducted among infertile couples suggest the contrary. Among the overall population, adoption is a socially desirable and worthy act. But for the infertile couples interviewed, ART is pre- ferred to adoption. Adoption usually represents a last-resort solution, chosen only when other means of becoming a family have failed, for example, after the three (or four) IVF trials covered by the general health insurance (Slepičková, 2010). Thus, the actual behaviors of infertile couples do not correspond to the declared attitude of the Czech population.

The voices of physicians

In 2012, a survey of Czech physicians was conducted with the aim to capture their opinions about the general situation within Czech medicine (Slepičková & Šmídová, 2014). Czech doctors were also asked about their opinions concerning the introduction of potential changes in reproductive medicine (see Figure 3.3). Attitudes towards the medical manipulation of DNA and embryos were also exam- ined. The attitudes of some doctors towards assisted reproduction techniques or changes in obstetric practices were supportive of changes – the introduction of ART for single women had the highest support, along with surrogate mother- hood. Moreover, approximately one-quarter of the physicians supported increas- ing the age of women eligible for financial coverage of assisted reproduction. Sex

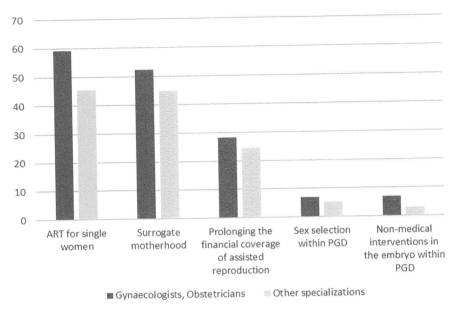

Figure 3.3 In your opinion, which of the following options should be accessible to Czech patients? (N = 1,200).

Source: Adapted from Slepičková and Šmídová (2014)

selection within PGD and non-medical interventions in the embryo, as the most ethically challenging practices, had almost no support. Gynecologists and obstetricians, who made up 13.25% of the sample, were generally more supportive of the changes to assisted reproduction in comparison to physicians, among other specializations.

The voices of patients

According to qualitative research conducted among infertile Czech couples, despite the wide range of procedures available to them, patients often perceive the reality of infertility treatment as restraining and discriminatory (Slepičková, 2010). The age limit is the biggest source of stress for women undergoing infertility treatment. Women, as the exclusive addressees of medical and media warnings about the age limit and the reproductive abilities of their bodies (Zamykalová, 2006), and as the sole representatives of age regulation for the availability of assisted reproduction, are more and more aware of their increasing age, which strongly affects their reproductive strategy (Bartošová & Slepičková, 2008). What is more, the fact that the age limit for treatment and the more general and informal age limits for parenting are related to formal and informal norms and sanctions directed exclusively at women can represent a basic source of conflict between partners (Slepičková, 2010). Women without a stable partner are declaring their maturity and preparedness for motherhood, but at the same time, they feel discriminated against and undignified within a system that denies them their independence. If they are not willing to conceive with an incidental acquaintance (as sometimes suggested by doctors), they have only one option to obtain treatment – undergo it abroad (Slepičková, 2010).[10]

Conclusion

Despite low fertility rates, high divorce rates and a growing proportion of children born outside marriage in the past three decades, Czech men and women repeatedly report strong positive attitudes toward family life and parenthood, exceptional even in the Central European context. Parenthood is considered the core of adult identity, and parenting children is the most important mission of marriage for the majority of Czech men and women, as shown by data from the most recent surveys, including the Value of Children or Marriage, Work and Family, which examine the attitudes of the general population toward parenthood and family (Rabušic & Chromková Manea, 2018). The high value of parenthood, together with low levels of religiosity and the high and stable prestige of the medical profession, referred to as "performing miracles" in the sphere of assisted reproduction, represent an environment in which infertility treatment is perceived as an automatic and doubt-free path towards parenthood for those experiencing fertility problems. However, its exclusivity, available only to a certain type of a parent-to-be, is a matter of political negotiation, and the result often represents quite conservative ordering.

Although the Czech Republic has liberal laws regarding the techniques of assisted reproduction, its legislation remains rather conservative in terms of access. Recent attempts to enable single women or women over 39 to use ART legally and with the coverage of health insurance as well as the idea of the introduction of non-anonymous donation of gametes for IVF provoked a heated discussion.

Even the government is not of a single opinion: the Ministry of Labour and Social Affairs (Czech Social Democratic Party) takes a permissive perspective and calls for an expert committee to review the regulation, while its party colleague, the Ministry of Health, bases its restrictive position on an analysis made by a traditionalist lobby organization. The supporters of more liberal policies argue with reference to the declining birth rate in the Czech Republic (and other demographic trends such as a high percentage of children born outside marriage and high divorce rate in the Czech Republic) and the fact that any intention to have a child should be supported, especially one made by mature and highly educated women. They also note that current regulation is frequently circumvented and forces women to use undignified ways to fulfill their wish to become mothers. The advocates of more restrictive legislation warn that the state cannot replace the father figure of the family and is not obliged to enable any woman to become a mother. They also object that the support of ART is not going to increase fertility.

Regarding final decisions in Parliament, the more conservative positions are repeatedly shown to be more powerful, supported by the Catholic institutions, that – surprisingly in the Czech Republic, with its low religiosity – have a traditionally high influence on Czech family policy.

On the level of practice and views of general population and physicians working in the field, we can observe more liberal attitudes than on the level of policies: the Czech population, according to representative surveys, is positive towards ART, and ART is used very often compared to internationally. Survey data also show support of gynecologists for more permissive regulations. What stands apart in all these debates is the position of infertile couples undergoing the process of fertility treatment who report that they feel stressed by the age limits, guilty about their own intimate relationship and reproductive decisions and discriminated against and undignified under current legislation (Slepičková, 2010).

Marginalization of the reproductive intentions and rights of women and sexual minorities is another common theme in the discussions of assisted reproduction. Women in particular are presented as foolish figures but at the same time fully responsible for reproduction and its connected problems, such as postponing parenthood and fertility issues, despite evidence showing that there are (especially young) men who hesitate to become parents (Kyzlinková & Šťastná, 2016) and who are the ones whose infertility is bringing couples to seek treatment. The reproductive intentions of women, especially single women or women outside the limits of "proper" motherhood, as well as homosexuals, are presented as a call for regulation for the sake of protecting the "traditional family" (or the "natural order"), which, considering the 50% divorce rate and 50% of children born outside of marriage, even now hardly represents the prevalent family form in the Czech Republic.

Notes

1 The number of clinics is increasing (from 27 clinics operating in 2007 to 43 in 2017). Based on the latest data available.
2 Four cycles are covered if in the first two cycles only one embryo is transferred.
3 The Czech Republic belongs among the countries with the highest ICSI usage (Kupka et al., 2014), with the proportion of the ICSI procedure greater than 80% of all IVF cycles.
4 Cycles initiated for reasons of surrogate motherhood are not differentiated in the official statistics, so we do not have any evidence on the diagnosis of the couple.
5 In May 2019, the Public Opinion Research Centre published the results of research on the tolerance of Czech society towards homosexual persons and their rights (Public Opinion Research Centre, 2019).
6 This reference was made several years before the former Czech prime minister (incumbent at the time this chapter was written; in office: 2017–2021), Andrej Babis, became the owner of a network of infertility clinics.
7 The Adam association called this change the "irresponsible experiment of social engineering" on its web pages and published an analysis supporting this claim.
8 In 2021, the change of the age limit for women undergoing IVF covered by health insurance from 39 to 40 was discussed in Parliament. The change was not approved.
9 In the section "news" on Adam's web pages, the following statement was published in April 2017: "We are glad that the bill including the right of single women to the access

to ART was not supported by Parliament. It is an extremely disputable step. Yes, the single woman has the right to have a baby when she is pregnant; no one has to force her to undergo an abortion or to take her child. But can she ask the state to fertilize her?"

10 There is an infertility treatment clinic in the Czech Republic, operating since 2011, focused on single women and explicitly promising them an IVF procedure involving donor sperm. "You can become a mother even without a partner", it advertises its services. The donors and patients are Czech, but the procedure itself occurs abroad during a 7–10 day stay in a country where assisted reproduction is legally accessible to single women.

References

Bartošová, M., & Slepičková, L. (2008). Problematické tranzice k mateřství. *Sociální studia/ Social Studies*, 5(2), 35–54. https://doi.org/10.5817/SOC2008-2-35

Czech Bishops´ Conference. (2008). *Stanovisko České biskupské konference k návrhu věcného záměru zákona o specifických zdravotních službách*. Czech Bishops´ Conference.

CzechTourism. (2021). *Reproductive medicine. In the Czech Republic, doctors can help virtually every couple*. www.czechtourism.com/a/reproductive-medicine/

Fenton, R. A. (2006). Catholic doctrine versus women's rights: The new Italian law on assisted reproduction. *Medical Law Review*, 14(1), 73–107. https://doi.org/10.1093/medlaw/fwi041

Hašková, H., Saxonberg, S., & Mudrák, J. (2012). *Péče o nejmenší: Boření mýtů*. Sociologické nakladatelství SLON.

Hašková, H., & Sloboda, Z. (2018). Negotiating access to assisted reproduction technologies in a post-socialist heteronormative context. *Journal of International Women's Studies*, 20(1), 53–67.

Institute of Health Information and Statistics of the Czech Republic. (2015). *Asistovaná reprodukce 2013*. www.uzis.cz/rychle-informace/asistovana-reprodukce-2013

Institute of Health Information and Statistics of the Czech Republic. (2019). *Asistovaná reprodukce 2017*. www.uzis.cz/index.php?pg=aktuality&aid=8356

Kopecký, J. (2017, April 26). Zbláznila se, řekla Marksová o Chalánkové, která odmítla právo na dítě. *IDNES.Cz*. www.idnes.cz/zpravy/domaci/zblaznila-se-rekla-marksova-o-chalankove-ktera-odmitla-pravo-na-dite.A170426_131005_domaci_kop

Kupka, M. S., de Mouzon, J., Erb, K., D'Hooghe, T., Castilla, J. A., Calhaz-Jorge, C., De Geyter, C., Goossens, V., Strohmer, H., Obruca, Strohmer Partnerschaft Goldenes Kreuz-Kinderwunschzentrum, Bogaerts, K., Biostat, I., D'Hooghe, T., Kyurkchiev, S., Antonova, I., Rezabek, K., Markova, J., Erb, K., . . . Baranowski, R. (2014). Assisted reproductive technology in Europe, 2010: Results generated from European registers by ESHRE. *Human Reproduction*, 29(10), 2099–2113. https://doi.org/10.1093/humrep/deu175

Kyzlinková, R., & Šťastná, A. (2016). Reprodukční plány mladých mužů v ČR. *Demografie*, 58(2), 111–128.

Ministry of Health. (2017). *Stanovisko Etické komise ministerstva zdravotnictví k některým otázkám asistované reprodukce*. https://socialnipolitika.eu/2017/05/stanovisko-eticke-komise-ministerstva-zdravotnictvi-k-nekterym-otazkam-asistovane-reprodukce/

Ministry of Health. (2020). *Komise pro reprodukční medicínu*. https://ppo.mzcr.cz/work Group/32

Ministry of Labour and Social Affairs. (2017). *Koncepce rodinné politiky*. www.mpsv.cz/files/clanky/31577/Koncepce_rodinne_politiky.pdf

Public Opinion Research Centre. (2019). *Czech public opinion on the rights of homosexuals – May 2019*. https://cvvm.soc.cas.cz/en/press-releases/other/relations-attitudes/4945-czech-public-opinion-on-the-rights-of-homosexuals-may-2019

Rabušic, L., & Chromková Manea, B. E. (2018). *Hodnoty a postoje v České republice 1991–2017.* Masarykova univerzita Brno.

Skoupá, A., Šrajbrová, M., & ČTK. (2017, April 26). Umělé oplodnění pro single ženy neprošlo. Mít dítě není základní právo, řekla Chalánková. *Aktuálně.cz.* https://zpravy.aktualne.cz/domaci/umele-oplodneni-pro-single-zeny-rozhadalo-politiky-mit-dite/r~d13e4ee02a8f11e7a8d6002590604f2e/

Slepičková, L. (2007). Vajíčko, spermie, zkumavka . . . A Gender. Postoje českých žen a mužů k asistované reprodukci a adoptivnímu rodičovství. *Gender – rovné příležitosti – výzkum, 8*(2), 68–75.

Slepičková, L. (2010). Couples undergoing infertility treatment in the Czech Republic: Broad range of possibilities in a traditional milieu. *Social Theory & Health, 8*(2), 151–174. https://doi.org/10.1057/sth.2009.25

Slepičková, L. (2015). Dokdy je možné fertilizovat ženu? Parlamentní debata o zákonné úpravě asistované reprodukce. *Gender Rovné Příležitosti Výzkum, 16*(2), 60–72. https://doi.org/10.13060/12130028.2015.16.2.221

Slepičková, L., & Šmídová, I. (2014). Postoje českých lékařů k medicíně a ke změnám v praxi reprodukční medicíny. *Data a Výzkum-SDA Info, 8*(1), 63–95.

Speier, A. (2016). *Fertility holidays: IVF tourism and the reproduction of whiteness.* New York University Press.

Thalerová, N. (2016). *Právní aspekty asistované reprodukce.* Univerzita Karlova.

Whittaker, A., & Speier, A. (2010). "Cycling overseas": Care, commodification, and stratification in cross-border reproductive travel. *Medical Anthropology, 29*(4), 363–383. https://doi.org/10.1080/01459740.2010.501313

Zamykalová, L. (2006). Mediální reflexe bezdětnosti v české společnosti mezi lety 1994–2004. In H. Hašková (Ed.), *Fenomén bezdětnosti v sociologické a demografické perspektivě* (pp. 95–144). SOÚ AV ČR.

4 Taming Technology

Assisted Reproduction in Denmark[1]

Janne Rothmar Herrmann

Introduction

The aim of this chapter is to outline the overall Danish legal framework for the regulation of assisted reproductive technologies (ART) and discuss how and why these particular regulations came about. The Danish regulation of ART contains numerous issues that could be highlighted (Adrian et al., 2021; Herrmann, 2013; Herrmann & Kroløkke, 2018; Kroløkke et al., 2019; Kroløkke & Herrmann, 2019); however, this chapter will focus on the history of ART regulation in Denmark in order to understand how and why the relatively prohibitive regulation came about in a country where 1 in 10–12 children is born through assisted reproduction.

The chapter relies on bills, parliamentary debates as the bills passed through the three readings in Parliament and the adopted acts, as well as preparatory documents such as public consultation responses, parliamentary questions, reports of the parliamentary health committee and reports by the Danish Council of Ethics (tasked specifically to advise Parliament on ART). The documents have been located using electronic and manual searches.[2] A number of non-electronically and non-publicly available files have been made available to me courtesy of the Library of the Danish Parliament. The legal doctrinal method has been applied to identify the relevant legal sources and to analyze what the law is. Drawing on inspiration from Bacchi's *What's the Problem Represented to be?* (WPR) approach (2009), the analysis is also critical. The WPR approach argues that policies contain implicit representations of the 'problems' they purport to address. The goal of the WPR approach is to treat these problem representations as problematizations that can be critically scrutinized. This chapter draws inspiration from this approach in also paying attention to what the problem is represented to be to understand how regulation was shaped and evolved over time. How and why did Danish regulation come about?

The Early Years of Debate

In 1948, a working group under the Ministry of Justice considered whether legislation on insemination was needed. However, their recommendations were been put forward as a bill by the government, and consequently assisted reproduction,

DOI: 10.4324/9781003223726-4

as with most medical procedures, did not attract regulatory attention. In 1956, the two Danes Fuchs and Riis published in *Nature* a feasible method for antenatal sex determination performed in the uterus. They flagged the potential ethical concerns relating to selection, stating that the method should not be used for mere curiosity. They further flagged it to the media and invited parliamentarians to a short briefing, but interest was low. In 1977, a working group under the Ministry for the Interior published a white paper considering prenatal testing from a predominantly scientific and economic perspective to assess if fetal diagnostics was to be expanded in the health care system. The political appetite for addressing the ethical issues relating to selection only emerged later in tandem with the emergence of ART.

The Beginning of Regulatory Interest: Assisted Reproduction as a Cause for Concern

1983 marked a fundamental change in available fertility treatments in Denmark. Fertility treatment, which had previously consisted of hormonal medication, surgery and insemination, was revolutionized with the introduction of in vitro fertilization (IVF) and consequently the birth of the first Danish IVF baby. The media called the baby boy a miracle. However, his birth also initiated regulatory interest in reproduction. Up until that point, assisted reproduction had not been subject to regulation, and the introduction of IVF as a treatment had thus been purely a medical decision, even bypassing the (non-binding) research ethics evaluation that would have been a stepping stone had IVF not been introduced directly as a treatment by medical professionals.

A few months after the birth of the first Danish IVF baby, the minister for interior (who belonged to the Conservative Party) formed a working group to consider the ethical and legal ramifications. These issues were not on the public agenda at the time. It was very much a decision based on the minister's personal troubles as a regular citizen in making head or tail of the technologies that were dawning on the horizon – difficulties sparked, inter alia, by a conference organized by members of the scientific community inviting the minister and the public to become aware of the emerging ethical issues. In October 1984, the working group published their report "The Price of Progress". The cover of the report depicted Adam and Eve holding the forbidden apple in the Garden of Eden, thus signaling the seriousness of what was at stake. The report stated that the issues at stake were central facets of our culture that transgressed normal disciplinary delineations and involved the public. As such, ethical considerations had to be balanced against scientific knowledge, the group recommended the establishment of a National Council of Ethics. It seems that the working group envisaged a body resembling the UK Human Fertilisation and Embryology Authority. The report also outlined some first thoughts on the potential of ART to select certain lives. The report thought it important to consider the nature of disease and at what point it became irreconcilable with leading 'a normal life'.

Parliament debated the report on April 10, 1985; the Socialists and the Christians in particular were skeptical of ART. The government at the time consisted of the Conservatives, the Liberals, the Christians and the Social-Liberals, and no one in the opposition was against subjecting ART to ethical reflection and subsequent regulation. In 1987, a Council of Ethics was established by Parliament with, inter alia, the task of considering ART, their ethical and legal implications and what regulatory measures were needed to protect fertilized eggs. Rather than being a regulatory or licensing body, the Council was to make recommendations to Parliament and initiate debate and dialogue with the public.

The Act instructed the Council to base its work on the assumption that human life began at fertilization, a point that had been highly debated. The Socialists, Labour and the Social-Liberals all expressed concern for the potential ramifications for on-demand abortion services. The Act's instruction to assume that life began at fertilization originated from the Christian Party and was introduced during readings in Parliament. It was not uncontroversial; among the opponents was the president of the Scientific Research Ethics Committee, who stated that fertilization was a necessary precondition of life but not an adequate condition for the development and subsequent birth of a child, emphasizing the equal importance of implantation and the following natural, biological deselection of non-viable embryos. The Act furthermore included a prohibition on conducting research on fertilized eggs. The prohibition was intended to last until the Council of Ethics had had time to deliberate.

A few years after the Council was established, it published its first reports, "Prenatal Diagnostics, Prenatal Screening, Genetic Counselling – A Discussion Paper" (1989) and "Protection of Human Gametes, Fertilized Eggs, Pre-Embryos and Embryos – A Report" (1989), reflecting that selection of lives was thought to be a pressing and important ethical issue. During the parliamentary debate on the first proposed legislation, preimplantation genetic diagnostics (PGD) was also one of the most debated issues; the Socialists were very skeptical, stating, "no matter what, preimplantation genetic diagnosis opens the flood gates to so many issues, that we will have to prohibit all sorts of things next time we look at the Act", but the Red-Green Alliance was more positive, emphasizing that the strain on the woman was considerably lower if selection could take place prior to implantation rather than as an abortion later in the pregnancy. The Conservatives emphasized that they did not want a scenario where there was "a right to receive all sorts of diagnostic tests for all sorts of diseases" without specific indications.

The Council's 1989 report on the protection of human gametes, embryos, pre-embryos and fetuses became part of the preparatory work that shaped the 1991 Bill on Biomedical Research Ethics Committees, which regulated some elements of ART when they were still considered experimental, and thereafter the Bill on Artificial Fertilisation that would later be adopted. One of the issues raised related to the storage of gametes and embryos (for subsequent self-donation). The Council observed that viability of gametes and embryos was hard to preserve and accordingly recommended a time limit for cryopreservation. A majority of the Council found "that cryopreservation of eggs should be allowed subject to the same conditions applicable to sperm, i.e. that cryopreservation should be allowed for a limited time and had to be destroyed at the time of the depositor's death" (p. 81). However, in the section dedicated to considerations on the cryopreservation of sperm, the Council found that the duration of storing of sperm should not be subject to any limitations except what medical or administrative grounds would call for as long as the sperm was destroyed when the depositor died (p. 60–61). Whereas male gametes had no storage limit, women's eggs were to be restricted with regard to the number of years that they could be cryopreserved. Another issue raised by the report was the question of access to treatment. The Council found that ART was to be likened to natural intercourse, and as such, no conditions should be posed in terms of parenting skills. There were two different majority groups within the Council; one found that a child should have one parent of each sex and that both parties should assume parental responsibility prior to treatment through an informed consent. In case of donor sperm, the social father would be the consenting father. Another majority group found that it was not paramount to secure the child a father from the beginning, thus finding that single and lesbian women should also be given access to treatment (p. 59).

Most of the issues considered by the Council of Ethics did not spark immediate regulatory response. The initial impact of the Council of Ethics' report was simply that it formed part of the background material for the 1991 Act on Biomedical Research Ethics Committees, which lifted the research ban on fertilized eggs in order to ensure adequate quality in the provision of fertility treatments. IVF was slowly becoming a recognized clinical treatment, which meant that research – as was the case in all other treatments offered – was integral in ensuring good quality. Thus, initially, the dominant perspective was on the research aspect of ART. However, section 14 of the act did address treatment aspects in that it authorized the health minister to issue a ministerial order regulating donation and cryopreservation of human eggs. In the travaux préparatoires to the authorization of the minister, the government stated that the authorization provided the basis for the regulation of questions of a more medical/scientific nature raised by the application of ART. This included first and foremost requirements regarding establishing egg banks and cryopreservation. But the authorization was in reality not solely for regulation of technical questions. A normative issue was intended to fall within the authorization, reflected in the fact that the government explicitly stated that it presupposed a maximum cryopreservation period of 12 months for eggs and embryos, but no reasoning for the limit was given in the comments included in the bill.[3] In this manner, eggs and embryos were regulated in ways that sperm was not (Herrmann & KrChapter 4Løkke, 2018), and the first regulation of ART was thus included in an act otherwise predominantly concerned with creating a legally binding framework with respect to research ethics.

The general regulation in medical law at the time was characterized by a high degree of professional self-regulation and covered primarily the legal and administrative framework for the healthcare system and some educational demands regarding healthcare personnel and issues of malpractice, torts and complaints, as well as the duty to provide information to patients. As a result, fertility treatment had also been left to develop within the healthcare system without regulatory interference. A working group on fertility treatment set up by the minister of health in 1992 (Sundhedsministeriet, 1992) argued that there was overall no need for special regulation "because the practice of insemination had evolved in such a way that it did not give rise to any worries". Insemination was performed by gynecologists and other medical specialists, and as such, the working group was satisfied that the standard of care met professional medical standards and that adverse risk of transferal of diseases through donation was managed in an appropriate manner.

However, the public was increasingly concerned that the medical community had introduced IVF as a treatment and that access to treatment was not based only on medical criteria but also on whether the couple had any common children (Larsen, 2007). In 1993, the government issued a press release outlining its intent to regulate ART.[4] The headline of the government's paper outlining its intent to regulate ART seemingly offered reassurance ("Clear Guidelines for Artificial Fertilization") and stated that the minister had asked the National Board of Health to issue guidelines based on the government's "comprehensive initiative to regulate". The initiative included limiting the maximum number of embryos to be implanted after IVF, a requirement to use cryopreserved sperm only in case of donation (for safety reasons, since cryopreservation would ensure adequate testing for HIV), to implement a national reporting system allowing the Board of Health to "control retrieved eggs" and supervise the quality of treatment and to set in place guidelines which "mirrored women's natural ability to bear children". Having in mind that said ability could end unnaturally early in some women (premature menopause), ART could always be offered to women up to 40 years of age. But on account of the maintenance and upbringing of the child, 45 years was to be the upper limit for women to receive fertility treatment, while no age limit existed for men. In a response to the parliamentary Committee for Health, the minister added that the increased risk in pregnancy and at birth for older women was also to be considered in setting the upper limit at 45 years.[5] This was the first step in subjecting fertility treatments to various guidelines and instructions.[6] Subsequent legal interpretation would also rely on the intention to *control* as the basis for denying eggs transnational mobility.

Thus, the government's paper outlined some boundaries but was hardly a comprehensive regulatory effort. It set the framing of the 1993 guidelines issued by the National Board of Health. The guidelines stated that assisted reproduction as a form of fertility treatment raised ethical questions, making it necessary for the Health Board to issue guidelines. The guidelines then listed the following decisive elements (which also illuminate what ethical issues were of concern for the regulator): that there were several different solutions to infertility which should be reflected in the physician's information to the couple; that there was a need to balance the risk of complications in relation to hormonal stimulation and multiple pregnancy with the desire to achieve pregnancy; that ART made pregnancy possible in female age groups where pregnancy and childbirth were rare; that it was timely to update the regulation of donation, making egg donation possible and limiting the use of donor sperm to cryopreserved sperm only for safety reasons; and that the pace at which ART was developing made it advisable to make these clarifications. In this way, when fast-paced technological developments transformed to treatments, they had to be controlled not only to protect patients from risk but also to balance the new technological answer to infertility with the other solution (adoption). At the time of ART being in its infancy, parliamentary debates often expressed concern that the technological answer to infertility would leave potential adoptive children without potential adoptive families. Control was also needed in order to codify what was seen as the "natural" reproductive age and make it normative. The guidelines noted in that respect that the average age for the onset of menopause was 52 years but that only a small number of women over the age of 45 years conceived naturally. Clinical experience with pregnancy and birth following ART in first-time mothers over 50 years old was limited, making the physician's duty to assess risk in relation to age especially important. As such, ART was seen to raise ethical and societal issues that challenged the image of the responsible and morally sound doctor which had prevailed previously.

The guidelines framed ART as a *treatment* for infertile heterosexual couples. The treatment perspective was underlined through the legalization of egg donation and the intention to provide legal clarity and foreseeability for physicians when making changes in existing treatment practice or introducing new treatments. The choice of the guideline as a means of regulation reflects that it was professional in nature, addressed to physicians from the supreme regulatory and supervisory authority and to be sanctioned within the professional disciplinary system and not within the criminal law system. Such guidelines were generally meant as professional best practices and are not instructive but support the decisions made by health professionals. As such, physicians could deviate from the guidelines on solid professional and scientific grounds. Conversely, a deviation that was ill founded would be a breach of the professional due care duty, and the National Board of Health would be able to take steps in its capacity as the authority issuing licenses to practice and supervising professional standards.

The chosen regulatory model ties in well with the predominant legislative view of that time. However, the trust in medical doctors to navigate the ethical issues raised by ART was under fire. In a parliamentary debate on January 25, 1994, on the topic "What are the government's plans in relation to following, regulating or prohibiting the use of current and future reproductive technologies?" Parliament agreed on a motion confirming that ethical assessments must be part of the ongoing development of ART in relation to both research and clinical applications. Parliament underlined explicitly that treatment could not be introduced if the underlying research was prohibited according to the 1991 Act on Biomedical Research Ethics Committees and that the Council of Ethics and Board of Health should be notified before the introduction of new treatments in order to advise on any ethical and health issues. Furthermore, the minister for health was to make sure that new treatments did not exceed what was ethically acceptable before they were introduced into clinical practice.

The Parliamentary motion was subsequently transformed into a Ministerial Order and guidelines by the National Board of Health.[7] A remarkable gendered implication of the Ministerial Order was the newly added restriction on transnational mobility. Increased mobility of human tissues had been a European political focal point for more than a decade with, for example, the Council of Europe's 1979 recommendation no. R (79) 5 concerning international exchange and transportation of human substances calling for member states to facilitate such exchange. Unfertilized eggs, embryos and sperm were, however, exempt. It is not clear why the Danish Ministerial Order restricted transnational mobility on eggs and embryos *only* (and not sperm). However, in a decision of March 22, 1993, the Health Ministry had denied a Danish woman permission to export nine cryopreserved embryos retrieved from a private hospital in Denmark to a private clinic in Germany where she lived, citing the legislature's premise of being able to *control* that the limitations on cryopreservation and the like were enforced. The decision was brought before the Ombudsman, who noted (opinion FOU 1993.277) that the legal basis for such a prohibition was inadequate. But since he could not refute that it had been Parliament's intention that eggs and embryos were to stay in the country for control purposes, there was insufficient ground for criticizing the Ministry.[8] Most likely, ethical concerns motivated the control of eggs and embryos. In 2002, the same argument was used as the reasoning for a provision to ensure that stem cell lines derived from embryos could only be imported into Denmark if the same requirements as those applicable in Danish law had been met abroad.[9] No longer residing in the safety of the female body, the eggs and embryos were discursively positioned as entities in need of state protection.

Moving From Professional Guidelines to Legislation

It was clear from the 1994 debate that Parliament was anxious for government to put forward comprehensive regulation of ART due to ethical concerns. In February 1996, a bill[10] was introduced to regulate "artificial fertilization", providing a legal basis for the prohibitions, which had previously been issued administratively.[11] This meant that the regulation of ART moved away from being an administrative regulation of physicians' professional activity to being a normative comprehensive act with criminal law sanctions. ART was now framed predominantly as a fertility treatment (which had to be tamed).

The bill's overall approach was to regulate in the language of prohibition. The prohibitions related to both research activities and clinical applications and introduced an approval system in terms of the introduction of new treatments. It included a provision on cryopreservation, which codified the limitation on the cryopreservation of eggs and embryos to 12 months. However, the National Health Board would have the possibility to grant permission to extend cryopreservation "in special cases, where the woman's health or other critical grounds" spoke in favor of an extension. Once again, no upper storage limit existed with regard to the cryopreservation of sperm. It is clear from the Parliamentary debate following the first reading in Parliament that the linguistic similarity in the Danish language between the words "unfertilized eggs" (*ubefrugtede æg*) and "embryos" (*befrugtede æg*) made it difficult to distinguish between the two. The spokesperson for the Socialdemocratic Party said: "At present no eggs are frozen, but technology may catch up. I find 12 months to be right. To me, there is something unethical about having embryos in storage maybe even to have twins in separate pregnancies".[12] The monstrosity of disrupting what appeared a normative kinship order ("twins in separate pregnancies") became pivotal in these debates (Herrmann & Krpløkke, 2018). The Conservative Party's spokesperson admitted that it was difficult to provide a rational reason for the 12-month limitation: "it is the thought of the artificial that scares me . . . after 2 or 3 years in the freezer . . . are the eggs in good condition? The foods we freeze have a shorter shelf life". The spokesperson for the Socialist Party was generally against ART, referring to them as "monstrous research".[13] However, the bill did not succeed in being read three times during the parliamentary working year, because the parliamentary Health Committee felt that there was insufficient time to debate and negotiate the bill. Consequently, it was automatically struck from Parliament's agenda. The government reintroduced the bill with slight revisions the following Parliamentary year.[14]

When the bill was put forward again the following parliamentary year, PGD was hardly debated at all. Minor revisions had already been included to address the original concerns, which meant that PGD was only to be used in case of a known risk of the child being born with severe genetic disorders or to diagnose or rule out chromosomal disorders. The regulation of PGD applied to both infertile and fertile women. The predominant concern during the debate now was taming "monstrous research", also reflected in the prohibitive language used to draft the act. As the 1997 Act on Artificial Fertilisation was adopted, certain techniques, which had previously been unregulated, became the object of legislative interest. This included PGD, and the provision remains unchanged since its adoption. Section 7 allows fertile couples with prior known risk of passing on a serious hereditary disease to use PGD, as well as infertile couples who are treated for infertility with IVF. In both cases, the preparatory work states that PGD is allowed in order to offer an alternative to subsequent abortion, stating that PGD could become the most acceptable alternative to a late induced abortion. The dominant perspective is thus that of wishing to spare the woman having to undergo an abortion at a later stage, reflecting a gradualist view of the ethical status of the embryo/fetus, which dominates Danish law in general, while limiting the use of PGD to the specific instances allowed in the act. The adopted act, which applied to treatment by medical doctors only, allowed only couples (married or in a marriage-like relationship) to access treatment. It further included an "objective" age limit of 45 years for women in replacement of the bill's suggested subjective limit of 40–45 years that was based on an *individual assessment* of the woman's reproductive capacity (meant to assess whether she was still able to reproduce 'naturally' or menopausal). This assessment was initially intended to apply to both men and women, but following public outcry from various men in the media, the adopted requirement related to women only. During the parliamentary Health Committee's deliberations, different constellations of party minorities, majorities and individual members proposed a large number of amendments. As for limiting cryopreservation, a proposition stated that it was offensive to have "the family in the freezer", which is why fertilized eggs should be allowed to be stored for two years only and the cryopreservation of unfertilized eggs should be extended to two years. Interestingly, cryopreserved sperm did not invoke the same kind of response.

The general extension of the one-year legal limit on cryopreservation was believed to address the concerns related to the woman and her family (having to rush the use of cryopreserved eggs), cases of illness in the woman and the physical and mental trauma of having to undergo renewed hormone stimulation and egg retrieval. The extension was meant to ensure the successful achievement of one pregnancy in legally accommodating further treatment cycles if the first attempt was unsuccessful. It was noted that the Ministry had received more than 100 applications asking for dispensation from the time limit and that longer cryopreservation limits abroad indicated that there were no safety issues in extending the limit. However, the limit was not to be extended beyond the two years out of consideration for the voiced ethical concerns including the Council of Ethics, which in its yearly report for 1995 had stated that scientific studies indicated that cryopreservation of eggs would likely damage the chromosomal material. Between readings, the parliamentary Health Committee considered the bill, and various members posed various suggestions for amendments. Their deliberations, the public consultation responses and the suggested amendments reflect a number of key concerns: Would the technology lead to unnecessary treatments (and burden the welfare state)? What were the consequences (for women's rights) of individualizing eggs and embryos in this way? What were the best interests of the child, and what was the appropriate age of mothers (Adrian et al., 2021)? It is clear that politicians could not look to existing party manifestos to form an opinion, and across the political spectrum, all parties (except perhaps the Progressive Party) had some form of concern relating to the aforementioned themes. The responses from public consultation show that it was predominantly the affected or involved actors who responded through their respective organizations (the Danish Society for Women, the Association for the Involuntarily Childless, the Association of Disability Organisations and various medical and healthcare professionals and societies).[15] Apart from a few private persons expressing general concerns, the organizations tended to support strict regulation on, for example, the maximum age of mothers and limitations on PGD while supporting the availability of ART as a treatment offer in general.

The adoption of the Act on Artificial Fertilisation in 1997 was followed by the adoption of the Patients' Rights Act 1998, reflecting a general legislative move away from self-regulation to taming health technologies. As noted, the regulators' perception of medicine as a scientific endeavor in the service of the moral good was changing.

According to the act's section 30, subsection 5, the government was obliged to consider if revisions to the Act on Artificial Fertilisation were needed. Consequently, in 2000, the government proposed an extension of the two-year cryopreservation period to four years. The travaux préparatoires stated that there were both medical and ethical reasons behind the regulatory limit. However, it is clear that the precautionary principle was also an important factor. The government emphasized that the experience from countries with more liberal limits for cryo-preservation indicated that the embryos would not be damaged by extended cryo-preservation. The extension was proposed to help the women who did not achieve pregnancy within the current limit, sparing them the procedure and possible complications of a renewed cycle of hormonal stimulation and egg retrieval. During the referral to the parliamentary Committee on Health, several supplementary amendments were made to the bill, including provisions on self-payment and assessment of parenting skills. A suggested provision demanding payment for fertility treatment was a fundamental deviation in the delivery of healthcare and, as such, seen as an attack on the Danish welfare state, which provides free and equal access to health care. For that reason, the minister advised Parliament to vote no to the amended bill. Consequently, cryopreservation continued to be allowed for up to two years only, and the suggested assessment of parental skills was held off.

In 2004, a further use of PGD was introduced requiring ministerial approval in each case. In case PGD was necessary to create a 'savior sibling' with a compatible tissue type to save an older sibling with severe disease, the use of PGD could be allowed. The amendment of the act followed media reports of several children where a savior sibling was perceived to be the only option left to the parents. Again, the Socialists were critical – especially of the number of supernumerous embryos that would be created as a result. They were joined by the Red-Green Alliance, which was concerned by the ethical dilemmas this put parents and children in. The minister (who belonged to the Liberals) emphasized that the introduction of this new measure had been recommended by the University Hospital of Copenhagen.[16] The Council of Ethics had been against it by a narrow majority, arguing that children were not 'spare parts' (Det Etiske Råd, 2003), but the amendment was nonetheless supported by a majority in Parliament.

Families (Forever)

In 2006, a bill[17] to reform the Act on Artificial Fertilization was more successful. The stated objective of 'modernization' set the tone for a relaxation in several respects. The act focused less on the fear of technologization of reproduction characteristic of the first act and more on the human aspects of assisted reproduction: making families. In an attempt to make egg donation more readily available in the clinic, it widened access for egg donation, allowing all women – not only those undergoing fertility treatment – to donate eggs. It included new provisions on assessment of parenting skills to ensure that technology would not help create children for unfit parents, obliging doctors to deny treatment or refer assessment to an appropriate authority in case of doubt. The assessment of parental skills was not to be an actual assessment of parental skills but more of an attempt to spot and block access to treatment for those who were obviously not competent to parent due to mental illness, abuse problems or previous removal of children by social services. Based on previous media accounts of couples who had been given access to treatment in spite of having several children already removed by the authorities, the main political concern was to ensure that those with an obvious lack of parental skills would not be able to reproduce with assistance. The act did not mirror the more thorough assessment of parental skills already in place in the regulation of adoption. Furthermore, it extended the maximum period of cryopreservation of eggs to five years and allowed single and lesbian women access to treatment. The accompanying remarks state that both the Ministry and the National Board of Health had continued to receive requests for dispensation from the time limit in order for the family to try for a second child with the cryopreserved eggs. Whereas the two-year limit had been about ensuring a successful treatment resulting in *one* pregnancy, the issue was now that of securing families more time in establishing *a second pregnancy*.[18] In this respect, the 'modernization' of the act actually supported the establishment of a traditional nuclear family with two children. Relying upon scientific knowledge that cryopreservation posed no risk, the government extended the cryopreservation limit to five years, successfully enabling the possibility of having two children from the same stimulation cycle. It was stressed, however, that cryopreserved eggs were subject to other legal limitations besides the length of the cryopreservation period, such as the requirements of destruction in case of death and divorce, the rules on donation to other women and the requirements of consent in case of donation to research. It was mainly to ensure enforcement of these rules and requirements that an upper limit for cryopreservation should still be in place. Meanwhile, no upper storage limit was in place on the cryopreservation of sperm. The introduction of assessments of parental skills followed media reports of a few instances of children born as a result of IVF treatment being immediately taken into care by social authorities due to the unfitness of the parents to care adequately for the child. The major element of modernization in the act was that it departed from the notion of ART to replace a natural function between a man and a woman and embraced new family forms to a wider extent than the original act. Because the act had previously applied to physicians only, single women and lesbian couples had only had access to simple insemination performed by, for example, midwives, but not to more sophisticated IVF treatments, which belonged to the domain of medical doctors. With the amendment, equal access to ART was granted, and, as such, ART was no longer seen solely as a cure of infertility but also as a means to make families for people who could not have a child for reasons other than infertility.

In 2010, a High Court judgment[19] allowed a widow access to her deceased husband's sperm on the grounds that as a security deposit prior to cancer treatment, the sperm had not been deposited as part of an ongoing fertility treatment and as such fell outside the scope of the Act on Artificial Fertilisation. In reference to this judgment, the Act on Assisted Reproduction was amended in three respects in 2011.[20] The requirement of the Act to destroy sperm in case of the man's death was removed. Furthermore, the ban on transnational mobility of eggs and embryos was lifted. Although legal scholarship had questioned the conformity of such a ban with EU law (Herrmann, 2008), the reasoning was linked to the risk of evasion of Danish law being low, especially following the abandonment of the requirement to destroy stored sperm in case of the depositor's death. Finally, the act now allowed for openness in donation, allowing women and couples a choice between anonymous donation and a known donor (Herrmann, 2013).

When the American Society for Reproductive Medicine (ASRM) in 2012 announced that egg freezing was no longer considered experimental, new clinical practices opened up. In the bill (2013/1 L32), a new possibility to deviate from the five-year limit on egg freezing was extended to the treating physician in order to accommodate adequate fertility preservation for women suffering from severe illnesses. The supporting comments stated that five years was not always sufficient to create pregnancies in cases of, for example, severe cancer with complications, but stressed that the woman's age (45 years) was still to be the upper limit. The possibility to extend cryopreservation applied to both unfertilized eggs and embryos, stressing that men and women should be equal, and a male partner's serious illness – even if it did not directly affect the ability to make his partner pregnant – could also be a legitimate reason for further cryopreservation. The bill did not raise any discussion during the readings in Parliament and was adopted. The adoption of the act also meant a change in the title of the law, as the previous name, "artificial" reproduction, was left behind in favor of "assisted" reproduction. The change in terminology had been suggested by the Danish Fertility Society (a medical association for fertility doctors) and the patient organization for the involuntarily childless and was supported by the government, which further motivated the change in terminology with changing perceptions: fertility treatment was no longer considered 'artificial' but rather a common and accepted process for women and couples desiring pregnancy.[21]

Egg Donation

Cryopreservation and donation of eggs and embryos was originally regulated in the Act on Biomedical Research Ethics Committees that authorized the minister for health to set in place regulation. The supporting motives given in the bill[22] stated that the minister could regulate issues of a medical nature raised by the use of ART. The authorization provided the basis for issuing Ministerial Orders nos. 650/1992[23] and 392/1994,[24] which both limited egg donation so that only women who were themselves undergoing IVF treatment could donate (supernumerous eggs). Based on the wording of the authorization, the motive for limiting egg donation was medically founded and thus must have related to the risk of undergoing hormonal egg stimulation.

In the following years, Denmark became known for having the world's largest sperm bank.[25] But donated eggs were in short supply. In 2006, the Act on Artificial Fertilisation introduced a relaxed provision on egg donation, allowing all women to donate. Although the number of donated eggs increased some, it still did not correspond to the demand. The Board of Health's guideline on compensation for egg donation limited the acceptable compensation to donors to 500 DKK (67 EUR), which was the rate applicable to sperm donors, too. Subsequently, the amount had been increased to 2,400 DKK (322 EUR). Following deliberations in the Council of Ethics (Det Etiske Råd, 2013), 2016 saw the level of compensation raised to 7,000 DKK (940 EUR). The increase was supported widely in Parliament and was expressly adopted to increase the number of egg donations,[26] acknowledging that previous efforts had raised the numbers somewhat but not sufficiently.

On October 5, 2017, the minister for health proposed a bill[27] amending the act's prohibition on double donation, which had previously required couples to be able to provide one set of gametes themselves. Following deliberations in the Council of Ethics, the act was adopted by Parliament, making double donation legally permissible if double donation was indicated on medical grounds. Because double donation is strictly limited to medically indicated cases, lesbian couples who would both like to create a connection to the child through one woman donating her egg in order for the other to carry the pregnancy are barred from doing so. This provision highlights the conflicting perspectives of the act; on the one hand, the 2006 modernization left behind the idea of ART being a cure for infertility only, allowing access to single women and lesbian couples, but on the other hand, the act's perspective on ART is still heteronormative, seeing fertility treatment as a treatment that replaces a natural function.

Surrogacy

Not long after the birth of the first Danish child born as a result of assisted reproduction, discussions on surrogacy arose. In 1986, an amendment of the Adoption Act introduced section 33, which prohibited the giving and receiving of help in relation to connecting an intended mother and a surrogate mother. The accompanying remarks[28] stated that the potential commercial exploitation involved gave rise to serious concerns necessitating regulatory response. Children should not be objects of commercial transaction. Section 33 criminalizes both the intermediary and the parties involved in such arrangements and is irrespective of the intermediary demanding a fee for his/her services. The regulation is meant to limit surrogacy to cases where there are such close ties (often familial ties) that no intermediary is needed.[29] It was a paramount concern that a family member or close friend should be able to help a childless person through altruistic surrogacy while at the same time adopting regulations that would make commercial surrogacy hard to navigate.

At the same time, the Ministry of Justice made it clear that transferal of parental rights could not be granted in cases where the parent(s) were offered any kind of fee or compensation.[30] A codification followed in 1999 with the adoption of the Children Act, with section 31 stipulating the legal invalidity of any agreements on the subsequent transferal of a child after birth.[31] Consequently, the woman who had given birth was not obliged to give up the child, and the receiving parents were not obliged to receive the child. The traveaux préparatoire remark that agreements on surrogacy made abroad cannot be recognized or enforced in this country.

Consequently, it is not prohibited to act as a surrogate or to enter into surrogacy agreements. However, the child of a surrogacy arrangement must be conceived by sexual intercourse or by home insemination. If ART is needed to establish a pregnancy in the surrogate, such treatment is prohibited under the Act on Assisted Reproduction. Altruistic surrogacy not requiring ART is legally possible through the legislation on recognition of paternity, adoption and transferal of parental rights and responsibilities. However, various acts try to set in place legal obstacles by rendering any prior agreements legally void and by criminalizing intermediaries.

As surrogacy cases in the Scandinavian countries began to be reported in the media (Herrmann & Pedersen, 2017) and Iceland considered whether new legislation should be introduced, the Nordic Committee on Bioethics held a workshop in the Danish Parliament in 2012,[32] but it seems to be perceived by most parliamentarians as a settled issue and has not attracted renewed legislative interest.

Overview of the Current Legal Framework

The consolidated Act on Assisted Reproduction (no. 93 of January 19, 2015) with subsequent amendments regulates ART. Originally, though, at the time of adoption in 1997, it was named the Act on Artificial Conception, thus framing ART as inherently unnatural. This framing is still visible in some of the contents of the act, as it is still – although some bans have been relaxed over time – formulated in a prohibitive language with a special emphasis on what was perceived as potential monstrosities (e.g. the creation of human-animal hybrids, the development of the human fetus in an animal or artificial uterus, etc.). The Act not only applies to ART clinics but also to any services performed by tissue centers when they relate to treatment, diagnosis or research in the context of assisted reproduction (such as preparation and sale of donor sperm). Research involving human gametes, pre-embryos and embryos is also covered by the act. The act warrants criminal sanctions in the form of fines or up to four months' imprisonment for health professionals.

The act regulates access to treatment in sections 1a and 7, subsections 1 and 3, allowing access to treatment to single women or couples without common children (i.e. children from former partnerships are no hindrance to access to treatment). However, couples who have cryopreserved embryos stored following a previous treatment cycle and wish for a second child and couples who by special permission from the National Board of Health need PGD to have a so-called "savior sibling" (who can act as a donor for an older sibling with a serious disease) are also granted access to treatment in spite of having a common child already.

Chapter 2 of the act outlines a number of prohibitions that limit treatment, diagnosis and research in assisted reproduction; assisted reproduction must only take place using a genetically unmodified ovum and a genetically unmodified sperm; identical ova or embryos may not be implanted in women with a view to conceive; donated gametes must not stem from children, parents or close relatives; treatment must not be offered or continued if the woman is older than 45 years of age; the intended parents must not give rise to doubts in terms of their ability to care for the child after birth (in which case the State Administration agency decides on access to treatment); sex selection must only take place in order to hinder a serious, gender-related disease in the child; the embryo must not be gestated outside the woman's uterus; and gametes and ovaries from deceased women must not be used. The chapter also includes provisions on the use of PGD; the details of the regulation have already been outlined previously.

Chapters 3 regulates egg donation and the sale and storage of eggs and embryos. Selling or assisting in the sale of eggs and embryos is prohibited. Providing treatment in surrogacy agreements is prohibited under section 13 of the act. Eggs and embryos that are being stored on 'medical indication' may be stored up until the woman's 46th birthday. This extension of the previous five-year limit was adopted in 2020 but only on medical indication, as the minister for health found it unnecessary to extend the limit for elective (or so-called social) freezing, as this would only 'pull the wool over women's eyes'. The act additionally authorizes the minister for health to set up further regulation in Ministerial Orders and guidelines on donation, storage, compensation and use.

Chapter 4 regulates donation, use and storage of sperm, prohibiting other than medical doctors to use manipulated (i.e. washed/purified) sperm and providing the legal basis for the minister of health to regulate further in ministerial orders on donation, use and storage.

In terms of research-related prohibitions, Chapter 7 stipulates that research on pre-embryos may only take place during the first 14 days from fertilization; the aim of the research must be to improve IVF, improve PGD or gain knowledge that will improve the possibilities of treating diseases in humans (stem cell research). However, a number of prohibited experiments are also listed in section 28, prohibiting experiments aimed at creating humans with identical DNA, experiments aimed at joining genetically different pre-embryos before implantation, experiments aimed at creating hybrids and experiments aimed at developing the fetus in a non-human uterus.

New methods for diagnosis and treatment in assisted reproduction must be approved by the minister for health on the basis of ethical and medical interests. This control measure, which is laid down in Chapter 5 of the act, is an exception to the general principle of physicians' methodological freedom (according to which the choice of diagnostic method or treatment falls under the medical/scientific discretion of the physician), framing ART as in need of independent ethical and medical review.

Finally, Chapter 6 stipulates a number of requirements that must be met when ART is offered as a treatment; a written informed consent from the woman (and in the case of couples, her partner) must be obtained prior to treatment. The health professional responsible for providing treatment must ascertain the continued validity of the consent when treatment commences. Information on the treatment and any risks or side effects must be given both orally and in writing. The information must include information on adoption and on the legal consequences of using donated gametes (in terms of legal paternity/maternity). In case donated gametes are used, an informed consent is also required from the donor.

Infrastructure

Denmark is home to the world's largest sperm banks, and over the years, the number of pregnancies resulting from ART has increased. In 2018, a total of 39,739 infertility treatments IVF and Intra Uterine Insemination (IUI) were performed from which 7,001 children were born (Sundhedsdatastyrelsen, 2018), compared to a total of 37,606 infertility treatments in 2016 from which 6,533 children were born (Sundhedsdatastyrelsen, 2016). In 2018, 21,314 in vitro fertilization treatments were initiated, resulting in 4,620 pregnancies (success rate of 21.7%); 6,870 frozen embryos were thawed and transferred, resulting in 1,951 clinical pregnancies (success rate of 28.4%); 1,625 IVF treatments with donated eggs were initiated, resulting in 371 pregnancies (success rate 22.8%); and 18,425 inseminations were carried out in total, 10,034 with partner sperm and 8,391 with donor sperm (success rates of 12.1% with partner sperm and 11.2% with donor sperm) (Sundhedsdatastyrelsen, 2018).

In 2016, 8% of the 61,614 births in Denmark were a result of assisted reproduction, compared to 11% of 61,273 births in 2018. There is a significant amount of ART tourism from women (notably from Sweden and Norway) traveling to Denmark to benefit from the possibility of anonymous donor sperm and treatment availability for single women and lesbian couples. In 2016, 20.1% of IVF/ICSI treatments performed at IVF clinics were performed on foreign women (Sundhedsdatastyrelsen, 2019).

The ART infrastructure is divided between a public and a private sector. Denmark provides full public funding for ART treatments as part of the National Health Plan.[33] Some treatments can be obtained in the private sector for free if the patient is referred by a general practitioner (e.g. hormone stimulation and insemination with partner's own sperm). Three cycles of IVF are offered for free in the public sector if the couple meets the legally and administratively set access criteria. The region of the capital area adopted an action plan in 2019 intended to raise this to six cycles, but only if all five regions of Denmark could agree to raise the service level. This agreement has as of yet not been made. According to the National Board of Health guidelines, a maximum of two fresh embryo transfers are allowed due to the risks associated with multiple pregnancy.

Anyone who does not meet the administratively set access criteria or who wishes additional cycles or to bypass public waiting lists can go to the private sector and pay out of pocket (Keane et al., 2017); however, there is reimbursement for the medication (International Federation of Fertility Societies, 2013).

There are 8 public fertility clinics, 4 public hospital departments, 27 specialist practices, 11 private fertility clinics and 2 midwife-run clinics. IVF is performed exclusively at fertility clinics, with 43% of IVF/ICSI being performed at public fertility clinics. Intra uterine insemination (IUI) is performed at all clinics with tissue licenses. Preimplantation genetic diagnosis is offered in two public hospital departments[34] and one private fertility clinic.[35] Ovarian cryopreservation is only performed at the Laboratory for Reproductive Biology at Copenhagen University Hospital Rigshospitalet.

A longitudinal cohort study has shown that the total costs per live birth in 2012 prices could be estimated as 10,755€ (Christiansen et al., 2014).

Conclusion

Although the initial fears associated with the 'artificialness' of ART that resulted in naming the act the Act on Artificial Fertilisation have lessened to such a degree that the act was renamed the Act on Assisted Reproduction, the legal model used by the act remains unchanged. It still regulates in prohibitive language, with a clear focus on the potential perceived monstrosities raised by ART, even though Danish regulation can be seen as comparatively liberal, with a considerable number of incoming infertility patients, not least due to the legality of using anonymous sperm and access to treatment for single and lesbian women.

Nonetheless, the legal model using prohibitive language and strict regulation of treatment dating from 1997 has on the whole been maintained over the last 20 years, with minor restrictions (e.g. parental assessment by the doctor, extension of the act's scope over time to encompass not only treatment by doctors but by all licensed health professionals) and some relaxations (e.g. extension of cryopreservation period, accommodation of new family forms, post-mortem use of sperm) added over time. No comprehensive/formal evaluation efforts or reports of the effect of the rules have been undertaken during that time. Rather the updating of the regulation has been piecemeal in response to, for example, media reports (on a couple unfit to parent who had their child removed by social services following IVF), requests from health professionals (updating the name of the act from artificial to assisted reproduction and allowing more women to donate eggs to address supply shortage) and so on. The single most important development over time has been the increased acceptance of alternative family forms. Today, not only heterosexual couples but also single women and lesbian couples have access to assisted reproduction in the public sector without charge. As a result, more than 1 in 10 births resulting from assisted reproduction are born to 'solo mothers'. In an analysis of the treatments in 2011, then chair of the Danish Fertility Society concluded that 1,900 woman without a male partner (single or lesbian) had received treatment, expectedly resulting in 750 births, of which approximately 400 would be born to single women and 350 would be born to lesbian couples (Jakobsen & Gunge, 2013). The legislative support of new family forms has been followed by the 2013 introduction of co-motherhood as a new legal term.[36] An agreement of co-motherhood ensures legal rights in terms of inheritance and visitation rights and establishes rights and duties in terms of the financial and emotional care for the child. Before the introduction of co-motherhood, a child born to a lesbian couple had one legal parent only until such time as the process of stepchild adoption could be finalized (after living together with the child for at least 1½ years). The recent amendment of the act allowing double donation (when donation of both sets of gametes is necessary on medical grounds) was criticized (Petersen, 2017) for denying lesbians double donation, since double donation could be a lesbian couple's only means of both establishing a connection to the child: one woman would donate her egg to the other woman, who would carry the pregnancy – not on medical grounds but to both be involved. Since the conception would in most cases require the use of donated sperm (except in cases where the lesbian couple used a male friend who was intended to be a father both legally, genetically and socially), such an arrangement would not be possible to count as double donation.

ART was introduced directly as a treatment by the medical community, thus sidestepping the (then non-binding) framework for biomedical research ethics had ART been deemed experimental. Legislative interest should probably be seen as a critical response to the introduction of ART by the medical community itself with a view to the societal and ethical implications they raise. It is, however, clear that Parliament and government were uneasy in regulating fertility treatment and thus began regulating by means of professional guidelines and subsequently in a comprehensive act with a dominant focus on the potential perceived 'monstrosities' raised by IVF.[37] Having established legal and ethical certainty about the perceived monstrosities (e.g. mixing the human and the animal, disrupting the normal kinship order), a process of increased trust in the technology has slowly started to appear in some areas, concurrent with the acceptance of new family forms, for example, while other areas have continued to be dominated by traditional and normative perceptions of, for example, the appropriate age of motherhood, leading to non-action in relation to social freezing. The fact that the legal regulation was primarily a response to the medical community introducing by itself a technology laden with ethical concerns is perhaps also the reason the legislature has never felt the need to assess or evaluate assisted reproductive technologies in terms of public perception or what effects the act has (had) from a treatment perspective.

Notes

1 The work in this chapter was supported by Independent Research Fund Denmark grant # 8019–00002B.
2 www.retsinfo.dk, www.ft.dk, Folketingets Forhandlinger and Folketingstidende.
3 L59 (23 October 1991) available at https://pro.karnovgroup.dk/document/7000281373/1
4 http://webarkiv.ft.dk/?/samling/19931/udvbilag/suu/almdel_bilag63.htm. Document is not electronically available but made available to the author courtesy of the Parliamentary Library.
5 http://webarkiv.ft.dk/?/samling/19931/udvbilag/suu/almdel_bilag137.htm. Document is not electronically available but made available to the author courtesy of the Parliamentary Library.
6 In the form of the Health Board's guidelines no. 15120 of 22 December 1993 on physicians' use of artificial fertilization and other forms of fertility enhancing treatments and the Health Board's circular no. 108 of 13 June 1994 and guidelines no. 109 of the same date, both on the introduction of new treatment methods within reproductive technologies.
7 Ministerial order no. 392 of 17 May 1994 and Guidelines no. 109 of 13 June 1994 on the introduction of new treatment methods in assisted reproduction.
8 The legal basis for the prohibition restricting transnational mobility of eggs and embryos was consequently provided with the adoption of the 1997 Act (§16 of the act).
9 2002/1 LF 209 (2 April 2003) www.retsinformation.dk/Forms/R0710.aspx?id=101976
10 1995/1 LSF 200 (7 February 1996) available in Danish at www.retsinformation.dk/Forms/R0710.aspx?id=112506

11 The Health Board's guidelines no. 15120 of 22 December 1993 on physicians' use of artificial fertilization and other forms of fertility enhancing treatments, the Health Board's circular no. 108 of 13 June 1994 and guidelines no. 109 of the same date, both on the introduction of new treatment methods within reproductive technologies.

12 Bill no. 200 of February 23, 1995 (Folketingets Forhandlinger page 4055) http://webarkiv.ft.dk/?/samling/19951/lovforslag_oversigtsformat/l200.htm

13 1996/1 LSF 5 debate following first reading on October 8, 1996, printed in Folketingets Forhandlinger page 244–257.

14 1996/1 LSF 5 (16 June 1997) www.retsinformation.dk/Forms/R0710.aspx?id=112035

15 The Ministry of Health, memorandum of November 15, 1995 (summation of incoming consultation responses).

16 http://webarkiv.ft.dk/Samling/20031/salen/L188_BEH1_69_3_(NB).htm

17 2005/1 LF 151 (26 January 2006) www.ft.dk/samling/20051/lovforslag/l151/index.htm

18 See also the health minister's speech during the first parliamentary debate www.ft.dk/samling/20051/lovforslag/l151/beh1-48/81/forhandling.htm?startItem=#nav

19 Judgment (unpublished) of December 16, 2010, High Court of Eastern Denmark.

20 www.ft.dk/ripdf/samling/20111/lovforslag/l138/20111_l138_som_fremsat.pdf

21 www.ft.dk/ripdf/samling/20131/lovforslag/l32/20131_l32_som_fremsat.pdf

22 www.retsinformation.dk/Forms/R0710.aspx?id=110656

23 www.retsinformation.dk/Forms/R0710.aspx?id=46403

24 www.retsinformation.dk/Forms/R0710.aspx?id=46280

25 According to the Guinness Book of Records, Cryos International is the world's largest sperm bank. See also https://dk.cryosinternational.com/about-us (accessed 27 April 2018).

26 Ministry of Health Press Release dated 18.05.2016 https://webcache.googleusercontent.com/search?q=cache:kPH4zUm8BpOJ:https://sum.dk/Aktuelt/Nyheder/Sundhedspolitik/2016/Maj/Minister-Ny-politisk-aftale-boer-give-flere-donoraeg.aspx+&cd=5&hl=da&ct=clnk&gl=dk&client=firefox-b-d

27 www.folketingstidende.dk/samling/20171/lovforslag/L60/index.aspx

28 www.retsinformation.dk/eli/ft/198512K00164

29 http://webarkiv.ft.dk/?/samling/19991/lovforslag_oversigtsformat/l197.htm general remarks section 5.

30 Ministerial orders 597/1986 and 994/1995.

31 http://webarkiv.ft.dk/?/samling/19991/lovforslag_oversigtsformat/l197.htm

32 www.ncbio.org/events/previous/2012rsnc (accessed 26 January 2021).

33 In January 2011, the Danish government cut funding for assisted reproduction treatments. Patients had to make a co-payment unless they required treatment that included preimplantation genetic diagnosis and this treatment had to be done in a public hospital. The out-of-pocket contribution amounted to €1,840 per cycle (Connolly et al., 2011). However, co-payment was abandoned in November 2011 with an amendment of the Health Act (see www.ft.dk/samling/20111/lovforslag/L37/som_vedtaget.htm)

34 www.rigshospitalet.dk/afdelinger-og-klinikker/julianemarie/fertilitetsklinikken/undersoegelse-og-behandling/Fertilitetsbehandling/Sider/aegsortering.aspx

35 www.aagaardklinik.dk/nyheder/nyt-tilbud-om-behandling-med-aegscreening-pgs

36 www.retsinformation.dk/Forms/R0710.aspx?id=152306 Act no. 652 of June 12, 2013.

37 The initial debate in Parliament directly used the term "monster research".

References

Adrian, S. W., Krøløkke, C., & Herrmann, J. (2021). Monstrous Motherhood – Women on the edge of reproductive age. *Science as Culture*, 30(4), 491–512. https://doi.org/10.1080/09505431.2021.1935842.

Bacchi, C. (2009). *Analysing policy: What's the problem represented to be?* Pearson Australia.

Christiansen, T., Erb, K., Rizvanovic, A., Ziebe, S., Mikkelsen Englund, A. L., Hald, F., Boivin, J., & Schmidt, L. (2014). Costs of medically assisted reproduction treatment at specialized fertility clinics in the Danish public health care system: Results from a 5-year follow-up cohort study. *Acta Obstetricia et Gynecologica Scandinavica, 93*(1), 64–72. https://doi.org/10.1111/aogs.12293

Connolly, M. P., Postma, M. J., Crespi, S., Andersen, A. N., & Ziebe, S. (2011). The long-term fiscal impact of funding cuts to Danish public fertility clinics. *Reproductive Biomedicine Online, 23*(7), 830–837. https://doi.org/10.1016/j.rbmo.2011.09.011

Det Etiske Råd. (1989). *Prenatal diagnostics, prenatal screening, genetic counselling – A discussion paper*. The Council of Ethics.

Det Etiske Råd. (1989). *Protection of human gametes, fertilized eggs, pre-embryos and embryos – A report*. The Council of Ethics.

Det Etiske Råd. (2003). *Etiske problemer vedrørende kunstig befrugtning, 3. Del. Mikroinsemination og præimplantationsdiagnostik*. The Council of Ethics. www.etiskraad.dk/~/media/Etisk-Raad/Etiske-Temaer/Assisteret-reproduktion/Publikationer/Del-3-Mikroinsemina tion-og-praeimplantationsdiagnostik.pdf

Det Etiske Råd. (2013). *Udtalelse om kompensation for ægdonation*. www.etiskraad.dk/~/media/Etisk-Raad/Etiske-Temaer/Assisteret-reproduktion/Publikationer/2013-02-01-Udtalelse-om-kompensation-for-aegdonation.pdf

Herrmann, J. R. (2008). *Retsbeskyttelsen af fostre og befrugtede æg*. DJØF Publishing.

Herrmann, J. R. (2013). Anonymity and openness in donor conception: The new Danish model. *European Journal of Health Law, 20*(5), 505–511. https://doi.org/10.1163/1571 8093-12341290

Herrmann, J. R., & Kroløkke, C. (2018). Eggs on ice: Imaginaries of eggs and cryopreservation in Denmark. *NORA – Nordic Journal of Feminist and Gender Research, 26*(1), 19–35. https://doi.org/10.1080/08038740.2018.1424727

Herrmann, J. R., & Pedersen, F. H. (2017). Barnets bedste ved omsorgsrelationer uden genetisk tilknytning – Nogle kommentarer i lyset af Paradiso & Campanelli v. Italien. *Nordisk Socialrättslig Tidskrift, 15–16*, 129–161.

International Federation of Fertility Societies. (2013). *IFFS surveillance 2013*. International Federation of Fertility Societies.

Jakobsen, S. B., & Gunge, U. (2013, July 11). Hvor er fædrene henne? *Belingske*. www.berlingske.dk/samfund/hvor-er-faedrene-henne

Keane, M., Long, J., O'Nolan, G., & Farragher, L. (2017). *Assisted reproductive technologies: International approaches to public funding mechanisms and criteria. An evidence review*. Health Research Board. www.hrb.ie/fileadmin/publications_files/Assisted_reproductive_technologies_evidence_review_2017.pdf

Kroløkke, C., & Herrmann, J. R. (2019). Slægtskabsreguleringer. Feministisk retsretorik som analyseramme og dens potentiale for at identificere lovens performative effekter. *Rhetorica Scandinavica, 79*, 44–65.

Kroløkke, C., Petersen, T. S., Herrmann, J. R., Bach, A. S., Adrian, S. W., Klingenberg, R., & Petersen, M. N. (2019). *The cryopolitics of reproduction on ice: A new Scandinavian ice age*. Emerald Group Publishing. https://doi.org/10.1108/978-1-83867-042-920191001

Larsen, E. (2007). Et tilbageblik på Etisk Råd og dets samspil med Christiansborg. In K. Kappel & A. Lykkeskov (Eds.), *Etik i tiden. 20 år med Det Etiske Råd* (pp. 71–86). The Council of Ethics.

The Ministry of the Interior. (1977). *Betænkning 803/1977 om prænatal genetisk diagnostik*. The Ministry of the Interior.

Petersen, T. S. (2017, December 20). Professor i etik: Nyt lovforslag spænder ben for lesbiske. *Politiken*. https://politiken.dk/debat/profiler/filosofferne/thomassoebirk/art6261422/Nyt-lovforslag-sp%C3%A6nder-ben-for-lesbiske

Sundhedsdatastyrelsen. (2016). *Assisteret reproduktion 2016. IVF-registeret – Tal og analyse.* https://sundhedsdatastyrelsen.dk/da/tal-og-analyser/analyser-og-rapporter/andre-analyser-og-rapporter/assisteret-reproduktion

Sundhedsdatastyrelsen. (2018). *Assisteret reproduktion 2018. IVF-registeret – Tal og analyse.* https://sundhedsdatastyrelsen.dk/da/tal-og-analyser/analyser-og-rapporter/andre-analyser-og-rapporter/assisteret-reproduktion

Sundhedsdatastyrelsen. (2019). *IVF-registeret (assisteret reproduktion).* https://sundhedsdata styrelsen.dk/da/registre-og-services/om-de-nationale-sundhedsregistre/graviditet-foedsler-og-boern/ivf-registeret

Sundhedsministeriet. (1992). *Behandling af ufrivillig barnløshed: En rapport afgivet af en arbejdsgruppe nedsat af sundhedsministeriet.* Sundhedsministeriet.

5 A Regulatory Jungle

The Law on Assisted Reproduction in Germany[1]

Sven Geyken

Introduction

Today, reproductive medicine includes various forms of assisted reproduction, and it is constantly being further developed. It can help couples accomplish their desire for a child when the woman is unable to get pregnant or bear the child in natural ways or when the man is infertile. Additionally, single women and couples of the same sex can be helped to fulfill their desire for a child.

To achieve this goal, the physician inserts spermatozoa (artificial insemination/AI) or spermatozoa and an egg cell (gamete transfer/GT) into the body of the woman. The insemination may take place inside the woman's body (in vivo), or it is carried out extracorporeally (in vitro) and the fertilized egg cell is then implanted into the body of the woman (embryo transfer). The semen used can stem from the intended father (homologous) or a semen donor (heterologous).[2] In addition, both egg donation and embryo donation are possible. Finally, surrogate motherhood is also a method to reach the goal of childbirth.

From a medical point of view, all these methods are possible but connected with different risks and chances of success. From a normative perspective, they are treated very differently by German law.

In regulating assisted reproductive technologies (ARTs), the German legislature is bound to the Basic Law for the Federal Republic of Germany (Grundgesetz – GG). He has to consider the protection of developing life (art. 2 sub. 2 GG) and its personality (art. 2 sub. 1 in conjunction with art. 1 sub. 1 GG), the best interests of the (born) child (art. 6 sub. 2 GG), its right to a family (art. 6 sub. 1 GG) and its right to knowledge of its parentage (art. 2 sub. 1 in conjunction with art. 1 sub. 1 GG). Additionally, consideration must be given to the intended parent's right to reproduction (art. 2 sub. 1 in conjunction with art. 1 sub. 1 GG) and their respective right to establish a family (art. 6 sub. 1 and 2 GG). Regarding the semen donor, egg donor and surrogate mother, they can refer to the general freedom of action (art. 2 sub. 2 GG) and the right to physical integrity (art. 2 sub. 2 GG). The physician is protected by the freedom of occupation (art. 12 GG) and the scientific researcher by the freedom of research (art. 5 sub. 3 GG). In the context of the European Convention on Human Rights (ECHR), the right of the child and the intended parents to respect for private and family life (art. 8 ECHR)

DOI: 10.4324/9781003223726-5

has to be considered. The German legislature and those applying the law have to respect these rights and bring them into balance. Therefore, they are bound to the principle of equal treatment (art. 3 GG and art. 14 ECHR).

Highly controversial is the question of whether the embryo is protected by the principle of human dignity (art. 1 sub.1 GG). In its judgments on abortion, the Federal Constitutional Court in Germany pronounced the opinion that after implantation, the embryo enjoys not only protection by the right to life (art. 2 sub. 2 GG) but also protection by the principle of human dignity. Other opinions range from granting human dignity to totipotent or even pluripotent cells or fertilized egg cells to radical refusal to grant this right to human beings without consciousness and subjectivity. Consequently, the unsolved nature of the debate gives the German legislature a margin of appreciation by the Federal Constitutional Court.

Current Regulation of ART[3]

Sources of Law on ART

German law on reproductive medicine stems from various sources, each covering a different aspect. The Embryo Protection Act (Embryonenschutzgesetz – ESchG), a criminal law statute enacted in 1990, is the one German act directly regulating reproductive medicine. It prohibits some ARTs or their use for specific purposes which are regarded as inacceptable. Furthermore, it prohibits commercial exploitation of, and experimentation with, the embryo; prohibits the creation of clones, hybrids and chimeras; and also restricts the performance of artificial reproduction to medical professionals. Any violation constitutes a criminal offence. In effect, the Embryo Protection Act outlaws a limited number of techniques and practices or their application for specific purposes.

Other techniques, or their application for other purposes, which are not banned by this act are legal. For these, the general rules (according to medical law) apply. Mainly these are the general rules on medical interventions and family law rules on parenthood, both contained in the Civil Code (BGB). Furthermore, ART is partly regulated by other federal and state laws, for example, the Transplantation Act (Transplantationsgesetz – TPG), the Medicines Act (Arzneimittelgesetz – AMG), or the Adoption Placement Act (Adoptionsvermittlungsgesetz – AdVermiG), and also by the guidelines and directives of State Chambers of Physicians (Landesärztekammer), which are highly relevant in practice but are mostly legally non-binding.

Prohibited Forms of ART

Several medical techniques of reproductive medicine are prohibited in Germany by criminal law. The transfer of foreign egg cells, gametes and embryos to another woman is outlawed (sec. 1 sub. 1 no. 1, 2, 6, 7 and sub. 2 ESchG) in order to avoid "split" motherhood where the childbearing (legal) mother is different from the genetic mother. As a result, for example, egg and embryo donations or surrogacies cannot be lawfully applied. There is only one exception when embryo donation is allowed: the Embryo Protection Act does not prohibit the transfer of embryos to another woman when the original embryos are created by extracorporeal fertilization in order to transfer them to the intended mother but this transfer no longer becomes possible. The legislation allowed this in cases where an embryo donation is the only way to save the embryo that was created with a lawful purpose but which can no longer be realized. Further, any assistance to surrogate motherhood by reproductive medical treatments (sec. 1 sub. 1 no. 7 ESchG) or its mediation in a public quest or offer for surrogate mothers and parents is forbidden (secs. 13c, 13d AdVermiG).

Nevertheless, these prohibitions are highly controversial in terms of legal policy, in view of both the German constitution and human rights. Particularly disputed are the different legal treatments of (forbidden) egg donation on the one hand and the (allowed) semen donation on the other hand. The Federal Constitutional Court has not taken a stand on this issue yet. The European Court of Human Rights has, however, considered an Austrian provision, which is similar to German law, as compatible with the European Convention on Human Rights.[4]

Furthermore, the prohibition of several medical techniques of assisted reproduction raises questions relating to civil law.

Contractual arrangements between the intended parents, the physician, the donor and the surrogate mother are valid, provided they stay within the legal limits of the law (sec. 134 and 138 BGB). A contract directly concerning illegal behavior (e.g. a contract between a woman wishing for a child and a physician on the implantation of a donated egg cell or a contract regarding the mediation of a surrogate mother) violates legal prohibitions, rendering it invalid (sec. 134 BGB). Since egg, gamete or embryo donations as such are not outlawed, contracts between a physician and a donor are not in violation of statutory prohibition. However, they may be invalid because of their relation to a prohibited method (sec. 138 sub. 1 BGB). In the case of an exceptionally allowed embryo donation, the contract between the intended parents and the donor, as well as the treatment contract with the treating physician, is valid.

The familial relationships of the children are subject to family law, which is mostly mandatory in order to protect the interests of the child. According to German family law, the legal mother of a child is the woman who gives birth to it (sec. 1591 BGB). This traditional rule has been put into the Civil Code by the "Kindschaftsreformgesetz" in 1998 with regard to medically assisted reproduction. The legislation deliberately did not add an option to challenge maternity. Another woman can become this child's mother through adoption only. "Genetic motherhood" is irrelevant for legal motherhood.

Homologous and Heterologous (Donor) Insemination

The Embryo Protection Act does not prohibit homologous and heterologous in vivo or in vitro insemination. Hence, these methods are legal. The enforcement follows the rules of the general law. The following distinctions have to be made:

Family Law

The mother of a child is always the woman who gives birth to the child (sec 1591 BGB). "Genetic motherhood", meaning the origin of the egg cell, is irrelevant for legal motherhood.

The allocation of a child to a man as its legal father is regulated in three stages. In order of priority, the mother's husband becomes father of the child (sec. 1592 no. 1); otherwise, fatherhood is assigned to the man who voluntarily acknowledges fatherhood in agreement with the mother (secs. 1592 no. 2, 1594 et seq. BGB). It is insignificant whether the legal father is the biological father. Thus, legal paternity is basically independent from biological. Biological paternity is only relevant if paternity is challenged. The legal father, the mother, the child and, under specific conditions, also the biological father, may challenge the legal paternity. In cases where the child has no legal father, paternity can be judicially determined on appeal from the mother, the child and the potential father (secs. 1592 no. 3, 1600d BGB).

Homologous artificial insemination does not raise any questions about legal parenthood. Either the intended father becomes the legal father by marriage with the mother, and respectively by acknowledgement of paternity, or by judicial determination. Challenge of paternity is not possible.

In the case of heterologous insemination, semen from a donor is used. The legal father of the child is usually the intended father: either because of marriage to the mother or, in the case of unmarried couples, because of acknowledgement of paternity with the consent of the mother (sec. 1592 no. 1 and 2 BGB). The acknowledgement of paternity is already possible before birth (sec. 1594 sub. 4 BGB) but not before conception. This also applies to artificial insemination. However, this bears the danger of a child being created by artificial insemination and the intended father denying his paternity afterwards. Since the intended father is not the biological father, a judicial determination of his paternity is not possible (secs. 1592 no. 3, 1600d BGB). Therefore, following the examples of other countries, a regulation is suggested which ties the acknowledgement of paternity to the intended father's agreement in the case of heterologous insemination.

In the case of heterologous artificial insemination, the legal father may challenge paternity (secs. 1599 et seq. BGB) because he is not the biological father. In order to avoid this, sec. 1600 sub. 4 BGB excludes the challenge of paternity by mother and legal father when they agreed to procreation of a child by artificial insemination using a sperm donation of a third person.

The child has an unrestricted right to challenge paternity. Upon reaching the age of majority, they can exercise their right themselves because the limitation period to this right starts anew (sec. 1600b sub. 3 BGB). After a successful challenge, the child can request the court determine paternity with all its consequences under family and inheritance law. The intended parents cannot waive these rights on behalf of the child. Nevertheless, they can promise the sperm donor to compensate the child's maintenance claims against him. As of the 1st of July 2018, children who from then on have been procreated by medically assisted artificial insemination with the help of a donor who has been donating sperm through a sperm bank can no longer legally have the donor's paternity determined.[5] Thus, mutual maintenance claims are excluded. If the donor himself wants to take on the role as legal father, he can acknowledge paternity.

Medical Law

The aim of reproductive insemination is to fulfill the intended parent's wish for a child. The contract between the intended parents and the physician is a treatment contract (sec. 630a sub. 1 BGB). Both the intended mother and the intended father are contractual partners of the physician. Reproductive treatments have to be performed lege artis (sec. 630 sub. 2 BGB), and the medical measures have to be indicated. The indication is to be assumed if the childlessness is based on sterility, infertility or reduced fertility of one or both partners. Since the use of donated semen is associated with higher risks, it is indicated only if the use of homologous semen is impossible or unlikely to lead to impregnation. Furthermore, the patient's informed consent regarding his treatment is required (secs. 630d, 630e BGB). The man and the woman are entitled to revoke their consent regarding the use of their reproductive cells until fertilization. The treatment has to be terminated then. After fertilization, the rules on abortion are applicable.

As to homologous reproductive insemination, all treatments apply to the intended parents, so that they are based on the treatment contract between them and the physician. The same basically applies to heterologous (donogen) insemination. However, in addition, a contract on semen donation is necessary. The semen donor does not provide the semen in his own interest but in the interest of the intended parents. Therefore, the contract on semen donation, between the semen donor and the physician (respectively the contract on extraction and storage of semen with the sperm bank), is not a common treatment contract. Rather, it is a contract on altruistic donation of body material; such is the case with blood donation. In addition, informed consent of the donor is required for the extraction and storage.

Since sperm (and egg) cells are regarded as tissue within the meaning of sec. 1a no. 4 TPG, their extraction, processing and dealings follow the rules on tissues contained in the Transplantation Act, the Medicines Act and the relevant ordinances.[6] In particular, the rules on tissue establishments (secs. 8d, 8e TPG, 20b et seq. AMG), documentation, traceability, reporting obligation and data protection (secs. 13 et seq. TPG) apply. The German Medical Association, in agreement with the competent federal authority, establishes in directives the generally recognized state of the art of medical science regarding the extraction of tissues (including germ cells) and their transfer[7] (sec. 16b sub. 1 s. 1 TPG).[8] Mandatory compliance with the state of the art in medical science is assumed if the directives of the German Medical Association have been observed (sec. 16 sub. 2 TPG). However, the special requirements for living donors of tissue (sec. 8 TPG) are mostly inapplicable, because sec. 8b sub. 2 TPG expressly excludes semen donations used for reproductive insemination. Accordingly, the informed consent of the sperm donor is sufficient (sec. 8 sub. 2 s. 1 and 2 TPG). Otherwise, the general rules on medical interventions apply.

In an anonymous donation scenario, the realization of the child's constitutionally guaranteed right to know its parentage is prevented. Since the child procreated by heterologous insemination may assert its rights against the semen donor, an anonymous semen donation is obviously of interest to donors.[9] The physician carrying out the heterologous reproductive insemination is obliged to respect this right. This obligation is part of the treatment contract with the intended parents. The child is also protected by this contractual obligation. Therefore, the physician has to provide information about the identity of the semen donor to the child, as well as documenting the information. The contracting parties cannot ignore these obligations. The Transplantation Act codifies the child's right to information (sec. 14 sub. 3 s. 1 TPG). As a result, anonymous semen donation is effectively barred. In the event that a physician carries out a homologous fertilization with an anonymous semen donation, he violates the child's right to knowledge of its parentage and is liable both in contract and tort. If, on the other hand, a semen bank and the respective attending physician promise anonymity to the donor, and the child later on asserts their right, the semen bank and physician are liable to the donor in contract.

Under the Law Regarding the Right to Knowledge of the Origin of Heterologous Use of Semen,[10] which entered into force on the 1st of July 2018, the legislation has prescribed documentation of the donor identity in a central register and regulated in detail with regard to the concerned child's right to information. According to sec. 2 Samenspenderregistergesetz (SaRegG), data on the identity of the sperm donor must be collected from the sperm banks. Name and surname, date and place of birth, nationality and address must always be documented (sec. 2 sub. 2 SaRegG). Sperm banks must ensure that donors are informed, inter alia, about the collection, storage and transfer of their data and the child's right to information. Also, donors must be informed about the importance of the knowledge regarding the affected child's descent and the legal consequences of a sperm donation (sec. 2 sub. 1 no. 1–7 SaRegG). The sperm must only be transmitted to so-called medical care facilities (sec. 3 sub. 1 SaRegG), which may be reproductive medical centers or general practitioners. If a heterologous artificial insemination is performed in such a facility, it must be ensured that the recipient of the sperm donation – much in the same way as the sperm donor – is informed about collection, storage and transfer of her personal data; the child's entitlement to information; and the significance of the child's knowledge of her own descent, as well as the legal consequences of a sperm donation (sec. 4 s. 1 no. 1–7 SaRegG). Semen from abroad may only be used if it is ensured that the prescribed information about the donor can be transmitted (sec. 5 sub. 1 s. 2 SaRegG). After fertilization is completed, the sperm donor register must be informed about the identity of the recipient, the identification number of the sperm donation used and the date of birth of the child or children. If the sperm donor register is informed of the birth of a child, it must request data on the identity of the sperm donor from the sperm bank (sec. 7 sub. 2 SaRegG) and must save it together with the data on the recipient and the child for a period of 110 years (sec. 8 s. 1 SaRegG). The sperm donor has to be informed about this storage process (sec. 7 sub. 4 s. 1 SaRegG), so that he becomes aware that a child was most probably born with the help of his semen. He does not receive further information about the child or the recipient. The core of the law regards the claim for information regulated in sec. 10 SaRegG. Thereafter, anyone who suspects that he has been conceived by heterologous use of semen in the context of a medically assisted artificial insemination is entitled to information from the sperm donor register (sec. 10 sub. 1 s. 1 SaRegG). From the age of 16, a person concerned can only request the information herself (sec. 10 sub. 1 s. 2 SaRegG); until that time, the parents, as the legal representatives of the child, can assert the claim for the child at any time (sec. 10 sub. 3 s. 3 and 4 SaRegG). The right to information relates to the communication of the stored personal data of the sperm donor whose semen has been used in the medically assisted artificial insemination of the mother. In substance, the scope of the law is subject to two significant limitations (sec. 1 sub. 2 SaRegG). The first limitation is that only cases of sperm donation are recorded. The second and probably more significant limitation is that only such donations are recorded which (quasi-officially) were made to a sperm bank and then used in the context of a medically assisted artificial insemination. So-called private semen donations using self-procured semen are thus not covered by the scope.

Preimplantation Genetic Diagnosis

The Embryo Protection Act basically prohibits PGD (sec. 3a sub. 1 ESchG). In the course of this, embryos produced outside the womb are examined for possible genetic defects in order to then transfer only suitable ones, for example, those without genetic deficiencies, or to carry out no transfer. However, it is not unlawful and therefore permissible if, due to the genetic disposition of the parents, there is a high risk of a serious hereditary disease in the child or a high probability of stillbirth or miscarriage (sec. 3a sub. 2 ESchG). PGD may then only be carried out under strict conditions. It may only be performed after given informed consent and advice on the medical, psychological and social consequences of the genetic analysis of embryo cells desired by the woman (sec. 3a sub. 3 s. 1 no. 1 ESchG). Further, it is necessary that an interdisciplinary ethics committee at the authorized preimplantation genetic testing center check compliance with the requirements of sub. 2 and submit a positive evaluation (sec. 3a sub. 3 s. 1 no. 2 ESchG). In addition, it may only be performed by a qualified physician in centers approved for PGD which have the necessary diagnostic, medical and technical facilities to carry out preimplantation genetic diagnosis (sec. 3a sub. 3 s. 1 no. 3 ESchG). Otherwise, the general rules of medical law apply. Thus, in addition to the indication and informed consent, a treatment contract between the woman and the physician is required, and the PGD has to be carried out lege artis. The measures taken in the context of PGD, including cases rejected by the ethics committees, are reported by the authorized centers to a central office in anonymous form and documented there (sec. 3a sub. 3 s. 2 ESchG). On the basis of this documentation, the federal government has to produce a report every four years on the experience gained with PGD. The report contains the number of treatments carried out each year and a scientific evaluation.

Law of the Medical Profession

Based on the statutory provisions and rules described previously, the medical profession has established professional rules on ART. The State Chambers of Physicians (Landesärztekammern)[11] have the competence to issue recommendations on the indication and execution of special medical measures or procedures. In the field of reproductive medicine, the German Medical Association has proposed a (model) Directive for Implementing Assisted Reproduction ([Muster-] Richtlinie zur Durchführung der assistierten Reproduktion), which was amended in 2006. The model directive has been implemented by most of the State Chambers of Physicians, making it part of professional law. It provides a guideline for the involved physicians by summarizing medical indications and contraindications of reproductive methods and setting out its requirements for practice. In addition, professional, personnel and technical prerequisites for specific methods of reproductive medicine are set out. The directive also explains the legal admissibility or inadmissibility of reproductive methods and techniques and informs about applicable law, particularly family law, embryo protection law and social security law. The directive also contains some additional professional regulations. For example, physicians are obliged to notify of their work on reproductive medicine as well as to prove they have the required skills and continued medical education.

To date, this directive has been extremely controversial: It has been said that the directive excludes single women and women in homosexual relationships from any reproductive treatments. Many people argue that the State Chambers of Physicians, by excluding these persons, exceed their competence and that the regulation violates the constitutional right to reproduction of those excluded by it. Others argue that this is a mere consequence of family law, and the law of parenthood in particular, so that it is not the regulation of the State Chambers which limits the access to ART but the statutory family law itself.

In February 2015, the executive board of the German Medical Association decided to set up a strategic working group and to clearly separate medical-scientific issues from socio-political aspects. Therefore, the (Model) Directive for the Implementation of Assisted Reproduction from 2006 was not updated any further. Instead, a directive was drawn up on the basis of the new legal basis created by the Tissue Act in accordance with sec. 16b of the Transplantation Act (TPG).[12]

Assisted Reproductive Treatments in Foreign Countries

Since several assisted reproductive treatments and techniques are outlawed in Germany (e.g. surrogate motherhood) but not in other countries, a number of intended parents go abroad to have the wish for a child fulfilled. This causes particular problems.

Several questions arise, such as whether contracts legally concluded abroad are also enforceable in Germany or who the legal parents are. In order to answer these questions, one first has to see whether there is already a foreign judgment on the issue at hand or whether German courts or authorities have to decide the issue themselves.

If there is already a foreign judgment, it is a matter of recognition and enforcement of foreign judgments in Germany. According to the relevant European and German law, foreign judgments will be recognized, except if it is against German public order (art. 45 sub. 1 lit. a Brussels I bis;[13] art. 23 lit. a Brussels II bis,[14] sec. 328 sub. 1 no. 4 ZPO,[15] sec. 109 sub. 1 no. 4 FamFG).[16]

If German courts or authorities should have to decide themselves, they have to clarify under the rules of private international law which law (German or foreign) is applicable. If foreign law is applicable, its application can still be precluded by Germany overriding mandatory provisions (art. 9 Rome I)[17] or German public order (art. 26 Rome I; Art. 6 EGBGB).[18] This has the following consequences:

Contracts for implementation of reproductive medical methods not allowed in Germany (e.g. surrogate motherhood), which are valid according to applicable foreign law, are regarded as invalid according to the prevailing opinion in Germany. These prohibitions are mandatory, or part of German public order. Likewise, foreign judgments concerning the enforcement of those contracts are not recognized according to the prevailing opinion, since this is against German public order.

A similar line of reasoning was applied to the family law issue on whether the allocation of the child to its intended parents by a foreign judgment or by foreign law, which has to be applied by German courts under art. 19 EGBGB, must be accepted by German law. If the child was procreated by a reproductive medical method not allowed in Germany, this was regarded as violating German public order. Since a recent decision by the German Federal Court (Bundesgerichtshof – BGH),[19] it depends on whether the allocation of the child in the individual case violates fundamental principles of German law. Therefore, it has to be taken into account that German law permits the intended father to acknowledge paternity regardless of the "genetic paternity" and thus adopt the child. In any case, priority must be given to the child's right to identity and continuity of family life (art. 8 ECHR, art. 6 GG). As a result, foreign judgments, or applicable foreign family law, respectively, which allocate the child to its intended parents should be corrected by the use of German public order only in exceptional cases.

Process of Legislation of Assisted Reproductive Technologies

Medical Profession

It was the medical profession that invented a new dimension of human reproduction by treating involuntary childlessness. Therefore, physicians recognized the opportunities and risks of assisted reproductive techniques very early. The 62th German Medical Assembly in 1959 had already focused on this issue. It considered a consensual homologous insemination carried out by a physician acceptable only in exceptional cases. It refused any forms of heterologous insemination on the grounds that these practices have medical, legal, ethical and psychological conse-quences, which the physician cannot clearly see but has to bear responsibility for.

The 73th German Medical Assembly in 1970 eased this strict position insofar as it considered consensual homologous insemination reasonable. However, due to many unsolved and related legal questions, the assembly did not recommend this procedure.

In 1985 the 88th German Medical Assembly (Deutscher Ärztetag) approved extracorporeal insemination and embryo transfer as a therapy to treat infertility and adopted directives on this issue. The State Chambers of Physicians (Landesär-ztekammern) implemented these directives, revolutionizing the law of the medical profession.

First Approach of Legislation

In 1962, German legislators had already thought of how to avert possible damage for social cohabitation as a result of artificial insemination. Thus, they wanted to penalize heterologous insemination by the new provision, § 203 StGB-E. The reasoning[20] was based, inter alia, on the following arguments. An "artificial child" is not the result of "love between two people"; that there is the danger of an emotional relationship between the wife and the donor; and that, in case of anonymous donation, there is a danger of "biologically unfavourable" or "incestu-ous insemination". Such practices might affect "the roots of moral order and the human culture". These attempts at justification caused an ethical dispute. Many critics pointed out that there are good reasons for heterologous insemination, for example, that heterologous insemination is able to overcome the emotionally dif-ficult situation of involuntary childlessness. Further, it is usually not carried out because of "exuberance" but because of failed or impossible homologous insemina-tion. In consequence of these opposing positions, the bill failed. In addition, the thinking in the second half of the 1960s radically changed towards the general trend of avoiding penal provisions that only target immoral conduct.

Growing Public Discussions

The birth of the first extracorporeal begotten child, Louise Brown, in 1978 in England, provided new grounds for discussion. The following are exemplary of the countless reactions: In 1983, the 25th annual meeting of the German Women Lawyers Association focused on questions of gene technology and reproductive medicine (Deutscher Juristinnenbund, 1984). A working group of this association published its theses in 1986 (Deutscher Richterbund, 1986). They rejected legal prohibitions of homologous and heterologous artificial insemination, in particular semen, egg and embryo donations. However, the future child's interests, such as its personal rights, including the right to knowledge of its parentage, should be observed. An anonymous donation of germ cells is therefore already constitution-ally inadmissible. Also, the German Judges Federation stepped into the discussion in its "Theses on Reproductive Medicine and Human Genetics" (Deutscher Richterbund, 1986). In these theses, heterologous insemination is generally not recommended. In particular, heterologous insemination by in vitro fertilization is completely unacceptable. Heterologous insemination poses many ethical, legal and psychological problems. In addition, any forms of surrogate motherhood and embryo donation should be rejected. The 56th German Lawyers' Conference (Deutscher Juristentag) in 1986 provided an important impetus for legal clarification of forthcoming issues concerning the consequences of reproductive medicine in civil law (Coester-Waltjen, 1986; Starck, 1986).

In 1985 and 1986, the Protestant Church took part in the debate (Evangelische Kirche in Deutschland, 1986). It rejected heterologous (donor) insemination as well as extracorporeal insemination. The main reasons were the protection of the children's well-being and the ethical dilemma of residual embryos. The restrictive "Instruction on Respect for Human Life in its Origin and on the Dignity of Reproduction" (Sekretariat der Deutschen Bischofskonferenz, 1987) of the Catholic Congregation for the Doctrine of the Faith caused intensive discussions. The instruction considered a natural conjugal act the only moral form of human reproduction. The congregation expressed its conviction that human dignity derives inter alia from human sexuality. Therefore, it rejected all forms of medical treatments replacing or bypassing the conjugal act.

Political Debates and Legislation

The Benda-Commission

In May 1984, the federal minister of justice and the federal minister of research and technology called for a joint interdisciplinary Work Group In-Vitro-Fertilization, Genome Analysis and Gene Therapy, which was named[21] the Benda-Commission after its chairman, Ernst Benda. The commission addressed the new techniques of IVF and genome analysis as well as the possibilities of future gene therapy, their related ethical and legal problems and the question of a legislative action. In its final report (Bundesminister für Forschung und Technologie & Bundesminister für Justiz, 1986) in November 1985, the commission recommended a number of legal provisions including punishable prohibitions. Regarding heterologous IVF, which was not recommended in general, the Benda-Commission had the opinion that, in principle, sperm and egg donation shall be allowed for married couples. However, it demanded that sperm or egg cells from the same donor may only be used successfully ten times in order to avoid incestuous reproduction in the future. Furthermore, anonymous donation shall be prohibited. IVF treatment relating to unmarried couples and singles shall be forbidden as well as all forms of surrogate motherhood.

Subsequent to the report of the Benda-Commission, the political debate on ART grew in federal and state parliaments. Bavaria and Rhineland-Palatinate, Lower Saxony and Baden-Wuerttemberg developed draft laws and tried to influence the federal legislation via the Federal Council (Bundesrat).

The Federal and State Working-Group Reproductive Medicine

Under pressure from the states in the German Federal Council and the 57th Conference of the ministers of justice, the Federal and State Working-Group Reproductive Medicine was set up to elaborate upon an overall concept regarding the need for federal state action in the field of reproductive medicine and to provide adequate proposals for a solution. In August 1988, the working group published a comprehensive report (Bundesminister für Justiz, 1988). This report recommended the permission of artificial insemination and IVF, including embryo transfer, only under certain restrictions. Homologous insemination should be allowed for married couples during the lifetime of the husband. Heterologous (donor) insemination should be permitted under restrictions, such as medical indication, consideration of the best interests of the child, general obligation to consultation, notarial certified declaration of consent of the husband, centralized documentation with the opportunity to provide information for the child about its genetic origin and performance of heterologous insemination only in authorized facilities for this purpose. Insemination with sperm of the partner should be permissible for unmarried couples in a stable relationship under the restriction of mandatory psychosocial counseling, whereas insemination with donated sperm should be banned. IVF should be allowed for married and unmarried couples under the conditions of medical indication and mandatory psychosocial counseling. However, the working group recommended a prohibition of egg and embryo donation as well as surrogate motherhood. For implementation of these recommendations, the working group suggested a comprehensive Reproductive Medicine Act, a criminal law statute based on concurrent legislative powers of the Federation to legislate criminal law. In addition, the states should enact flanking health law and executive regulations. The state ministers of justice and the responsible minister for public health appreciated this report and considered it a remarkable basis for a closed system of federal and state regulations concerning reproductive medical issues. They recommended rapid implementation of this legislative proposal.

Salient Points of Contention

Though the report of the Federal and State Working-Group Reproductive Medicine was very well received, there was still contention about the admissibility of heterologous (donor) insemination and access to ART for unmarried couples.

The responsible state ministers for public health demanded a prohibition of heterologous insemination in contrast to the report's advice to allow it for married couples. Furthermore, in November 1988, a draft law proposed by Bavaria in the Federal Council wanted to restrict all forms of artificial reproduction to the homologous system under threat of punishment. Hence, the equal treatment of married and unmarried couples was rejected as well. A following draft law of the parliamentary group Social Democratic Party of Germany (SPD)[22] also intended to punish any artificial insemination carried out with donated sperm.

The critics of heterologous (donor) insemination argued that the unit of genetic, natural and social parenthood is very important for the best interests of the child and its development.[23] In the case of heterologous insemination, a third person, the donor, breaks this unit. The separation of social and genetic paternity could endanger the best interests of the child and the partner relationship, in particular if the child is disabled or its development does not meet the expectations of the parents. In addition to this, opponents feared a gateway for eugenic selection by the possibility of selecting donated sperm according to favorable donor characteristics. It was pointed out that foreign experience suggests such approaches.

The main argument of those who wanted to prohibit artificial insemination outside marriage also relates to the best interests of the child. It is indispensable for the child's welfare that such partnerships be stable and long-lasting. It was said that this basic condition, however, can be verified neither by the physician nor by anyone. In their view, only marriage can largely guarantee this condition.

These views did not meet with sufficient support in the committees of German Parliament and the Federal Council. The Committee on Legal Affairs had the opinion that heterologous insemination should not be banned in general. The minister of justice[24] considered that a prohibition under criminal law did not seem to be necessary. Recent experience from abroad has shown that parents usually fully accept the child and care for its well-being. A general ban of heterologous insemination was considered unenforceable due to its wide toleration abroad. Besides, such a penal provision would impede the German legislature from providing provisions to protect children, for instance in civil and health law. In addition, the Committee on Legal Affairs and the Health Committee declared themselves in favor of equal treatment of married and unmarried couples concerning reproductive medical issues. The majority in the Committee on Legal Affairs expressed that a criminal prohibition of artificial insemination with respect to unmarried couples might be in breach of the German Constitution. To date, no final decision has been made on both draft laws in the German Parliament.

The Embryo Protection Act

In July 1989, the federal government consisting of the Christian Democratic Union of Germany (CDU), Christian Social Union in Bavaria (CSU) and Free Democratic Party (FDP), introduced a draft law for the protection of embryos (Embryo Protection Act).[25] The draft law confined itself to the potential abuse of assisted reproductive techniques and provided penal prohibitions which were indispensable to protect the most important legal interests. In addition to the criminal prohibition of embryo research, the law indirectly banned only those assisted reproduction techniques whose prohibition was subject to consensus in Parliament, such as egg and embryo donation and surrogacy. In the course of the legislative process, it became clear that all parties concerned had the opinion that the legislator must not confine himself to criminal law. It was necessary to include the fields of family, social, medical and health law in order to regulate reproductive medical issues comprehensively. However, since the federal legislature did not have legislative powers for such a law, a constitutional change was needed. From the point of view of the federal government, a change of the basic law would have taken too much time. On the one hand, urgent questions of reproductive medicine ought to be regulated as soon as possible; on the other hand, the eleventh legislative period was to end very soon. So the federal government supported quick adoption of the penal provisions provided by the draft. Finally, the government coalition used their votes in the Parliament to pass the Embryo Protection Act in October 1990. On the 1st of January 1991, the Embryo Protection Act came into force. However, due to its fragmented nature, it was the unanimous opinion of all participants in the legislative process that the Embryo Protection Act should be further developed into a comprehensive Reproductive Medicine Act regulating all issues connected with reproductive medicine.

Legal Fragmentation Instead of a Reproductive Medicine Act

It was not until 1994 that the legislative power of the federal government was extended by a constitutional change.[26] The new article 74 sec. 1 no. 26 of basic law included the concurrent legislative powers to legislate "artificial insemination in humans", so that from then on, the federal Parliament had the power to exhaustively regulate reproductive medicine issues. The further course of discussion about a broad revision of the Embryo Protection Act focused on creating a – continually claimed[27] – comprehensive Reproductive Medicine Act. Subsequent to a highly regarded academic symposium on reproductive medicine,[28] organized by the Federal Ministry of Health, these considerations were specified in an internal key issues paper of the Ministry dated November 2000.[29] The law should have the purpose of helping couples to fulfill their desire for a child in the case of infertility, protecting the right to life of embryos in vitro, protecting the welfare of the future child and finally of preventing abuse of medical reproductive techniques. The transformation of the Embryo Protection Act into the Reproductive Medicine Act should primarily eliminate the criminal character of individual rules but should not lower the provided protection level of embryos. Thus, material amendments of the Embryo Protection Act were not intended. However, in the subsequent period, this key issues paper was unpursued. Also, recommendations of the Enquete Commission on "Law and Ethics in Modern Medicine" of the German Federal Parliament from 2002 and the Bioethics Commission of Rhineland-Palatinate from 2005 sought to create a comprehensive Reproductive Medicine Act. This should have brought a fundamental rights position into fair balance but did not lead to federal regulatory activities.

Instead of adopting an independent law on reproductive medicine, regulations were issued in a very scattered manner. Regarding family law, single questions like the legal relationship between the mother and the child were regulated in 1998,[30] followed in 2002 and 2008 by rules on the challenging of paternity by the child.[31] However, the legislation has not been able to fully reform family law on the challenges of reproductive medicine.[32] The so-called Tissue Act[33] of 20 July 2007 issued a substantial amendment to the Transplantation Act (TPG) and the Medicines Act (AMG) regulating the extraction, processing and dealings of human germ cells. Sec. 14 sub. 3 s. 1 TPG codified the right of the child to knowledge of his parentage, which had already been recognized by the Federal Constitutional Court since 1989.[34] For the purpose of traceability, this law was the first to regulate the documentation of donor data over 30 years. However, the right of a child to make a claim against the physician about access to information regarding the identity of the donor was first recognized in a court decision in 2013, further developing the law by the judges.[35] The "Samenspenderregistergesetz", which entered into force on 1 July 2018, further strengthens this right.

To date, the creation of a Reproductive Medicine Act is primarily discussed in scientific literature (Beitz, 2009; Damm, 2013; Dethloff & Gerhardt, 2013; Katzorke & Kolodziej, 2001; Laufs, 2003; Rosenau, 2012). In 2013, a number of researchers from Augsburg and Munich published a draft of a Reproductive Medicine Act (Gassner et al., 2013), which was not taken up further by policy. Most recently, an interdisciplinary expert group of the National Academy of Sciences Leopoldina restarted the discussion on the need for a law on reproductive medicine (Leopoldina Nationale Akademie der Wissenschaften, 2017, 2019).

Preimplantation Genetic Diagnosis

Preimplantation genetic diagnostics was established as a method in the 1990s. This procedure could not be properly subsumed under the prohibition provisions of the Embryo Protection Act, resulting in controversial discussions over whether PGD is permissible in Germany (Günther et al., 2008). It was mostly regarded as incompatible with the Embryo Protection Act (ESchG). The prohibition of PGD was derived from various provisions of the ESchG, in particular prohibitions on the fertilization of an egg cell for purposes other than the production of a pregnancy, the use of human embryos for purposes other than their preservation and the cloning of human embryos (Deutscher Bundestag, 2002; Günther et al., 2008). The directive of the German Medical Association (Bundesärztekammer, 2006) was content with the statement that PGD would not be carried out in Germany.

Several institutions dealt with possible future regulation of PGD. The medical profession had been contributing to the socio-political discussion since the beginning with a "Discussion Draft for Preimplantation Genetic Diagnosis" (Bundesärztekammer, 2000). In the draft issued in 2000, it was stated:

> If majority of the society wants the pre-implantation diagnostics, then legal certainty and a high level of protection can only be achieved through eligibility criteria, which must be strict and extremely restrictive. . . . Moreover, it is indispensable that the non-medical aspects of this procedure in civil and criminal law must be regulated by the federal legislator.

In 2004, a progress report from the Office for Technology Assessment at the German Bundestag provided comparative information on the practice, legal situation and public debate on PGD (Hennen & Sauter, 2005). In the same year, the Friedrich Ebert Foundation submitted another expert opinion with a country-comparative approach to PGD. However, the legislature remained inactive in the subsequent period

In a judgment dated 6 July 2010, the Federal Court of Justice (BGH) ruled that PGD carried out after extracorporeal fertilization by means of blastocyst biopsy, and subsequent examination of the pluripotent cells removed due to severe genetic damage, did not constitute criminal liability under the Embryo Protection Act.[36] With this judgment of the BGH, the social discussion was revived, after the court stated "that a clear legal regulation of the matter would be desirable".

The reactions to the judgment of the BGH were different. Against the background of the current socio-political debate, the Leopoldina – National Academy of Sciences – issued a statement in January 2011 entitled "Preimplantation Genetic Diagnosis (PGD) – Effects of a Limited Permission in Germany" (Leopoldina Nationale Akademie der Wissenschaften, 2011), in which the scientists argued in favor of limited permission for PGD. On 8 March 2011, the German Ethics Council published an opinion in which controversial recommendations were included as a contribution to the discussion on future regulations on PGD (Deutscher Ethikrat, 2011). The Ethics Council was unable to agree on a majority opinion. Thirteen of its 26 members voted in favor of permitting PGD under strictly limited conditions, 11 voted against, 1 member abstained, and another recommended in a special vote the general admission of PGD to identify viable embryos. On 1 June 2011, the 114th German Medical Assembly dealt extensively with PGD on the basis of a memorandum (Bundesärztekammer, 2011). As a result of this intensive discussion, 204 out of a total of 250 delegates confirmed the memorandum, with 33 votes against, and thus revised the current position of the medical profession. According to the decision of the German Medical Assembly, PGD should only be performed for diseases for which the couple has a high genetic risk.

In April 2011, the German Parliament also took up the concerns of the Federal Court of Justice. In the Bundestag, three bills were introduced – on a cross-party basis – to regulate PGD. While two draft laws pleaded for limited PGD admission,[37] a draft sought to ban PGD and sanction it.[38] The counterparts of the PGD argued that the system of values in the Basic Law explicitly states that every person has the same right to dignity and the same inalienable rights to participation. This value structure would be permanently damaged by the approval of PGD. For ethical and socio-political reasons, PGD should therefore be rejected.[39] Proponents of limited PGD approval felt that an explicit ban on PGD, which made it virtually impossible for genetically predisposed couples to have their own genetically healthy children, was constitutionally questionable. The prohibition of PGD would be in conflict with the possibility of the woman having her pregnancy terminated if a prenatal diagnosis determined serious genetic damage to the embryo or if there were a medical indication.[40] After a broad discussion, limited approval of PGD was finally decided upon by a narrow majority of votes, and section 3a was included in the Embryo Protection Act.[41]

Infrastructure

In Germany, there are about 136 approved[42] fertility centers offering reproductive medical treatment (Blumenauer et al., 2017). To date, 11 centers have been approved for PGD treatment. The costs of reproductive medical treatments are rarely covered in full by the German health insurance system. The reimbursement of costs depends on different conditions. In addition, some state subsidies can be claimed.

Statutory Health Insurance

Childlessness can be due to illness. Then the insured person receives benefits in accordance with sec. 27 Volume V of the Social Insurance Code (Fünftes Buch Sozialgesetzbuch – SGB V), which are aimed at establishing fertility or conception. Even if the infertility of the couple cannot be medically clarified (so-called idiopathic sterility), the statutory health insurance assumes the costs of an artificial reproduction according to sec. 27 a SGB V as "medical treatment benefits". This is an independent insurance claim that is subsidiary to sec. 27 SGB V.[43] To be eligible, the following legal requirements must be met: The claimants are married. Only the egg and sperm cells of the claimants are used (homologous fertilization). The minimum age of the claimant is 25 years, the maximum age of the woman is 40 years and the maximum age of the man is 50 years. The treatment must be medically indicated and have sufficient prospects of success. The treatment may take place only after medical consultation. The health insurance pays 50% of the costs for a maximum of three treatment attempts and only after a previously approved treatment plan. The details are regulated by the guidelines of the Joint Federal Committee of Physicians, Health Insurances and Hospitals (G-BA). According to these guidelines, the standard methods of artificial insemination, IVF and intracytoplasmic sperm injection (ICSI) are possible – usually with prior hormonal stimulation.

Since 2012, in order to increase competition in the public health system, statutory health insurances have expanded their scope by offering their insured persons additional benefits by statute according to sec. 11 sub. 6 SGB V. This applies expressly for measures of artificial reproduction according to sec. 27 a SBG V. For example, many health insurances grant their insured persons higher subsidies, some extending the age limits according to sec. 27 a sub. 3 SGB V. However, in the view of the Federal Social Court of Germany, health insurances exceed their scope when covering the costs of fertility treatment of unmarried couples.[44] Basically, the law, as a higher-ranking rule, determines the benefits of the statutory health insurance. The wording of sec. 27 a SGB V is clear and conclusive as far as the status of the couple is concerned. The legislation deliberately limited the claim to married couples on objective grounds. The Federal Social Court of Germany joined the judgment of the Federal Constitutional Court of 2007,[45] which declared the restriction to married couples constitutional. The preference for marriage over a "long-term" cohabitation was justified with the fact that it is a life-long, legally constituted coupled relationship of men and women, "in which the mutual solidarity is not only lived in practice as long as it is pleased but can be legally demanded" and is continued in the post-marital law. This legal frame-work provides better conditions for both the burden of artificial insemination for the couple and the well-being of the child. In the court's opinion, this typifying consideration is allowed regarding benefits legislation. The restriction to married couples and homologous insemination are thus "basic conditions". They may not be undermined by a change in the statutes of a health insurance company. By contrast, a statutory increase in the grant is within the legal scope.

PGD, in contrast to ART, has no benefits of the statutory health insurance.[46] Parents have to bear the costs for PGD-IVF, because it is not a medical treatment in the sense of the statutory health insurance. The artificial production of embryos and their evaluation by PGD prior to the pregnancy makes it possible to reject those embryos that carry a serious hereditary disease. Thus, PGD serves to prevent future suffering of a human being but not the treatment of existing suffering of the parents.

Private Health Insurance

Unlike in statutory health insurance, artificial reproduction in private health insurance is not regulated by law. Instead, childlessness is treated like a disease. Only if an organically caused disorder of the insured person causing the infertility of the couple is medically determined does the health insurance company assume the cost of artificial insemination as "medically necessary treatment". The obligation to pay benefits to the statutory health insurance is lower: If no medical reason for childlessness can be found, there is no obligation to cover the costs. However, the other prerequisites are not as strict in private health insurance: There are no age limits. In order to be a medically necessary treatment, the probability of success of pregnancy must be higher than 15%.[47] In addition, private health insurance covers the entire cost. It is not determined whether the couple must be married and has so far not been decided by the highest court. The jurisprudence is uneven, ranging from the restriction to married people[48] to the obligation to pay even without marriage and even for a heterologous insemination.[49] The costs for PGD are generally not covered by private health insurance, since this is not a treatment for a disease.

Government Grants

As part of the federal initiative "Assistance and Support in Case of Involuntary Childlessness", the federal government also provides financial aid for fertility treatment. The basis for this support is the Federal Directive on the Granting of Subsidies to Promote Measures of Assisted Reproduction.[50] Since the 1st of April 2012, the federal government has provided involuntarily childless couples with subsidies for fertility treatments (reproductive medical treatments). Since 7 January 2016, couples who live in a non-marital partnership have also been supported. The allowances supplement the benefits of health insurance for married couples and thus reduce the total treatment cost for couples. The granting of the subsidies by the federal government requires that the respective federal states in which the couples concerned have their main residence also have their own state programs for the promotion of fertility treatments. In addition, regardless of the existence of a marriage, the requirements of § 27a SGB V must be met, and the treatment must take place in Germany. Further, the treatment must consist of an IVF or ICSI treatment and covers up to four treatments. Under these conditions, subsidies for married couples of the first four treatments amount to up to 25% of their contribution after settlement with the health insurance. For unmarried couples, up to 12.5% and for the fourth treatment up to 25% of their remaining cost is covered.

Use of ART

In April 1982, the first child procreated in Germany through IVF was born at Erlangen University Hospital. Since then, medical and scientific knowledge has grown steadily, and the methods for diagnosis and therapy in the context of assisted reproduction have been refined. Meanwhile, a variety of treatment options for the unfulfilled desire to have children have become available. According to the Yearbook 2019 of the German IVF Register (Blumenauer et al., 2020), a total of 110,786 treatment cycles were carried out in 131 centers in Germany in 2019, and 65,328 women were treated. There were 261 treatments without a male partner and 345 treatments in lesbian couples. The birth rate after medically assisted reproductive treatments is increasing rapidly in Germany. In 2017, 22,282 children were born after IVF, ICSI or cryo-transfer. This is 1,500 children more than in 2016 (20,754). For comparison: In 2010, around 13,000 children in Germany were born. Almost 3% of all children born alive in 2017 were born after fertilization outside the body. In addition, it has been shown that more children were born in the federal states, where financial subsidies are granted for reproductive medical treatment (Blumenauer et al., 2017). From 2009–2015, a total of 2,360 more children were born in these federal states. While the average of other federal states has also increased, this increase is clearly above average. This may also be related to the willingness of some public health insurance companies to voluntarily reimburse 100% of the costs of medical reproductive treatments.

Regarding sperm donations, there are no reliable figures published. However, it is estimated that nearly 1,000 children are born each year due to medical reproductive treatments using donor sperm (Wehrstedt et al., 2012).

The procedure of PGD has been established much more slowly in Germany than expected by the legislature. Against the background of experiences in other European countries, it was expected that permitting PGD would lead to an estimated 200 to 300 applicants per year.[51] In fact, in 2014, only 13 applications for PGD were reported nationwide.[52] Of these, four applications were approved by the ethics committees and carried out. In the following years, the number of preimplantation diagnosis procedures performed increased significantly. In 2015, there were twice as many; in 2016 around 100, in 2017 around 200 and in 2018 over 300 performed procedures.[53]

Conclusion and Outlook

In Germany, ART is only regulated directly by the Embryo Protection Act, a criminal law statute enacted in 1990. As a result of its provisions, egg and embryo donations, as well as surrogacies, are forbidden. These were the only reproductive medicine procedures on whose prohibition there was consensus after a comprehensive debate on the admissibility of ART around 1990. With the exception of the limited admission of PGD in 2011 after the ruling of the Federal Constitutional Court, this law has not been revised in the last nearly 30 years. Homologous and heterologous in vivo or in vitro insemination are not prohibited by the EschG and hence are generally allowed. The enforcement follows the rules of the general law, such as family and medical law, including several special laws. As a result, inter alia, anonymous semen donation is effectively barred in order to respect the child's constitutionally guaranteed right to knowledge of its parentage. Due to the fragmented approach of legislation, the legal regulations for reproductive medicine have so far developed neither systematically nor congruently. Individual questions were regulated by isolated statutory provisions without regulating the overall context in a clear and concise manner (Hübner & Pühler, 2017). It has become a complicated network of regulations that is difficult to manage. A comprehensive Reproductive Medicine Act, which has been continually debated since the adoption of the Embryo Protection Act and which the constitution was changed for in 1994, has never been enacted. Thus, many questions of reproductive medicine have not been explicitly regulated[54] but left to general rules of civil law, criminal law and public law and also in the practice of the medical profession over access, especially for single and same-sex couples. In practice, therefore, reproductive health treatments are reserved only for married couples and unmarried couples in a stable relationship. A large part of the costs is covered by the healthcare system and government grants, whereby only married couples can claim health insurance benefits. While, on the one hand, the use of reproductive medical procedures has steadily increased in recent years, on the other hand, due to the prohibitions of the Embryo Protection Act and the prevailing legal uncertainties, more and more predominantly same-sex couples and single women go abroad to fulfill their wish for a child. At the same time, in recent decades, social values in Germany regarding homosexuality and new family models have changed considerably and led to liberalization. Some of these have found their way into legislation. For example, marriage for same-sex couples was opened in October 2017, equating this to traditional marriage.[55] Against this background, the legislature will have to examine again in the future whether same-sex partnerships or marriage preclude the best interests of the child. Further, a broad revision of family law has already been initiated to take account of the increasingly frequent divergence of social and biological parenthood. The family law department of the 71th German Lawyers' Conference in 2016[56] and a working group of the Federal Ministry of Justice and

Consumer Protection on the law of parentage (Bundesministerium der Justiz und für Verbraucherschutz, 2017) have elaborated far-reaching reform proposals. As a result, a "partial discussion draft" of the Federal Ministry of Justice was recently presented (Bundesministerium der Justiz und für Verbraucherschutz, 2019). These developments could serve as an opportunity to question the existing regulations of reproductive medicine and to discuss their unresolved questions in a broad manner.

Notes

1 This chapter takes into account the legal situation and related developments up to July 2021.
2 The term "homologous" is used inconsistently in Germany. By all means, it refers to the intended father being the donor and the husband of the treated mother, because it can be rightly assumed that he becomes the legal father. Whether the term also includes the donor who intends to become father but is not married to the future mother and therefore has to acknowledge paternity in order to become the legal father is viewed very differently.
3 See Lipp (2021).
4 ECHR decision of 3.11.2011–57813/00, published in: Neue Juristische Wochenschrift (NJW) 2012, p. 207.
5 Sec. 1600d sub. 4 BGB, entered into force on 1 July 2018; see Article 3 of the "Gesetz zur Regelung des Rechts auf Kenntnis der Abstammung bei heterologer Verwendung von Samen (Law Regarding the Right to Knowledge of the Origin in Case of Heterologous Use of Seeds) of 17 July 2017, Bundesgesetzblatt 2017 I p. 2513.
6 „TPG-Gewebeverordnung" (TPG-GewV) and „Arzneimittel- und Wirkstoffherstellungsverordnung" (AMWHV).
7 In particular, guidelines on the requirements for the evaluation of the medical suitability as a tissue donor; the examination of tissue donors; and the extraction, transfer and use of human tissues.
8 "Richtlinie zur Entnahme und Übertragung von menschlichen Keimzellen im Rahmen der assistierten Reproduktion" (Directive on the Extraction and Transfer of Human Germ Cells in the Context of Assisted Reproduction) of 6 October 2017, last amended 20 April 2018.
9 For medically arranged sperm donations which take place from 1 July 2018, the determination of the sperm donor as legal father is no longer possible.
10 "Gesetz zur Regelung des Rechts auf Kenntnis der Abstammung bei heterologer Verwendung von Samen" (Law Regarding the Right to Knowledge of the Origin in Case of Heterologous Use of Seeds) of 17 July 2017, Bundesgesetzblatt 2017 I p. 2513.
11 The State Chambers of Physicians (Landesärztekammern) are corporations under public law and are set up in accordance with the law of the respective state. The German Medical Association (Bundesärztekammer) is the joint association of the 17 State Chambers of Physicians. As the central organization in the system of medical self-administration in Germany, it represents the interests of all physicians working in Germany in matters relating to professional policy.
12 See previously, "Richtlinie zur Entnahme und Übertragung von menschlichen Keimzellen im Rahmen der assistierten Reproduktion" (Directive on the Extraction and Transfer of Human Germ Cells in the Context of Assisted Reproduction) of 6 October 2017, last amended 20 April 2018.
13 European Council Regulation (EC) No. 1215/2012 (Brussels I bis).
14 European Council Regulation (EC) No. 2201/2003 (Brussels II bis).

15 German Code of Civil Procedure (Zivilprozessordnung – ZPO).
16 German Code of Procedure in Family Matters and Non-Contentious Matters.
17 European Council Regulation (EC) No. 593/2008 (Rome I).
18 Introductory Act to the Civil Code (Einführungsgesetz zum Bürgerlichen Gesetzbuch – EGBGB).
19 BGH, decision of 10/12/2014 – XII ZB 463/13; published in: Neue Juristische Wochenschrift (NJW) 2015, p. 479.
20 Bundestag document XI/32, p. 357
21 Ernst Benda (* 15th of January 1925 in Berlin; † 2nd of March 2009 in Karlsruhe) was a German lawyer and politician (CDU). In 1968/69, he was the federal minister of the interior, and from 1971 to 1983, he was the president of the German Constitutional Court.
22 Bundestag document 11/5710.
23 Plenary Protocol of 595th Session of the Federal Council, p. 13.
24 Plenary Protocol of 595th Session of the Federal Council, p. 24.
25 Bundestag document 11/5460.
26 Act for amendment of the Basic Law of 27 October 1994, Bundesgesetzblatt I, p. 3146.
27 See Bioethik-Kommission Rheinland-Pfalz (2005), Deutscher Bundestag (2002) and Nationaler Ethikrat (2003).
28 Documented in Arndt et al. (2001).
29 Reference number 312–4080/17.
30 Sec. 1591 BGB.
31 Sec. 1600 sub. 5 BGB, sec. 1598a BGB.
32 Compare Bundestag Documents 13/4899, p. 52, 166; 13/8511, p. 69.
33 Gesetz über Qualität und Sicherheit von menschlichen Geweben und Zellen (Act on the quality and safety of human tissues and cells), Bundesgesetzblatt I p. 1574.
34 BverfG, Judgement of 31.01.1989–1 BvL 17/87, published in: Neue Juristische Wochenschrift (NJW) 1989, p. 891.
35 OLG Hamm, Zeitschrift für das gesamte Familienrecht (FamRZ) 2013, p. 637.
36 BGH, Judgement of 6.7.2010, – 5 StR 386/09, published in: Neue Juristische Wochenschrift (NJW) 2010, p. 2672 et seq.
37 Bundestag documents 17/5451 and 17/5452.
38 Bundestag document 17/5450.
39 Bundestag document 17/5450, p. 2.
40 Bundestag document 17/5451 p. 3.
41 Bundestag document 17/5451 with the appropriate stipulations of the recommended resolution of Bundestag document 17/6400.
42 See Hübner and Pühler (2017) for the details of authorization.
43 Settled case-law of the Federal Constitutional Court, BVerfGE 117, p. 316 = NJW 2007, p. 1343.
44 BSG, NJW 2015, p. 1903.
45 BVerfGE 117, p. 316 = NJW 2007, p. 1343.
46 BSGE 117, p. 212 = MedR 2017, p. 156.
47 See BGHZ 99, p. 228 (235) = NJW 1987, p. 703.
48 LG Düsseldorf, decision of 8.2.2007–11 O 297/06; LG Cologne, decision of 17.1.2007–23 O 196/06.
49 LG Berlin, judgment published in: Recht und Schaden (r + s) 2004, 203; LG Dortmund, judgment published in: Neue Juristische Wochenschrift – Rechtsprechungsreport (NJW-RR) 2008, p. 1414.
50 Directive of the Federal Ministry for Family Affairs, Senior Citizens, Women and Youth on the Granting of Subsidies to Promote Measures of Assisted Reproduction from 29.03.2012, last amended on 23.12.2015.
51 Bundestag document 17/5451, p. 3.

52 First report of the Federal Government on the experience with Preimplantation Genetic Diagnosis, Bundestag document 18/7020, p. 4.
53 Second report of the Federal Government on the experience with Preimplantation Genetic Diagnosis, Bundestag document. 19/16925, p. 37.
54 Regarding major open questions, see Bundesärztekammer (2017).
55 "Gesetz zur Einführung des Rechts auf Eheschließung für Personen gleichen Geschlechts" (Law on the Introduction of the Right to Marry for Persons of the Same Sex), 20.7.2017 (Bundesgesetzblatt I, p. 2787).
56 Resolutions are published in: Ständige Deputation des Deutschen Juristentages (2017).

References

Arndt, D., Obe, G., Bundesministerium für Gesundheit, & Robert Koch-Institut. (2001). *Fortpflanzungsmedizin in Deutschland. Wissenschaftliches Symposium des Bundesministeriums für Gesundheit in Zusammenarbeit mit dem Robert Koch-Institut vom 24. Bis 26. Mai 2000 in Berlin*. Nomos.

Beitz, U. (2009). *Zur Reformbedürftigkeit des Embryonenschutzgesetzes. Eine medizinisch-ethisch-rechtliche Analyse anhand moderner Fortpflanzungstechniken*. Peter Lang.

Bioethik-Kommission Rheinland-Pfalz. (2005). *Fortpflanzungsmedizin und Embryonenschutz. Medizinische, ethische und rechtliche Gesichtspunkte zum Revisionsbedarf von Embryonenschutz- und Stammzellgesetz*. https://jm.rlp.de/fileadmin/mjv/Themen/Bio-Ethik/2005-12-12_Fortpflanzungsmedizin_und_Embryonenschutz.pdf

Blumenauer, V., Czeromin, U., Fehr, D., Fiedler, K., Gnoth, C., Krüssel, J. S., Kupka, M. S., Ott, A., & Tandler-Schneider, A. (2017). D·I·R annual 2016 – The German IVF-registry. *Journal Für Reproduktionsmedizin Und Endokrinologie, 14*(6), 272–305.

Blumenauer, V., Czeromin, U., Fehr, D., Fiedler, K., Gnoth, C., Krüssel, J. S., Kupka, M. S., Ott, A., & Tandler-Schneider, A. (2020). D·I·R annual 2019 – The German IVF-registry. *Journal Für Reproduktionsmedizin Und Endokrinologie, 17*(5), 199–239.

Bundesärztekammer. (2000). Diskussionsentwurf zu einer Richtlinie zur Präimplantationsdiagnostik. *Deutsches Ärzteblatt, 97*(9), 525–528.

Bundesärztekammer. (2006). (Muster-)Richtlinie zur Durchführung der assistierten Reproduktion. *Deutsches Ärzteblatt, 103*(20), A1392–A1403.

Bundesärztekammer. (2011). Memorandum zu Präimplantationsdiagnostik (PID). *Deutsches Ärzteblatt, 108*(31–32), 1701–1708.

Bundesärztekammer. (2017). Für Rechtssicherheit bei unerfülltem Kinderwunsch. In Bundesärztekammer (Ed.), *120. Deutscher Ärztetag. Beschlussprotokoll. Freiburg, 23. Bis 26. Mai 2017* (pp. 123–125). Bundesärztekammer.

Bundesminister für Forschung und Technologie, & Bundesminister für Justiz. (1986). *In-vitro-Fertilisation, Genomanalyse und Gentherapie. Bericht der gemeinsamen Arbeitsgruppe des Bundesministers für Forschung und Technologie und des Bundesministers für Justiz*. Bundesminister für Forschung und Technologie, & Bundesminister für Justiz.

Bundesminister für Justiz. (1988). *Abschlussbericht der Bund-Länder-Arbeitsgruppe „Fortpflanzungsmedizin"* (No. 4a; Bundesanzeiger). Bundesminister für Justiz.

Bundesministerium der Justiz und für Verbraucherschutz. (2017). *Arbeitskreis Abstammungsrecht Abschlussbericht. Empfehlungen für eine Reform des Abstammungsrechts*. www.bmjv.de/SharedDocs/Downloads/DE/News/Artikel/07042017_AK_Abstimmung_Abschlussbericht.pdf

Bundesministerium der Justiz und für Verbraucherschutz. (2019). *Diskussionsteilentwurf des Bundesministeriums der Justiz und für Verbraucherschutz. Entwurf eines Gesetzes zur Reform*

des Abstammungsrechts. www.bmjv.de/SharedDocs/Gesetzgebungsverfahren/Dokumente/
DiskE_Reform_Abstammungsrecht.pdf?__blob=publicationFile&v=1

Coester-Waltjen, D. (1986). Die künstliche Befruchtung beim Menschen – Zulässigkeit
und zivilrechtliche Folgen. 2. Teilgutachten: Zivilrechtliche Probleme, Gutachten B. In
*Ständige Deputation des Deutschen Juristentages, Verhandlungen des 56. Deutschen Juristent-
ages.* C. H. Beck.

Damm, R. (2013). Fortpflanzungsmedizin als Gesetzgebungsprojekt – am Beispiel eines
Literaturprojekts. *GesundheitsRecht, 12*(10), 587–591. https://doi.org/10.9785/ovs-gesr-
2013-587

Dethloff, N., & Gerhardt, R. (2013). "Ein Reproduktionsmedizingesetz ist überfällig".
Zuordnung des Kindes zu den Wunscheltern, nicht zum Samenspender. *Zeitschrift Für
Rechtspolitik, 46*(3), 91–93.

Deutscher Bundestag. (2002). *Schlussbericht der Enquete-Kommission „Recht und Ethik der
modernen Medizin"* (12/9020). http://dip21.bundestag.de/dip21/btd/14/090/1409020.pdf

Deutscher Ethikrat. (2011). *Präimplantationsdiagnostik. Stellungnahme.* www.ethikrat.org/
mitteilungen/2011/deutscher-ethikrat-legt-stellungnahme-zur-praeimplantationsdiag
nostik-vor/

Deutscher Juristinnenbund (Ed.). (1984). *Juristinnen in Deutschland: Eine Dokumentation
(1990–1984).* J. Schweitzer Verlag.

Deutscher Richterbund. (1986). Thesen des deutschen Richterbundes zur Fortpflanzungsmedizin und zur Humangenetik – Beschluß der Bundesvertreterversammlung. *Deutsche
Richterzeitung,* 229–230.

Evangelische Kirche in Deutschland. (1986). *Von der Würde werdenden Lebens, Extrakor-
porale Befruchtung, Fremdschwangerschaft und genetische Beratung* (No. 11; EKD-Texte).
Evangelische Kirche in Deutschland.

Gassner, U. M., Kersten, J., Krüger, M., Lindner, J. F., Rosenau, H., & Schroth, U. (2013).
Fortpflanzungsmedizingesetz. Augsburg-Münchner-Entwurf. Mohr Siebeck.

Günther, H.-L., Taupitz, J., & Kaiser, P. (2008). *Embryonenschutzgesetz. Juristischer Kommen-
tar mit medizinisch-naturwissenschaftlichen Einführungen.* Kohlhammer. http://ub-madoc.
bib.uni-mannheim.de/25047

Hennen, L., & Sauter, A. (2005). Präimplantationsdiagnostik zwischen Verbot und Markt-
freigabe. Praxis und Regulierung der PID im Ländervergleich. In A. Bora, M. Decker, A.
Grunwald, & O. Renn (Eds.), *Technik in einer fragilen Welt. Die Rolle der Technikfolgenab-
schätzung* (pp. 267–276). Nomos.

Hübner, M., & Pühler, W. (2017). Systematische Rechtsentwicklung für die Reproduktionsmedizin. *Medizinrecht, 35,* 929–935. https://doi.org/10.1007/s00350-017-4784-9

Katzorke, T., & Kolodziej, F. B. (2001). Perspektiven eines geänderten Fortpflanzungsmediz-
ingesetzes. *Reproduktionsmedizin, 17,* 325–333. https://doi.org/10.1007/s00444-001-
0310-6

Laufs, A. (2003). *Auf dem Wege zu einem Fortpflanzungsmedizingesetz? Grundfragen der artifi-
ziellen Reproduktion aus medizinrechtlicher Sicht.* Nomos.

Leopoldina Nationale Akademie der Wissenschaften. (2011). *Ad-hoc-Stellungnahme.
Präimplantationsdiagnostik (PID) – Auswirkungen einer begrenzten Zulassung in Deutschland.*
www.leopoldina.org/uploads/tx_leopublication/201101_natEmpf_PID-DE.pdf

Leopoldina Nationale Akademie der Wissenschaften. (2017). *Ein Fortpflanzungsmedizingesetz für Deutschland.* www.leopoldina.org/uploads/tx_leopublication/2017_Diskussion_
Fortpflanzungsmedizin.PDF

Leopoldina Nationale Akademie der Wissenschaften. (2019). *Fortpflanzungsmedizin in
Deutschland – Für eine zeitgemäße Gesetzgebung.* www.leopoldina.org/uploads/tx_leopubli
cation/2019_Stellungnahme_Fortpflanzungsmedizin_web_01.pdf

Lipp, V. (2021). Fortpflanzungs- und Genmedizin. In A. Laufs, C. Katzenmeier, & V. Lipp (Eds.), *Arztrecht* (8th ed.). C. H. Beck.

Nationaler Ethikrat. (2003). *Genetische Diagnostik vor und während der Schwangerschaft. Stellungnahme.* www.ethikrat.org/fileadmin/Publikationen/Stellungnahmen/Archiv/Stel lungnahme_Genetische-Diagnostik.pdf

Rosenau, H. (Ed.). (2012). *Ein zeitgemäßes Fortpflanzungsmedizingesetz für Deutschland.* Nomos.

Sekretariat der Deutschen Bischofskonferenz. (1987). *Instruktion der Kongregation für die Glaubenslehre über die Achtung vor dem beginnenden menschlichen Leben und die Würde der Fortpflanzung. Antworten auf einige aktuelle Fragen.* Sekretariat der Deutschen Bischofskonferenz.

Ständige Deputation des Deutschen Juristentages (Ed.). (2017). *Verhandlungen des 71. Deutschen Juristentages Essen 2016. Band II/2; Sitzungsberichte (Diskussion und Beschlussfassung).* C. H. Beck.

Starck, C. (1986). Die künstliche Befruchtung beim Menschen – Zulässigkeit und zivilrechtliche Folgen. 1. Teilgutachten: Verfassungsrechtliche Probleme, Gutachten A. In *Ständige Deputation des Deutschen Juristentages, Verhandlungen des 56. Deutschen Juristentages.* C. H. Beck.

Wehrstedt, S., Thorn, P., Werdehausen, K., & Katzorke, T. (2012). Vorschläge zur Vorgehensweise bei Auskunftsersuchen nach donogener Zeugung. *Journal Für Reproduktionsmedizin Und Endokrinologie, 9*(3), 225–231.

6 Assisted procreation in Italy

A long and winding road

Ines Corti

Introduction

Scientific knowledge in the bio-medical field and its application have a profound influence in the procreative sphere, offering various options to people who are unable to pro-generate: assisted reproductive technology (ART) allows those people who cannot have children the chance to fulfill this otherwise unattainable and deep-rooted wish for maternity and paternity.

For years, sterility and infertility have been on the rise.[1] Medical intervention, which is not always able to prevent or cure these pathological conditions, can, however, overcome these difficulties in various ways. Resorting to reproductive treatment is also helpful for people who are ill or are carriers of hereditary genetic diseases. Through pre-implantation genetic diagnosis (PGD), it is possible to identify a diseased or malformed embryo and therefore decide whether to proceed with the pregnancy or prevent the birth of a seriously ill child. Moreover, assisted procreation can also meet the wishes of those who, while not suffering from any pathology, do not have the opportunity to become parents, such as single men and women and same sex couples.

The aim of this chapter is to describe the Italian legal framework as characterized by the very restrictive Law no.40 of 2004, which has been completely "rewritten" by the Constitutional Court. By declaring the illegitimacy of most of its norms, the court has transformed the initial content of the law. The chapter focuses on both the long complex political and legal path that has led, years after the first jurisprudential decisions, to Law no. 40 and the period following the law, with attention paid to the most problematic issues within the Italian experience. Analysis of the various issues will shed light on the impact of the specific regulatory provisions and the law as a whole. In order to scrutinize the system in its entirety, data relating to the number of treatments, infrastructures and cost in the country will be given.

Social and political debate

The debate on ART in Italy follows the first judicial cases. The earliest decision goes back to 1956[2] and regards a case of disavowal of paternity following

DOI: 10.4324/9781003223726-6

heterologous insemination: the judges accepted the father's request to disavow his son born following donor insemination despite previously giving his consent. The same decision was taken in the 1990s by other courts.[3] Meanwhile, there was a case of surrogacy in which the surrogate mother changed her mind after the birth of the child, refusing to give her to the intended couple. In this case, the court established that the surrogacy contract was void and therefore unenforceable.[4]

In the years immediately following the first decision on ART, several bills[5] were drawn up, all of which were in favor of prohibiting artificial insemination, even to the point of making it a criminal offence. These bills reflect the sociocultural climate of those years in which the "family" was based exclusively on marriage and in which Art. 559 of the Criminal Code still considered adultery a crime. Only at the end of the 1960s did the Constitutional Court declare this article illegitimate.[6]

From the first experiences, the debate split into two opposing camps. One was based on the right/freedom to procreate and therefore on the principle of self-determination concerning the most personal choices of the individual, and the other was based on the rights and interests of the future child, defined within the sphere of traditional family relationships.

This first view sees reproductive technologies as a further opportunity, offered by science, to become a parent. The opposing view considers these technologies simply as a remedy for sterility within the limits imposed by the family model mentioned previously. The debate has always been swayed by the thinking of the Catholic Church expressed in the "Instruction on Respect for Human Life in Its Origin and on the Dignity of Procreation" by the Catholic Congregation for the Doctrine of the Faith (1987). This instruction rejects all forms of ART and considers only natural relations between wife and husband ethical.

The opinion of the Church has strongly influenced the Italian debate, which has been particularly ideological (Rescigno, 2002, p. 198; Rodotà, 2009, pp. 77–78), based on Catholic and non-Catholic confrontation. This situation, based on preconceptions and not on personal experiences, has influenced the political parties regardless of their differences. While it is true that the left-wing parties have always seemed more open to freedom of choice for everyone, some politicians among them have not been immune to Church influence. Likewise, in the right-wing parties, closer to the standpoint of the Church, there are those who have sided in favor of ART.

Regardless of the news reported in the media on the decisions of the courts on some casesthe debate on ART has been limited to legal experts and politicians. Moreover, the discussion has focused not on the concrete experiences of people, particularly women, but on the borderline cases associated with fantasies and fears generated in the collective imagination (Valentini, 2004, p. 44). Situations have been exacerbated by media representation, which has almost always presented them in a distorted way.

The issue of ART was considered a matter for few people, not a matter of general interest. At the same time, there was a fear of subverting values intrinsic to the family culture of the time. Even the feminists, at the beginning, did not involve the general public in this debate. In fact, for a long time, the debate remained within the bounds of the political feminist context.[7]

The first restrictive bills regulating heterologous insemination were followed by more liberal ones which, albeit within the limits of the right to health, legitimized both homologous and heterologous procreation, in vivo and in vitro.[8]

In 1984, the first Ministerial Commission was set up to regulate ART.[9] It presented two proposals, one on homologous insemination, the other on heterologous insemination and on the treatment of the gametes and embryos. While affirming the principle that babies should preferably be born from an act of love between their parents or be adopted, the Commission admitted the possibility of recourse to homologous and heterologous insemination, both in vivo and in vitro, although only in cases where health issues were involved.[10] Access was limited to just two cases: when the couple suffered from sterility that could not be overcome in other ways and when there was the possibility of a serious threat to the health of the parents or the baby. The fertilized embryos were to be restricted to those needed for the success of embryo implantation, and if there should be any remaining, they were to be preserved for a further implantation or allocated to other sterile applicants who were considered suitable. The proposal banned all forms of surrogate motherhood.

In 1995, a second Ministerial Commission[11] reorganized the subject matter and, with a very similar outlook, reaffirmed access to homologous insemination for married couples. Again, heterologous insemination (with donor gametes and also with embryo donation) was closely tied to health, and any form of surrogate motherhood was banned.

The work carried out by the two commissions was an attempt to find an answer to particularly complex questions ruled on by different courts, often with conflicting interpretations. These were questions such as those concerning the disavowal of paternity following heterologous insemination and surrogate motherhood, above all regarding the recognition of the *status filiationis*. The law was considered necessary because the existing lack of legal certainty gave judges extensive discretionary power in their decisions. The law was invoked to put an end to what, according to some, had become the real "wild west" of assisted procreation, a situation of anarchy in which people did as they pleased, often to the detriment of others.

A little earlier, in 1994, the National Committee of Bioethics[12] had drawn up a document on artificial insemination in which, despite the conflicting opinions of its members, agreement was reached on some aspects, such as the lawfulness of homologous insemination; the need for consent to the treatment and the ensuing responsibility as parents; the guarantee regarding the status of the baby, that is, who is legally the mother and the father; the prohibition of commercial and industrial exploitation of gametes and embryos; the prohibition of the production of embryos solely for experimental purposes; and the prohibition of surrogate motherhood (there was unanimous agreement on this matter if surrogacy was done for commercial gain). Differing views were held regarding access to heterologous insemination and concerning the nature and protection of the embryo (Comitato Nazionale per la Bioetica, 1994).

In 1995, the Medical Association thought it appropriate to intervene with regulations of an ethical nature. In the Code of Medical Deontology,[13] the following procedures are forbidden "also in the best interest of the minor": all forms of surrogate motherhood, forms of assisted insemination for those not in a steady heterosexual relationship, practices of insemination for menopausal women who do not have premature menopause and forms of assisted insemination after the death of a partner. In addition, it prohibited all assisted insemination inspired by racial prejudice; selection of gametes; commercial, advertising and industrial exploitation of gametes; and embryos and embryonic and fetal tissue, as well as the production of embryos solely for research purposes and the practice of assisted insemination in medical surgeries, practices or health facilities without the appropriate requirements. These regulations have put obstacles in the way of people who wish to procreate by preventing doctors from intervening. However, these are regulations for professionals that concern their work and responsibility. They are, by their very nature, unsuitable for regulating questions regarding people's fundamental rights.[14] The judges, for this reason and despite the prohibition of the Medical Code, accepted the requests of those who wished to procreate: the Court of Palermo[15] authorized a doctor to implant embryos in the body of a mother after the death of her husband, and the Court of Rome[16] authorized a doctor to carry out the implantation of an embryo in the uterus of a surrogate mother.

In 1999 came the first attempt at drawing up a law, which was approved by the Chamber of Deputies but rejected by the Senate.[17] It was a restrictive bill, which, although extending the opportunity to have recourse to reproductive technology to cohabitants, limited it to homologous insemination while excluding heterologous insemination and surrogate motherhood.

After a long and troubled procedure, on the 10th of February 2004, Parliament approved Law no. 40 on "Rules on Medically Assisted Procreation", which is notable for being particularly prohibitive, strict and punitive. The attempt to repeal some of the more restrictive regulations through an abrogative referendum on 12–13th June 2015 met with failure, as the quorum requirement was not reached.[18]

Law 40: Rules on Medically Assisted Procreation

Purpose of the law

Article 1 of the law allows access to ART only "in order to facilitate the resolution of problems stemming from sterility or reproductive human infertility" and "if there is no other effective treatment to remove the causes of sterility or infertility". Recourse to assisted procreation, defined as a "therapeutic method", is legitimized therefore in the sphere of safeguarding the right to health, with the implicit exclusion of freedom of choice between natural and assisted procreation. The very rubric of the law, "Rules on Medically Assisted Procreation", gives the idea of procreative techniques as therapies or at least as solutions to a couple's pathological condition. Moreover, according to Article 4, access to ART is permitted "only when it is found impossible to otherwise remove causes impeditive to procreation" and when the causes of sterility or infertility or unexplained infertility are documented or certified by a medical act.

According to the official guidelines, as provided in Article 7 of the law by the Ministry of Health, the causes of sterility and infertility can be as follows: genetic and biological but also social and environmental, deriving, for example, from stress, pollution or the advanced age of the couple who decide to have a child.[19] The law lays down, and not without criticism from many members of the medical profession,[20] that "in order to avoid the use of interventions that have a degree of technical and psychological invasiveness that are burdensome for the recipients", ART techniques should be applied gradually, "guided by the principle of the least invasiveness". However, over time, the updating of the guidelines[21] has recognized that it is up to the doctor "to define the gradualness of the techniques" taking into account a series of conditions linked to specific cases.[22]

The legislation, by limiting recourse to ART to people not able to procreate, excludes those couples who, although neither sterile nor infertile, have or are carriers of serious genetically transmissible diseases. As we will show, prohibiting these couples from access to reproductive technology is combined with the strong protection that the law as a whole reserves for the unborn child. In relation to this aspect, the Constitutional Court intervened with Sentence no. 96, 14th May 2015, in which it declared that part of the law that excludes fertile couples who are carriers of genetically transmissible diseases from recourse to assisted procreation is constitutionally illegitimate.[23]

Bearing in mind the therapeutic nature of the procreative techniques, the law in Article 4, paragraph 2, letter b) accounts for the principle of informed consent. The legislation's reference to the need for informed consent from anyone who undergoes reproductive technology is almost superfluous, since in the medical field it is an acquired principle in the Italian legal system. Consent to health care is based on specific regulations found in the Italian Constitution: in Article 2, which recognizes the inviolable rights of the individual, from which derives the freedom of self-determination; in Article 13, which safeguards personal liberty; and in Article 32, which safeguards the right to health and states that no one can be forced to have a health treatment except under provisions of the law, which may not violate the limits imposed by respect for the human person. The Convention of Oviedo on Human Rights and Biomedicine[24] outlines this principle more clearly, affirming in Article 5 that no health intervention may be carried out without the free informed consent of the patient. Furthermore, the need for informed consent is provided for in Article 33 of the Code of Medical Deontology,[25] which establishes what information a doctor must give a patient so that he/she may be fully aware of the health issue.

Article 6 lays down that no less than seven days must elapse between the manifestation of consent and the ART treatment and that the decision to have that treatment may be revoked up until the time of fertilization of the egg. The doctor in charge may decide not to proceed with ART for exclusively medical-health reasons, for which he must provide his motives in writing to the couple. The consent governed by Article 6 of Law 40 is in actuality more wide ranging than normally required for those undergoing a health treatment. The regulation requires that the doctor not only inform the couple of the medical-health aspects, including psychological aspects, but also bioethical considerations and the legal consequences of ART for mother, father and baby, as well as the cost of the treatment when it is carried out in authorized private healthcare facilities. The doctor must also propose the possibility of adoption or foster care procedures as an alternative to medically assisted procreation.

The reference to the institutions of adoption and foster care in this context does not seem justifiable. These institutions meet needs that are different from those of assisted procreation. Under Italian law, adoption and foster care are aimed at fulfilling the right of a minor to a family and not fulfilling the wish of those who want a child of their own. Nor should it be forgotten that adoption and fostering are quite particular and call for parenting skills capable of coping with the often problematic experiences of abandoned children or children with serious difficulties due to their past and or due to being from a different culture.[26]

The provision for conscientious objection is also linked to medical practice. Article 16, paragraph 1, allows the doctor and the auxiliary personnel to abstain from taking part in ART treatment if, in advance, they have raised a conscientious objection.

Homologous assisted procreation

Among the various forms of parenthood made possible by the new procreative techniques and within the scope of the purposes of Article 1, the law allowed access only to homologous insemination, namely that which facilitates procreation within the couple through the union of gametes belonging to both partners. This type of parenthood does not cause any particular problems since the child is genetically linked to both parents.

Ten years after Law 40 was passed, a Constitutional Court sentence ruled that the prohibition of heterologous insemination was illegitimate and also ruled in favor of heterologous insemination both for sperm and egg donation.[27]

Personal requirements

According to Article 5, only couples who are of age may have recourse to this type of insemination. Both partners must be living, of different sexes, married or cohabiting and at a potentially fertile age. Consequently, some categories are excluded such as singles, same-sex couples and people over the age of potential fertility. The forms of parenthood accepted by the law are in this way limited to a traditional model.

The age of majority

Article 5 of the law lays down that couples who are of age can have access to ART. The regulation must be understood such that the requirement to be of the age of majority applies to both parents. Although the legislation is not explicit, this interpretation is confirmed in Article 12, paragraph 2, which states that a doctor who has used assisted procreative techniques on a couple, one of whose members is a minor, will be fined.

The decision of the legislature to limit access to this technology to those who have reached their majority is not unanimously endorsed. In fact, this restriction has been regarded as inconsistent with that capacity of self-determination found in the Italian legal system. For example, the minor can recognize his/her child. Undoubtedly, the legislature considered the decision to have access to ART to be of greater consequence, also from the point of view of health, compared with that of procreating naturally.

Married or cohabitants

Under Article 5, married or cohabiting couples can have access to assisted procreation. This article, however clear it may appear on a first interpretation, does not resolve doubts concerning the possibility of a separated couple having recourse to ART. Separated spouses and cohabitants will still have to appeal to the judges.

Prior to the law, the Court of Bologna[28] refused the request made by a separated woman to have a frozen embryo belonging to herself and her husband implanted in her uterus. Her husband was against the implantation, hence her appeal to the judge. The court stated that the right to procreate is subject to reconciliation with other fundamental rights, first of all the right of a child to have two parents. Furthermore, according to the court, insofar as the pregnancy had not begun, one parent's right of freedom of choice as to whether to procreate must be balanced with the same right of the other parent.

Recently, giving a different interpretation, the Court of Santa Maria Capua Vetere[29] upheld a mother's request for embryo implantation despite separation from her husband and his refusal. The reason given for decision was the preeminent protection of the embryo's life that can be deduced from the whole legislative text that recognizes the embryo as a subjectivity (art. 1). In the court's opinion, this protection is also guaranteed by the Constitution (Article 2), and it can be limited only in case of conflict with other fundamental rights (such as women's health rights). Moreover, the rule on consent to assisted procreation foresees the possibility of revoking it until the moment of fertilization (Article 6).

Regarding access to ART for cohabiting couples, in contrast with the severity and inflexibility that permeates the entire text, the legislation takes a position of openness given the fact that at the time there was no law on civil unions, as this did not enter into force until 2016. According to the legislation, limiting access to procreative technology to couples can only be justified by the wish to safeguard the right of the minor to have a two-parent family.

In reality, although the presence of both parents must be considered beneficial for a child, it is not included in the Italian Constitution as a fundamental right. A two-parent family seems to be perceived as necessary only in the sphere of assisted procreation, since the law, in the case of "natural" procreation, provides for the possibility of only one parent recognizing a child, and the same regulations regarding adoption state that in some specific cases a child can be adopted by just one adult. Thus, the right to a two-parent family is not part of the Italian legal system, which raises suspicions that the rule preventing a single woman from having recourse to ART is unconstitutional.

The prohibition for a single person to have access to assisted reproductive technology conflicts with a series of fundamental rights, such as the right to procreation (Article 2 Const.), the right to personal liberty (Article 13 Const.) and the right to health (Article 32 Const.).

It is precisely this last aspect which deserves further consideration. The law, by permitting recourse to ART solely to facilitate solving the problems of sterility and infertility, operates within the sphere of the right to health. The right to health is a fundamental right to which every person is entitled under the legal system. Therefore, forbidding a sterile single woman access to some "therapeutic methods" based on her personal condition exacerbates the doubt concerning unconstitutionality.

Couples of different sex

Law no. 40 (article 5) posits a further condition for those wishing to have access to ART, namely that the couple must be of different sexes. Same-sex couples cannot have access to ART. The lack of a specific provision for same-sex couples is a problem that could be overcome by the legal possibility for a single person to have recourse to heterologous insemination regardless of their sexual orientation. This, however, is forbidden under the Italian legal system. Moreover, article 12 establishes high administrative fines (from 200,000 to 400,000 euros) for anyone applying these technologies to same-sex couples and interdiction measures (disqualification from practicing or running activities) for doctors and healthcare facilities.

The prohibition does not seem consistent with Article 21 of the Charter of Fundamental Rights of the European Union that forbids discrimination based on sexual orientation and also with Article 3 of the Italian Constitution. The issue is also highly debated at the jurisprudential level, where there are conflicting decisions between the courts.

The Constitutional Court, with a decision of October 2019,[30] ruled that the prohibition for same-sex couples is not unconstitutional. More specifically, the court does not consider Articles 3 and 117 of the Constitution have been violated (the latter relating to Articles 8 and 14 of the ECHR). Contrary to what was stated in the referral orders, the court considers the exclusion of same-sex couples does not imply discrimination based on sexual orientation since the "physiological" infertility of the couple (in this case female) is not comparable to the total and irreversible infertility of the heterosexual couple affected by reproductive disorders. Also, with respect to the possible conflict with Articles 8 and 14 of ECHR, the court points out that the Strasbourg Court itself ruled that a national law that reserves access to ART solely to sterile heterosexual couples cannot be considered unequal treatment of same-sex couples given that the respective situations are not comparable.[31] In the view of the Constitutional Court, therefore, the right to procreate using any method other than the natural one does not exist under the Italian legal system.

For similar reasons, the court considers inadmissible the question of constitutional legitimacy raised following the refusal by a civil registrar to issue a birth certificate certifying the double maternity of a baby boy born in Italy to a foreign gestational mother (American, and therefore the child was also an American citizen) and an intentional Italian mother (married to each other in America).[32]

Nor, recently, does the Court of Cassation seem to offer any favorable interpretations for same-sex couples. With two decisions, no. 7668 and no. 8029 of 2020,[33] the court confirms the legitimacy of the civil registrar's refusal to specify the double maternity on the birth certificate of children born in Italy as a result of assisted procreation carried out abroad.

These decisions raise a question regarding the cases of babies also conceived using ART but born abroad for whom double parenthood has been specified at the time of transcribing and obtaining the birth certificate. An example is the 2017 sentence that accepts the request for the "correction" of the birth certificate of a minor born abroad to two married mothers (transcribed in Italy in the civil registers with reference to only the birth mother), as, according to the judges, this was not in contrast with the "public order".[34] A similar evaluation was made in 2016 regarding the request for the transcription of a foreign birth certificate of a son born to two mothers, one of whom had donated the egg and the other of whom had given birth.[35]

Regarding these differing interpretations, the Court of Cassation[36] itself has underlined that in the case of babies born abroad, a different legal parameter is applied, that of the principles underlying the legal system: what is evaluated is the principle of continuity and the preservation of *status filiationis* as well as the principle relating to the circulation of legal documents drawn up abroad (for specific questions about the cases of male same-sex couples who turn to surrogate motherhood, please refer to section "Surrogate Motherhood")

Potentially fertile age

Under Law no. 40, anyone who undergoes ART must be of potentially fertile age. The aim of this is to avoid creating so-called mummy-grannies, a situation considered harmful for the minor. The law is vindicated also in its aim to reduce the greater medical risks connected with the use of ART for pregnancies in older women.

The lack of a pre-established age over which it is not possible to have recourse to ART is seen as positive, since in nature, it is not possible to pinpoint a definite procreative age. It is clear that this could lead to some problems in interpretation and applications of the regulation differing from case to case, from healthcare center to healthcare center.

Problems of interpretation arose after the Constitutional Court sentence on the illegitimacy of the prohibition of heterologous insemination,[37] which has again made possible the use of this technique in the national territory. In particular, doubts have arisen both with regard to the different age limits established by individual regions and with regard to a differentiation between homologous (50 years) and heterologous (43 years) techniques within the same region, motivated by the higher difficulty of success of the latter compared to the former. In this regard, the Council of State has recently deemed illegitimate the provision of a different discipline for heterologous procreation regarding the age limit, as it is considered unreasonable and discriminatory.[38]

The vagueness of the law also leads to the conclusion that only one member of the couple must not be over the potentially fertile age. It is undeniable that the limit is related to the condition of the woman, since it is difficult to apply to the man, who by nature can father a child until a late age.

Living parents

Progress in research and technology has made it possible to fulfill the wish for a child after the death of the partner. This is done through the retrieval of gametes, the formation and transfer of the embryos to the uterus and the cryopreservation of genetic material.

The law opposes this possibility by establishing that both partners must be living to have access to ART. It establishes a general prohibition of what is called *post-mortem* insemination without making any distinction between different methods for procreating after the death of a spouse or cohabitant, for example, by using the frozen sperm of the dead partner or retrieving the sperm from the body immediately after death. Or, again, finding a surrogate mother, if the female partner dies after the formation of the embryo.

Despite the various possibilities, the legislature's requirement of "both living", referring to the people involved, is vague and does not define the limits of the prohibition. In other words, it is not clear if it is delimited by the hypothesis of the death of one member of a couple occurring before or after the fertilization of the embryo.

Prior to the law, the Court of Palermo had ruled in favor of the request of a woman to be able to continue her procreative plan by implanting other embryos after having been widowed following the first attempt at homologous insemination.[39] Even in this case, there could be further similar requests today which would again leave the job of interpretation to the judges. Following the adoption of the law, the courts seem to be more favorable to accept the requests of the widows for the transfer of the embryos fertilized rather than of cryopreserved gametes.[40] The Court of Cassation however, with decision no. 13000 of 2019, established that the consent of husband or partner to assisted procreation ia an adequate basis to attribuite to the child the legal status of filiationis even if the husband or partner has died.[41]

Rules on heterologous insemination: the prohibition and the sentence of the Constitutional Court

Article 4, paragraph 3, Law 40/2004, in its original version, absolutely prohibited heterologous insemination, namely the use of donor gametes, and hence any form of parenthood not dependent on a genetic link. Recourse to the use of gamete donation by a third person is still, however, the subject of discussion. On the one hand, claims are made for the right to have a child to love and raise, whereas on the other hand, the participation of an outsider in the procreative process is seen to have a negative effect on the couple's relationship and on that between parents and children.[42]

Legally, those who maintain that recourse to heterologous techniques is legitimate base their arguments on those referring to fundamental rights such as the right to procreation, the right to respect for one's own personal and family life, the right to have a family and those principles of liberty and autonomy that shape the governing of personal and family relationships, all of which are an expression of the evolution of law marked now by a significant reduction in public interference in family matters.

On the other hand, there are several objections to this view on heterologous techniques, which also became clear in the parliamentary debate during the passage of Law 40. The most traditional viewpoint in this line of argumentation goes as far as to suggest that the intervention of a third-party donor is at variance with the duty of fidelity laid down in Article 143 of the Civil code and with the protection of the legitimate family.

As far as the principle of protection of the legitimate family is concerned, the legislation on filiation had already eroded the foundations of this principle by giving the couple the right to recognize a child born from an extra-conjugal relationship.

On the children's side, one of the objections concerns the risk of psychological damage that could occur when the child learns that he/she is genetically linked to someone else. This risk could increase following a separation by the parents or if there is a worsening in the conflictual relationship between the parents themselves. Currently, however, pathological conditions stemming from this parent-child relationship do not seem to have been observed.

Another objection concerns the right to know one's origins, which is violated by the rules that establish the anonymity of the gamete donor. More specifically, the knowledge of one's biological descent is thought to be indispensable for reasons concerning the safeguarding of the health of the child, as in the case of a pre-disposition to possible illnesses. This objection could be overcome, as it has been in other countries,[43] by not giving the donor the right to anonymity or through the setting up of a data bank where it would be possible to trace useful information without necessarily discovering the identity of the donor.

Moreover, under Italian law, the right to know one's origins does not seem to be established in absolute terms, not even regarding natural procreation. It is linked with the principle of truth which, although characteristic of the current legislation on filiation, does have several limits. In some circumstances, it is the principle of the interest of the minor that prevails over the principle of truth. However, the current regulations on heterologous insemination do show some kind of opening.

It should also be emphasized that, prior to Law no. 40, heterologous insemination was permitted without particular restrictions. It was regulated by circulars from the Ministry of Health. The first (1st March 1985) forbade the practice of this type of insemination in national healthcare facilities; the second (27th April 1987) regarded the protocol for using gametes and rules for the registration of couples and donors; and the third (10th April 1992) the methods of retrieval, preparation and cryopreservation of the gametes, as well as the screening which the recipient woman had to undergo to protect the potential unborn baby. The last was a ministerial ordinance (5th March 1997) relating to the prohibition of selling and publicizing gametes and human embryos.

An important question was raised regarding the *status filiationis* and the possibility for the father to disavow paternity based on the lack of a genetic link with the child. In addition to the already mentioned 1956 sentence of the Court of Rome, in 1994, the Court of Cremona upheld the request of a father to disavow his son born following heterologous insemination.[44] Unlike these interpretations, the Supreme Court affirmed that once a husband has given his consent to the insemination of his wife with the sperm of a third party, he cannot then disavow the child.[45]

In accordance with the Supreme Court's decision, Law 40 established (Art. 9.1, Law no. 40), despite prohibiting heterologous insemination, that in the case in which the couple had resorted to heterologous insemination, disavowal of paternity (Art. 235. c.c.) and the action against the recognition of children born out of wedlock (Art. 263 c.c.) were precluded if the spouse or the partner had given their consent to insemination of his wife or partner. This is a way of protecting the babies: legislative prohibition introduced by the law has not stopped people using these procreative techniques in other countries where they are permitted. It should also be pointed out that heterologous insemination in vivo (hence male) can be done with a "Do it yourself" kit without medical assistance. These rules (Art. 9.1, Law no. 40) relating to the protection of the child remain in force even after the decision of the Constitutional Court declared that the prohibition of heterologous fertilization was illegitimate.

The Constitutional Court, with the 2014 decision,[46] recognized that the prohibition of heterologous insemination was a violation of the fundamental right of the couple, to whom Law no. 40 was addressed, to form a family with children. Furthermore, the absoluteness of this law was not justified by the need to protect the baby. It was a prohibition that implied unequal treatment for sterile couples based on their financial situation since the fundamental right to health was denied to those not able to afford a trip to a foreign country.

Following this sentence, the Permanent Conference for Relations between the State, Regions and Autonomous Provinces has adopted a document for the regulation of heterologous insemination. It stipulates, among other things, the age of the male and female donors (18–40 for the former and 20–35 for the latter), the maximum number of donations per person (not more than 10), the gratuitousness and willingness of the act of donation and the anonymity of male/female donors. The force of this last regulation on anonymity has been attenuated by successive guidelines issued in 2018, which affirm the right of the child to trace his/her origins using the law on adoption as a model. Therefore, if the donors agree to reveal their identity, the children born following heterologous insemination may know their origins once they reach the age of 25.

Nevertheless, today around 10,000 couples resort to heterologous insemination and over a third go abroad for it.[47]

The greatest problem faced by all centers today is obtaining gametes, both male (sperm) and female (oocytes). The ten-year prohibition imposed by Law 40 (2004/2014) has led to a situation in Italy in which there are no reproductive cell donors (Conferenza delle Regioni e delle Province autonome, 2014).

Surrogate motherhood

Surrogate motherhood, that is, when a mother gives birth to a child not for herself but for another woman or couple, is prohibited by Italian law.

Before Law 40 came into force, there were no specific rules, and courts, called upon to resolve questions regarding the validity of a surrogacy contract and the attribution of paternity and maternity, came up with differing interpretations, thus highlighting the complexity of the issue. From the standpoint of the validity of the contract between the client couple and the surrogate mother, the courts considered the profit motive[48] in a negative light, while from the viewpoint of the attribution of parenthood, the question of the underlying relationship was considered irrelevant.[49]

The legislature, however, has not taken this complexity into consideration: overlooking the various problems, the law not only does not make any distinction between the different types of surrogate motherhood, but it does not even attempt to define it, "restricting itself" simply to establishing the penalty. Article 12, paragraph 6, lays down that anybody who, in any form, carries out, organizes or publicizes surrogacy (the selling of gametes or embryos) will be punished by imprisonment for a period of three months to two years and a fine from 600,000 to 1,000,000 euros.

At the same time, Article 9, paragraph 2, prohibits the surrogate mother from renouncing the legal attribution of maternity in order to favor the procreative project of another person: the rule prevents the woman who has undergone ART from declaring her wish to remain anonymous, which is actually recognized in the context of "natural" procreation.[50] This regulation was inserted in order to prevent a practice that had crept in, endorsed by juvenile court judges before the law came into force. This practice allowed the surrogate mother to not legally recognize the baby, while the father would recognize it as his child, and then the wife of the father would ask to adopt the baby under Article 44, paragraph 1, letter b, 1 184/1983. These judges, aside from their evaluation regarding the legitimacy of the surrogacy agreements, on the basis of the best interest of the minor, had indirectly permitted the reproductive wish of the social parents.[51]

Surrogate motherhood is a procreative modality that raises many objections, especially when it is carried out for commercial purposes. Surrogacy undermines a fundamental certainty, the identity of the mother. Maternity, the bedrock of absolute certainties, no longer stands firm in the face of today's subdivision of the genetic, gestational and social roles.[52]

Those who oppose this technique maintain that it is not consistent with human dignity that a woman should use her uterus for financial gain and treat it as an incubator for someone else's child. It is potentially degrading for women, as it reduces them to the status of reproductive objects. It raises the question of the serious risk of commercial exploitation of women, above all the poorest, who may be resident in other countries. These days, the number of those resorting to surrogate motherhood has increased mainly due to the availability of women living in countries where the practice is permitted.[53] This has caused a storm of protest on behalf of the surrogate women and babies from the poorest countries, with opponents calling for an international moratorium on the practice in the hope of making it an international crime.[54]

Others interpret it differently, maintaining that it is the surrogate woman's freedom of choice and her consent that legitimizes this relationship independently of whether she is paid. Some people think that there is greater exploitation if the woman is not paid.[55]

Even if Italian law does not distinguish between surrogacy based on solidarity or commercial gain, today there seems to be an openness towards the former. The National Committee of Bioethics, in a motion of 18th March 2016, expresses a negative opinion on surrogate motherhood solely for payment.[56] It considers a surrogate motherhood contract injurious to the dignity of the woman and of the child, who, like an object, is subjected to a purchase agreement, and because the notion of commercialization and exploitation of the body of a woman for its reproductive capabilities is in stark contrast with the fundamental bioethical principles laid down in the Convention of Oviedo and the European Charter of Fundamental Rights.

According to the Court of Appeal of Milan,[57] the regulatory ban would only be valid in the case of surrogacy for commercial ends since it is necessary to guarantee the fundamental rights of the woman whose "dignity is violated if she is bound in a 'pregnancy for others' for reasons of exploitation and commercialization of her body. This motivation is particularly evident in the case of more vulnerable women from developing countries". Otherwise, surrogacy cannot be considered a violation of the dignity of women if it is not based on commercial exchange and if it also guarantees the woman the possibility to rethink, keep and recognize the child. It is not possible to impose on a woman by contract (or by law) the use of her body for reproductive ends and to be, or not to be, a mother.[58]

As far as protection of the baby is concerned, some argue that the relationship between mother and child is itself distorted: it is considered an unnatural practice, as a woman deliberately allows herself to become pregnant with the intention of giving up the child to which she will give birth, and this is not the way to approach pregnancy. It is also potentially damaging to the child, whose bonds with the carrying mother are held to be strong.[59] While not denying the very close connection between a pregnant woman and her fetus, however, it should be underlined that at this moment, there are no studies that demonstrate psychological damage to children born via surrogacy.[60]

Some see surrogacy as involving selling babies, but others hold that this is not the case and see the technique as an aid to procreation. The surrogate mother makes her body available (often the embryos come from the intended parents) not from a procreative wish of her own but of others.

In addition, there are fears of the unexpected during the pregnancy and after the birth. For example, the surrogate mother may change her mind and decide to keep the child; she may opt to interrupt the pregnancy; the intended parents may also change their minds if the child is born with a disease, if the couple gets a divorce or if one of them dies.

On the other hand, for others, surrogate motherhood is a positive experience offering the chance to those who want a child but cannot withstand a pregnancy to fulfill their wish for parenthood.

The absolute prohibition of surrogacy by Italian law does not solve the problems and, above all, does not stop people from going abroad: this situation could be resolved by the recognition of legal models that safeguard, above all, the women involved and their dignity. Despite the lack of official data on the number of babies born abroad by using surrogacy, there have been many sentences in recent years regarding requests to register births of children born using surrogacy in countries where it is permitted. Although the jurisprudence is not unanimous on the question, many judges have indirectly accepted this form of reproduction, justifying the transcription of the birth certificate (with indication of the parenthood of the contracting couple if the surrogacy took place according to the laws of the foreign country) based on the principle of the best interests of the child.[61]

However, the Court of Cassation in its May 2019 decision[62] rejected the registration of the intended father who had no genetic links with the baby as the child's parent, affirming that a man who was not the biological father of the child could not be registered in Italy as the parent even if he had been recognized as such in the state where the child was born. According to the court, the prohibition of surrogacy stated by Italian law is a principle of "public order". The court added, however, that the non-biological father could become the child's parent through "adoption in particular cases" established by Law no. 184/83.[63]

This decision did not put an end to the contrast. In April 2020, after a first ruling in accordance with the United Sections,[64] the judges of the Court of Cassation raised the question of the constitutional legitimacy concerning the legal regulations in the part where they do not allow the possibility of recognizing the foreign provision that affirms the parenthood even of the intentional father, as it is against the "public order".[65] According to the judges, the interpretation outlined previously does not appear compatible with the rights of the child set out in the constitution and with international norms

In sentence no. 33 of 2021, the Constitutional Court, while deeming the questions of constitutional legitimacy raised inadmissible, recognizes that adoption, in special cases, as deemed feasible by the 2019 sentence, constitutes a form of protection that is not fully in line with constitutional and supranational principles regarding children's rights.

With this decision, the court does not offer a decisive answer to the question but through a long interpretative process refers to the legislature, which, the judges say, has the task of adapting the law to the requirements of protection of the interest of children born abroad to a surrogate mother, in the legal recognition of the relationship with the non-biological parent.

The subject is controversial, and there are now some bills designed to consider surrogacy a crime even if carried out in countries where it is legal.[66]

A different viewpoint is evident in the proposal presented by the Luca Coscioni Association that legitimizes surrogate motherhood by laying down the obligation for the woman who lends her uterus for the embryo of others to renounce all parental rights to the born child and the right to receive a reimbursement of the expenses sustained during pregnancy, directly or indirectly connected with it (Associazione Lucacoscioni, n.d.).

Protection of the embryo

Chapter VI of Law 40/2004 is dedicated to the protection of the embryo. It includes articles 13 and 14, which are entitled "Experimentation on Human Embryos" and "Limits to the Application of Techniques on Embryos" respectively.

Article 1 of the law already establishes strong protection of the embryo, as it states that in order to facilitate the solution to reproductive problems, recourse to assisted procreation is permitted under the conditions and in the manner prescribed by the law "that guarantees the rights of all the individuals involved including the unborn child".[67]

The law establishes the prohibition of any experimentation on a human embryo (Art. 13, clause 1), permitting clinical and experimental research "on the condition that it is exclusively for therapeutic and diagnostic purposes associated with it for the protection of the health and development of the embryo itself, and if no alternative methods are available" (Art. 13, Clause 2). Also prohibited is the creation of embryos for the purposes of research (Art. 13, Clause 3, Letter a).

The Italian law is very restrictive even when compared with the Convention of Oviedo, which does not prohibit experimentation as such, nor the use of already formed embryos but only the creation of embryos for the purposes of research (Art. 18).

However, if many appear to agree with the prohibition of creating embryos for the purposes of research for ethical reasons, doubts are raised concerning the prohibition of experimentation and research on already formed embryos which are preserved and destined for certain death. These are embryos which cannot be used for procreative purposes for a series of reasons: for the expressed wish of the couple, because under the new law they cannot be donated or because for scientific reasons they cannot be preserved beyond a certain time. These are embryos that could advance useful research aimed at finding new cures in the future for people who are seriously ill.

However, attempts to get the prohibition lifted have not been successful. Regarding the prohibition of utilizing the surplus embryos for purposes of research, the Constitutional Court in 2016 stated that it is the legislator who must achieve the necessary balance between the right of the embryo and the right of scientific research.[68] Earlier, the European Court of Human Rights ruled that the prohibition of research on cryopreserved embryos established in Law 40/2004 with Art. 8, ECHR, which recognizes that everyone has the right to respect for his private and family life.[69]

Furthermore, the law prohibits all forms of selection of embryos or gametes for eugenic purposes or interventions that are intended to alter the genetic heritage of the embryo or gamete or to predetermine genetic characteristics. Only interventions for diagnostic and therapeutic purposes undertaken for the health and development of the embryo are possible (Art. 13, clause 3, letter b). The Constitutional Court also ruled on this prohibition by declaring that the banning of PGD of embryos was illegitimate (sentence no. 96/2015), as was the related crime of selection of embryos (sentence no. 229/2015) established by the law. The court had previously also considered illegitimate Article 14, where it established a limit to the number of embryos for implantation (maximum three) and the obligation to implant them all at the same time (sentence no. 151/2009).

In addition, the law forbids cloning both for reproductive purposes and for research (Art. 13, clause 3, letter c); it also prohibits the fertilization of a human gamete with a gamete of a different species and the production of hybrids or chimeras (Art. 13, clause 3, letter d). Punishments for the violation of these prohibitions are severe, including imprisonment and, in the case of a practitioner in the healthcare profession, the suspension of the exercise of the profession.

Facilities, cost and administrative procedures

Law 40 lays down further obligations: the Higher Institute of Health must prepare an annual report for the Ministry of Health based on the data collected on the activity of the authorized facilities, with reference to the epidemiological assessment of the techniques and treatments carried out. Following this, the Ministry of Health must present its report to Parliament on the implementation of the current law (art. 15).

The data cited in the following is from the latest report presented to Parliament in 2020 and refer to the situation as it was in 2018.[70] Under Law 40, treatments for ART are carried out in public or private facilities authorized by the regions and entered in the designated register (art. 10). Data relating to 2018 confirm the tendency of couples to opt for public facilities or private centers that are part of the state-run healthcare service, even though private healthcare facilities are more numerous.

Regarding the comparison with previous years, the Ministry of Health Report gives some indications. Considering all the techniques – homologous and heterologous, both at Level I (insemination) and at Level II (insemination in vitro) – from 2017 to 2018, there was an increase in the couples treated (from 78,366 to 77,509), stability in the cycles initiated (from 97,888 to 97,509) and an increase in the babies born alive (from 13,973 to 14,139).

However, there is a significant increase in the application of gamete donation techniques. The average age of women receiving insemination with fresh semen remains constant: 36.7 years old (the latest data published by the European register gave an average age of 34.9 years old for 2015). Women using heterologous insemination are older (41.6 years old) if the donation is of oocytes and younger if the donation is of sperm (34.8).

The fact that older women make use of the donation cycles seems to indicate that this technique is chosen mainly on account of physiological infertility due to the age of the woman rather than because she is suffering from any specific disease.

Twin and triplet pregnancies have dropped, the latter in line with the European average despite a persistent variation in numbers between the centers.

Regarding the cost, there are differences between Italian regions.[71] In fact, despite all the services relating to assisted procreation being included by the National Health System in the essential levels of assistance (LEA),[72] their application and related costs depend on the regional health organization, as there is still no shared indication at national level.

Putting aside the varying cost in private structures, the differences determined by the regional health system appear to conflict with the right to equal access to health care. The law recognizes the so-called conscientious objection of members of the healthcare services, namely the right to be exempted from the performance of procedures and activities relating to medically assisted procreation. This point has been particularly criticized and, as has already been pointed out, seems to demonstrate the legislature's aversion to the use of reproductive technologies. There are no data regarding this.

Conclusions

In its original form, the Italian law on ART lays down a multitude of prohibitions and even criminal penalties, which is unusual from a technical legal viewpoint, since it deals with the regulation of fundamental rights relating to the life of a person.

It was underlined years ago that it would be dangerous to bring in punitive, repressive regulations in the area of personal rights where the general principle is that of freedom (Perlingieri, 1989), and by virtue of this idea, some jurists pointed out that the only possibility would be "soft" regulation which offers guarantees and safeguards for the individuals involved without restricting their choices and fundamental rights (Rodotà, 1989), whereas the law currently in force reveals a strong aversion to ART.

Law 40, which has been almost completely "rewritten" by the Constitutional court, has penalized the lives and wishes of many people who have taken legal action to achieve their procreative plans. This situation is very painful both on psychological and financial levels. The economic aspect also affects the possibility for the couple to fulfill their wishes abroad, an opportunity reserved only for people financially able to meet all the expenses. In its decision regarding the illegitimacy of the prohibition on heterologous insemination, the Constitutional Court affirmed that it creates discrimination based on the economic resources of individual people. This topic is still unresolved, as is that concerning surrogacy.

Most importantly, Law 40 has infringed on many fundamental individual rights, such as the right to procreate, the right to found a family and the right of each person to the respect for private and family life. The exclusion of single people and same-sex couples seems unreasonable in light of the Italian legal system itself, as is demonstrated by the decisions regarding the recognition of homosexual parenthood, which the courts are gradually conceding.

The issues surrounding Law 40 have highlighted the relations between law and the life of the individual and between law and procreation, in other words, how far the law can go in regulating relationships and personal choices and to what extent it can be imposed on our personal decisions as individuals. Against the background of the diversity of family models now accepted by society, there is no place for imposed prohibitions. The restrictive, penalizing model of this law has demonstrated its ineffectiveness and limits. The rewriting of part of it by the judges is not, however, sufficient to provide a coherent and definitive framework. The legislature has the duty to deliver a new law, a "soft" law that many jurists have supported and which over time has been proven right.

Notes

1 According to Ministry of Health data (Quotidiano Sanità, 2015), one in five couples is not able to have children: around 20% of couples actually have difficulty in procreating naturally. Twenty years ago, the percentage was about half of this figure.
2 Court of Rome, 31st April 1956, in *Foro it.*, 1956, I,1212.
3 Regarding other decisions following this, starting with the decision of the Court of Cremona, 17th February 1994, in *Nuova giur. comm.*, 1994, I, 54, see paragraph 3.3.
4 The Court of Monza, called upon to decide the validity and enforceability of the surrogacy contract, ruled on 17th October 1989 in favor of the pregnant mother. Regarding the subsequent cases; see paragraph 3.4.
5 Bill C. 585, 25th Nov., 1958, Gonella and Manco; Bill C. 1017 Riccio, Spena and Frunzio; Bill S. 754, 2nd July, 1969, Falcucci.
6 Constitutional Court sent. no. 126/1968 (unconstitutionality of the first two clauses of Art. 559 Penal Code), and no. 147/1969 (unconstitutionality of the other two clauses of the same article.)
7 For an analysis of the Italian feminist debate, see Corti (2000).
8 Two bills Lanfranchi – Cordioli and others (Parliamentary Act no. 852, 16 November and Parliamentary Act no. 3694, 17th April, 1986); bill Malagodi (Senate Act no. 1304, 17 April 1985); bill Artioli and others (Parliamentary Act 3740, 9th May, 1986).
9 Ministry of Health decree 31st October 1984. The Commission was headed by F. Santosuosso. See the final proposals: *Norme sui procedimenti non naturali per la fecondazione con seme del marito e Norme sulla fecondazione artificiale umana e sul trattamento di gamete ed embrioni*, in *Giur. it.*, 1986, IV, c. 33 s.
10 The first proposal admitted only homologous insemination, the second also heterologous insemination.

11 Ministry of Justice decree, 1995. The Commission was headed by F. Busnelli. See the final proposal: *Fecondazione assistita. Relazione e proposta della commissione di studio per la bioetica*, 10th May 1996, in *Dossier Camera dei Deputati*, no. 42/3 p. 203.

12 The Italian Committee for Bioethics (ICB) was established by a decree signed by the president of the Council of Ministers on 28th March 1990 with the task of expressing opinions and also for the purpose of preparing legislative proposals to address the ethical and legal problems that may arise as a result of the progress in scientific research and technological applications on life. Committee members are appointed by the president of the Council of Ministers.

13 Code of Medical Deontology by the National Federation of the Orders of Physicians, Surgeons and Dentists, 1995, and subsequent amendments: it is a body of self-regulation concerning the medical profession, binding for members.

14 On the debate concerning ethical standards, see Belelli (2002).

15 Court of Palermo 8th January, 1999.

16 Court of Roma, 17th February, 2000.

17 Bill no. 4048 approved by the Chamber of Deputies 26th May, 1999. The bill grew out of an earlier and more liberal proposal (Bolognesi) drawn up at the Commission of Social Affairs of the Chamber of Deputies which also provided for heterologous insemination. The procedure demonstrates the failure of an initial compromise between Catholics and the laity. For views against the restrictive approach of the prohibition, see Rodotà (1995, p. 147) and Caporale et al. (1998). For a historical analysis, see Piccinini (1999, p. 219).

18 The organizing committee of the referendum was composed of Radicali Italiani, Associazione Luca Coscioni Democratici di sinistra, Socialisti Italiani, Rifondazione comunista and members of other parties. The four referendum proposals aimed at canceling the limit placed on clinical and experimental research on embryos; the rules on access limits; the rules on the purposes, on the rights of the subjects involved, on the limits of access; the prohibition of heterologous fertilization.

19 Ministry of Health Decree of 21st July 2004, published in Gazzetta Ufficiale, 16th August 2004.

20 Among the many critics of the law, also from a strictly medical viewpoint, see Flamigni (2011).

21 Art. 7 of Law no. 40 foresees that the minister of health periodically emanate guidelines concerning the techniques and procedures of ART that are "binding for all authorized facilities". The latest guidelines were issued in July 2015.

22 The doctor must take into account the age of the woman, the specific problems and the risks inherent in individual techniques both for the woman and the baby, how long she has been trying to get pregnant, and the specific pathology diagnosed in the couple with due regard for the ethical principles of the couple themselves and in compliance with the provisions of the law.

23 Constitutional Court sent. no. 96, 14th May 2015. See paragraph 4.

24 Convention for the Protection of Human Rights and Dignity of the Human Being with regard to the Application of Biology and Medicine, Council of Europe, opened for signature on 4th April 1997 in Oviedo.

25 Code of Medical Deontology by the National Federation of the Orders of Medical Surgery and Dentistry 2014.

26 See Italian Law on Adoption: Law 4th May 1983, no.184 "Disciplina dell'adozione e dell'affidamento dei minori".

27 Constitutional Court, sent. no.162, 10th June 2014. See paragraph 3.3.

28 Court of Bologna, ord. 9th May 2000.

29 Court of Santa Maria Capua Vetere, ord. 27th January 2021 and ord. 25th November 2020.

30 Constitutional Court, sent. no. 221, 23 October 2019. The decision followed two similar ordinances of the Court of Pordenone and the Court of Bolzano which raised the

question of the constitutional legitimacy of articles 5 and 12 of Law no.40. It referred to female same-sex couples who had requested access to ART but had been denied it by the local health authorities. See also Constitutional Court, sent.no.32, 28 January 2021. The Court shifts attention to the lack of protection of child born of same-sex couples, inviting Parliament to identify forms of legal recognition of parenthood not present in the system. According to the Court this lack is no longer tolerable.

31 European Court, 15th March 2012, *Gas and Dubois v. France*.
32 Constitutional Court, sent. no. 237, 15th November 2019.
33 Court of Cassation, 3rd April 2020, no. 7668, and 22nd April 2020, no. 8029. See the different interpretations of Court of Brescia,11th November 2020; Court of Genova, 4th November 2020; Court of trento 27 maggio 2020.
34 Court of Cassation, 15th June 2017, no.14878.
35 Court of Cassation, 21st June 2016, no.19599.
36 Court of Cassation, 3rd April 2020, no. 7668.
37 See Paragraph 3.3.
38 Council of State, 24th November, 2020. The case regards the regional provisions of the Lombardy region, which establish that the maximum age limit for woman to undergo heterologous insemination is 35 years of age, while for homologous insemination, it is 50. The appeal confirms the decision of the TAR (Regional Administrative Court) of Lombardy of 23rd July 2019. The regulatory framework is very confused. The judges reconstruct a composite framework starting from the "Document on the problems relating to assisted heterologous insemination following the Constitutional Court sentence no. 162/2014" adopted by the Conference of Regions and autonomous Provinces (the political body of co-ordination between the regions and the autonomous provinces) and the DCPM (Prime Ministerial Decree) of 12th January 2017 (see paragraph 4).
39 Court of Palermo, 8th January, 1999, *in Fam. e dir.*, 1999, 52.
40 In accordance with the decision of the Court of Palermo: Court of Bologna, 16th January, 2015; against post mortem transfer of cryopreserved gametes: Court of Bologna, 31th May, 2012 and Court of Appeal, 11th December 2013; Court of Modena, 8th May 2020.
41 Court of Cassation, 15th March 2019, no. 13000.
42 See the different opinions in the document of the National Bioethics Comitato (1996).
43 See, for example, Swedish law.
44 Court of Cremona, 17th February 1994.
45 Court of Cassation 16th March 1999, no. 2315. The petition to the Supreme Court was filed after the decision of the Court of Appeal of Brescia, 14th June 1995, which had confirmed the sentence handed down at the first instance by the Court of Cremona.
   Following an ordinance of the Court of Naples, 14th March 1997, on the same subject, the Constitutional Court also had the opportunity to give a ruling, 9th October 1998, no. 348, declaring the question inadmissible, since a birth resulting from ART did not come under the law on disavowal of paternity of Art. 235 c.c., which referred exclusively to a child born from an adulterous relationship.
46 Constitutional Court, sent. no.162, 10th June 2014.
47 G. Baldini, director of the ART Foundation Italy, points this out: "The Foundation underlines that in Italy there is no applicable regulation for reimbursement of costs, expenses and to cover the donor's absence from work. This makes it necessary to purchase gametes from foreign banks at high prices. To this situation can be added the waiting lists which are long in the few centers where heterologous insemination is available"; among the main problems is the lack of homogeneity among regions (Redazione ANSA, 2018).
48 The Court of Monza, called upon to decide the validity and enforceability of the surrogacy contract, ruled on 17th October 1989 that it was void for several reasons, among which "the subject in hand lacked the prescribed requirements of possibility and lawfulness" and the conflict with the principle of unavailability of personal status and with Art. 5 of the Civil Code in which acts of disposition of one's own body are forbidden

and are "contrary to the law, public order and morality". It was a classic case: after the birth of a baby girl following a contract with a surrogate mother, the birth mother changed her mind and did not give the baby to the client couple, who took the decision to go to court. The contract provided for the payment of the surrogate mother. Another case was filed to the Court of Rome, 17th February 2000. The court upheld the request for the authorization of the implantation of an embryo in the body of a surrogate who was willing to lend her body out of a spirit of solidarity. The request was filed because the doctor was forbidden by the Medical Code of Deontology to carry out any form of surrogacy. The case was unusual, as it was filed before the pregnancy. A married couple unable to have children because of the woman's illness was forced to ask the judge for a provision in order to fulfil the obligation previously taken on by the doctor on the basis of the serious harm that would be caused to the life of the embryos with the passage of time.

49 For example, both the Juvenile Court and the Court of Appeal of Salerno, Juvenile section, although admitting the unlawfulness and therefore the invalidity of surrogate motherhood agreements, considered that this did not affect the request for adoption, which should be judged on the basis of the interest of the minor. The Juvenile Court of Rome also made the same judgment, although it did not consider the surrogacy agreement illegal.

50 Art.30, clause 1, D.P.R 3 November 2000, no. 396.

51 For example, decree 25th February 1992, in *Nuova giur. comm.*, 1994, I, 177 and Juvenile Court of Rome, decree 31 March 1992, in *Dir. fam.*, 1993,188. For further information on the decisions of the courts, see Corti (2000).

52 For a close examination of the concept of maternity as traditionally based on the principle *mater semper certa est*, see the different views in Niccolai and Olivito (1997).

53 In this regard, see interesting reflections by Pozzolo (2016) and an in-depth critical study of the subject by Danna (2015).

54 The reference is to the Charter of Paris, presented in February 2016 for the prohibition of surrogacy on a global scale. It is a political document drawn up by some feminist personalities and associations in contrast with other parts of the feminist world. In the same way, the Association "Se non ora quando" (SNOQ) has presented an appeal against surrogacy: it is not possible, it states, to accept that in the name of the rights of the individual, women go back to being the object of the will of others: no longer of patriarchy but of the market. Marchi (2017) holds a different opinion; the author has collected a series of interviews with surrogate mothers that tell of their decision and the freedom to use their uterus as they wish.

55 For example, this is the view held by Shaley (1989). More recently: Lalli (2004) and Gattuso (2017). For a different opinion, see Pateman (1988).

56 18th March 2016, in http://bioetica.governo.it/media/170978/m17_2016_surroga_materna_it.pdf.

57 Court of Appeal of Milan, ord. 25th July 2016. www.articolo29.it/wp-content/uploads/2017/06/app-milano-25-luglio-2016.pdf.

58 Valongo (2016) tackles the subject of the difference between surrogate motherhood in the spirit of solidarity or for financial gain.

59 See Danna (2017).

60 Gattuso (2017) underlines that the many scientific studies on babies born of surrogate mothers exclude repercussions on their psychological well-being.

61 Jurisprudential contrasts emerge above all with regard to "public order limits". See Juvenile Court of Bologna, 7th July 2017; the preceding jurisprudence had accepted, also for a same-sex couple, the request for the transcription of the birth certificate of a baby born abroad specifying both parents (Court of Appeal Trento 23rd February 2017; Court of Venice 28th June 2018; contra Court of Appeal Milan 28/12/2016; Court of Rome, July, 2018).

62 Decision of the joint sitting of the Court of Cassation, 8th May 2019, no. 12193. See Court of Appeal of Trento, Ordinance 23rd February 2017 that recognized the double

paternity of twins born as a result of same-sex parenting by validating the birth certificate registered in another state attesting the double paternity.

63 Article no. 44 (d) Law no.184/1983.

64 Court of Cassation no. 8029, 22nd April 2020.

65 Ordinance of the Court of Cassation no. 8325/2020, 29th April 2020. The judges refer to the *advisory opinion*, adopted on 10th April, 2019 by the European Court of Human Rights, where the Grand Chamber of the Strasburg court called on EU member states to give legal recognition, in the interest of the minor, to the parent-child relationship with the intentional mother (not biological) specified as "legal mother" on the birth certificates of other countries.

66 Bill no. 3684 presented to the Chamber of Deputies 18th March 2016 and no. 3770 presented to the Chamber of Deputies 21st April 2016: Bill no. 2270 presented 3rd March 2016 and no. 2296 presented 23rd March 2016.

67 The assertion of the recognition of legal status of the embryo has been at the center of a heated debate, even if, for the time being, it has not led to any concrete outcome so that many consider it to be a claim devoid of any efficacy.

68 Constitutional Court, sent. no. 84, 13th April 2016.

69 European Court of Human Rights, *Parrillo v. Italy*, ric. no. 46470/11, 27th August 2015.

70 See the annual report presented by the Ministry of Health to the Italian Parliament in June 2020 on the implementation of Law no. 40/2006: www.salute.gov.it/imgs/C_17_pubblicazioni_3023_allegato.pdf.

71 For the last cycle of treatments carried out, the 2016 Censis survey (Vaccaro, 2016) shows that for 14% of the couples, the cost of ART was covered entirely by the regional healthcare service; 49% of the couples paid the healthcare service fee; 35% paid for the whole procedure out of their own pockets, particularly in regions where there are many private facilities, such as in central Italy where the percentage of couples paying out of their own pockets rises to 67%, and in the South, where it reaches 51%. For couples who paid the full fee, the average cost of the last cycle is on average around €4,000 (€4,200 in the north, €5,200 in the center and €2,900 in the south).

For those who paid the healthcare service fee in public facilities or private centers that are part of the state-run healthcare service, the average cost is €340 (€280 in the north, €700 in the centre and €370 in the south).

72 DCPM, 12th January 2017. On the participation of the State in the cost of the heterologous fertilization, see: Conferenza delle regioni e delle province autonome 14/121/CR7c/C7, www.iss.it/documents/20126/0/Definizione_Tariffa_unica_eterologa_allegato6898409.pdf/b9746137-f4f5-d262-dc19-29c92cf6008e?t=1606993549916.

References

Associazione Lucacoscioni. (n.d.). *Proposta Di Legge Sulla Gestazione Per Altri in Italia*. Retrieved 4 February 2021, from www.associazionelucacoscioni.it/sites/default/files/documenti/Stesura%20GPA%20con%20relazione.pdf

Belelli, A. (2002). Il problema della giuridicità delle regole deontologiche in materia di procreazione assistita. In C. A. Graziani & I. Corti (Eds.), *Verso nuove forme di maternità?* (p. 89). Giuffrè.

Caporale, C., Massarenti, A., Petroni, A. M., & Rodotà, S. (1998, March 1). Così aumentano le chances della vita. *Il Sole 24 Ore*.

Comitato Nazionale per la Bioetica. (1994). *Parere sulle tecniche di procreazione assistita. Sintesi e conclusioni*. Istituto Poligrafico e Zecca dello Stato http://bioetica.governo.it/media/1911/p16_1994_tecniche-procreazione-assistita_it.pdf

Comitato Nazionale per la Bioetica. (1996). *La Fecondazione assistita. Parere del 17 febbraio 1995*. Istituto Poligrafico e Zecca dello Stato. https://bioetica.governo.it/it/pareri/pareri-e-risposte/la-fecondazione-assistita/

Conferenza delle Regioni e delle Province autonome. (2014). *Documento Sulle Problematiche Relative Alla Fecondazione Eterologa A Seguito Della Sentenza Della Corte Costituzionale Nr. 162/2014*. www.sierr.it/images/normativa_naz/Conf_Stato-Regioni_2014.pdf

Congregazione per la dottrina della fede. (1987). *Istruzione sul rispetto della vita umana nascente e la dignità della procreazione*, edizioni Dehoniane, Bologna. https://www.chie sacattolica.it/documenti-segreteria/il-rispetto-della-vita-umana-nascente-e-la-dignita-della-procreazione/

Corti, I. (2000). *La maternità per sostituzione*. Giuffrè.

Danna, D. (2015). *Contract children. Questioning surrogacy*. Ibidem Press.

Danna, D. (2017). *"Fare un figlio per altri è giusto": Falso!* Laterza.

Flamigni, C. (2011). *La procreazione assistita*. Il Mulino.

Gattuso, M. (2017). Gestazione per altri: Modelli teorici e protezione dei nati in forza dell'articolo 8, legge 40. *Giudicedonna.It, 1*. www.giudicedonna.it/2017/numero-uno/arti coli/forum/maternit%C3%A0/Gestazione%20per%20altri%20-%20Gattuso.pdf

Lalli, C. (2004). *Libertà procreative*. Liguori editore.

Marchi, S. (2017). *Mio Tuo Suo Loro. Donne che partoriscono per altri*. Fandango Libri.

Niccolai, S., & Olivito, E. (1997). *Maternità filiazione genitorialità. I nodi della maternità surrogata in una prospettiva costituzionale*. Jovene Editore.

Pateman, C. (1988). *The sexual contract*. Cambridge Polity Press.

Perlingieri, P. (1989). L'inseminazione artificiale tra principi costituzionali e riforme legislative. In G. Ferrando (Ed.), La procreazione artificiale tra etica e diritto. Cedam.

Piccinini, S. (1999). *Il genitore e lo status di figlio*. Giuffrè.

Pozzolo, S. (2016). Gestazione per altri (ed altre). Spunti per un dibattito in (una) prospettiva femminista. *BioLaw Journal – Rivista di BioDiritto, 2*, 93–110–110. https://doi.org/10.15168/2284-4503-155

Quotidiano Sanità. (2015, May 27). *Fertilità e natalità. Tutti i dati italiani e le previsioni per il futuro*. www.quotidianosanita.it/governo-e-parlamento/articolo.php?approfondimento_id=6290

Redazione ANSA. (2018, April 24). Eterologa, su 10 mila coppie un terzo va ancora all'estero. *Salute & Benessere*. www.ansa.it/canale_saluteebenessere/notizie/lei_lui/medicina/2018/04/24/eterologa-su-10-mila-coppie-un-terzo-va-ancora-allestero_566e7a00-e528–41c7–9453-d585824ba0fb.html

Rescigno, P. (2002). Una legge annunciata sulla procreazione assistita. *Corriere Giuridico, 8*, 981.

Rodotà, S. (1989). Diritti della persona, strumenti di controllo sociale e nuove tecnologie riproduttive. In G. Ferrando (Ed.), *La procreazione artificiale tra etica e diritto*. Cedam.

Rodotà, S. (1995). *Tecnologie e diritti*. Mulino.

Rodotà, S. (2009). *Perché Laico*. Laterza.

Shaley, C. (1989). *The birth power*. Yale University Press.

Vaccaro, C. M. (2016). *Diventare genitori oggi Il punto di vista degli specialisti*. Centro Studi Investimenti Sociali. www.ibsafoundation.org/wp-content/uploads/2018/05/becoming_parents_today_2017_the_point_of_view_of_medical_specialists_in_canton_ticino.pdf

Valentini, C. (2004). *La fecondazione proibita*. Feltrinelli.

Valongo, A. (2016). *La gestazione per altri: Prospettive di diritto interno*. BioLaw Journal – Rivista di BioDiritto, 2, 131–155. https://doi.org/10.15168/2284-4503-157

7 Avoiding ideological debate

Assisted reproduction regulation in the Netherlands

Heleen Weyers and Nicolle Zeegers

Introduction

From the 1950s onwards, innovations in assisted reproduction brought new opportunities for parenthood but also raised questions concerning the conditions under which the law could facilitate the application of such innovations, including the technological aspects. Together with changes in societal values – such as sexual self-determination, gender equality, and the upsurge of forms of cohabitation alternative to the traditional family – such new opportunities destabilized the existing cultural norms concerning procreation and family life. The central questions of this chapter are: What new norms developed out of the use of these new possibilities, how and when have such changes in norms been translated into legislation, and what did this mean in practice?

To investigate the changes, we start with a short introduction to the Dutch political system (first section). The heart of the chapter is the second section. This section addresses the societal and political debates concerning various assisted reproductive techniques (ART). Here the processes of rule formulation regarding four technologies will be described: assisted insemination (AI), in vitro fertilization (IVF), surrogate motherhood, and pre-implantation genetic diagnosis (PGD)[1]. Furthermore, the content of the regulations and the research into their effects are described. In the third section, we describe the infrastructure and use of ART. The chapter concludes with some reflections.

The chapter is based on previous work of the authors (Weyers, 2015, 2016; Zeegers, 2007, 2011). It relies on the analysis of bills, parliamentary debates, and preparatory documents such as publications of political parties and advisory bodies, reports by professional organizations, and the literature on ART in the Netherlands in general. The information was retrieved by systematic research on the internet (by key concepts) and by looking at references.

A country of minorities and political fragmentation

The Netherlands is a centralized consensus democracy (Lijphart, 1999) with a bicameral Parliament in which the Second Chamber is elected directly and

DOI: 10.4324/9781003223726-7

therefore more important than the indirectly elected First Chamber. Because of the proportional party list system and the low electoral threshold, many parties are represented in the Dutch Parliament. Another consequence of this system is that Dutch governments are always coalition governments. Until the early 1990s, the Christian Democrats had a pivotal position in these coalition governments, reflecting the well-known strong position of Christian parties in countries with a mixed Protestant and Catholic population.[2] However, since 1994, this supremacy has ceased to exist.[3] Ten years later, the entirety of the Dutch political landscape was in flux. In this new century, not only the Christian Democrat Party (CDA) but also the Social Democrats (PvdA) no longer count on solid support. Populist parties like the Freedom Party (PVV) and Forum for Democracy (FvD) have gained importance. Besides these parties, a number of smaller ones ranging from the left (left liberals – D66 and Green Left – GL) to right-wing religious parties (Political Reformed Party – SGP, Reformed Political Alliance – GPV – and Christian Union – CU) also contend for voters.

Advisory bodies play a prominent role in Dutch political decision making. Much policy is partly pre-cooked in a subsystem of policymaking where various interests and professionals are represented in semi-public bodies, such as the tripartite Economic and Social Council, with members from government, employers, and employees.[4] The Health Council and the Public Health Insurance Council are semi-public bodies that deal with the medical, ethical, and financial aspects of health policy (Timmermans, 2004). The Health Council is an independent scientific advisory council with the legal task of advising government and Parliament in the broad field of public health and health care. Based on the state of the science, the council provides government and Parliament with advice, both solicited and unsolicited, on issues across the entire spectrum of public health: from health care, prevention, and nutrition to the environment, working conditions, and innovation and the knowledge infrastructure.[5]

The coming into being and the content of ART regulations

Lifting donor anonymity: an unexpected turn

In the Netherlands, the development of ART started in the 1950s. AI was the first form of doctor-assisted reproduction that became available to couples with fertility problems. At the time, only a few doctors were willing to apply AI[6] and only in cases where the semen of the husband could be used. This fitted quite well into the Dutch cultural outlook at that time: a traditional religious country with rather strict views on family and morals.

At the end of the 1950s, public debate on the topic arose; in the 1960s and 1970s, views on AI quickly changed, and assisted insemination with donor semen (AID) became an accepted practice. This change started in medical practices where doctors were willing to help couples who could not become pregnant because of the poor quality (or total lack) of the husband's semen. The more general acceptance of this change among medical professionals is illustrated by the following statistic:

In the late 1950s, 94% of gynecologists opposed AID, whereas in the early 1980s, a majority (58%) was in favor (Kirejczyk et al., 2001).

Next, in the 1970s and 1980s, access to AID in fertility clinics was no longer restricted to married couples. This reflected the societal change of marriage losing its dominant position, co-habiting without marriage and giving birth to children in such a relationship becoming more normal.[7] Subsequently, feminist organizations took the position that refusing treatment to single and lesbian women should be considered a form of discrimination. Some doctors were willing to treat them, too. The first inseminations of single women and lesbian couples took place in the late 1970s.[8]

Another important change in the mid-1980s concerned the question of whether children should be informed about being donor offspring. Professionals such as psychologists and educationalists argued that it was in the best interests of the child to be informed about the way it was conceived. One, Professor Hoksbergen, stressed this importance by calling AID 'hidden adoption' (1985, pp. 21–22).

Through these developments, AID turned out to be a practice that rocked the foundation of marriage and the family. It is, therefore, no wonder that religious organizations started to problematize its consequences. However, they did so not directly by rejecting the practice as such (as they used to do) but by pointing to one of its consequences: The existence of children who do not know their biological father. In the early years of AID, it was seen as obvious that children should not be told that they were donor offspring (Takes, 2006). Informing them was supposed to raise many problems in education and family. In the late 1980s, those who opposed new family structures abandoned this view (Wetenschappelijk Instituut voor het CDA, 1988). In the Dutch Parliament, the Christian Democrats were the first to propound this view. At the end of the 1980s, the Christian Democrats argued for a mandatory sperm donor registry in Parliament, arguing that this would serve the best interests of the child. Non-denominational parties, for example, VVD and PvdA, did not have a firm position on this issue. They apparently did not oppose the practice. And before considering changing the law, they asked for scientific proof about whether conveying the artificial nature of their conception would be in the best interests of the donor offspring, or at least that not knowing their genetic origins would cause suffering.

The government (a coalition of Christian Democrats and right-wing liberals) decided to propose a bill in which a sperm donor registry would be mandatory. Notwithstanding the reluctance of the VVD mentioned previously, the explanandum accompanying the legislative proposal states quite firmly:

> Not knowing and not be able to know who is your father and mother, affects many heavily, especially those who don't and aren't. Knowledge of genetic origins offers human beings a footing. Without this footing, human beings lack materials which can offer a deeper insight into oneself.[9]

The Christian parties, not only the CDA but also the small Christian parties (SGP, GPV) were happy with the bill. On the other side of the political spectrum, the social democrats (PvdA) stressed that in the Netherlands, people do not have a right to know their origins. They nevertheless were willing to take into consideration that some persons are troubled by not knowing. They again asked for research into this question. The VVD supported this request and added that adopted children (seeking their roots) differ from donor offspring and therefore cannot be referred to as evidence in this matter. Donor offspring, for instance, genetically relate to one of the parents, and these children are not abandoned but very much wanted. In addition, D66 doubted the necessity of the proposed legislation and asked for more substantiation. Why do only donor offspring obtain the right to information and not, for example, children born out of wedlock? Clearly, the government was not intending to grant such a general right.

Shortly after the parliamentary debate, the Dutch Supreme Court issued the so-called Valkenhorst I ruling (1994). This ruling concerns a woman born in a home for single mothers back in the thirties. She wanted to have information about her biological father, but the institution refused to give it to her. The institution, called Valkenhorst, rejected her claim on the ground that it owed a duty of confidentiality to the mother. According to this duty, the information about the presumed biological father could only be disclosed with the mother's consent. The mother had refused to give this. Whereas the District Court and the Court of Appeals ruled against the daughter by holding that the duty of confidentiality owed by Valkenhorst towards the mother prevailed over the daughter's interest in knowing her paternity, the Supreme Court overturned these decisions and accepted the claim of the daughter against Valkenhorst. The judgment is interesting because the Supreme Court introduced the right to personality as the legal basis, ruling in favor of the daughter. According to the court:

> The point of departure for deciding the case is that the general right to personality, which lies at the roots of such constitutional rights as the right to respect for one's private life, the right of freedom of thought, conscience and religion and the right of freedom of expression, also includes the right to know one's parents. . . . This right gives a person in circumstances such as those of the woman concerned a claim against an institution such as Valkenhorst as to the disclosure, at her request, of the information about her parents.[10]

At the end of 1997, the debate on the legislative proposal was reopened, most probably because of the Supreme Court's judgment.[11] Without this judgment, the installment of the 'purple' government in 1994 (the first government without Christian Democrats) could have led to the silent death of the proposal to prohibit anonymous sperm donation. After all, the three coalition partners had been skeptical about it. However, after the Valkenhorst ruling, D66, one of the architects of the new government, turned out to have changed its position radically. Now D66 took the position that children not only have an interest in knowing their origins but also have the right to know who their biological father is. VVD and PvdA also appeared to have changed their position. They no longer deemed empirical proof necessary but simply assumed that children can have an interest in knowing their origins and that for those children who have this interest, the possibility of choice should be available. The consequence was that a majority in Parliament now was in favor, and the bill was accepted.[12] In 2004, the Artificial Insemination Donor Data Law came into force. Since then a couple of small – mostly administrative – changes have been adopted.

The basic structure of this law prohibits clinics from working with anonymous donors and provides a structure (an organization that makes sure that donor data are collected and stored) by which children can lay their hands on donor data.

The institution that takes the semen for insemination collects donor information.[13] These institutions must send the information to the national donor data institute. The data collected involve medical data, physical features, education, occupation, data regarding personal characteristics, family name, surnames, date and place of birth, and address. Donor offspring of 16 years and older can receive all the donor information. Donor offspring less than 16 years[14] old can receive data regarding physical (length, hair color, color of the eyes) and social (living situation, education, profession) characteristics.

There are no provisions in the law to limit the kind of patients who can receive donor semen and no formal requirements regarding the situation of the parent's life.[15] The law lacks a provision that makes informing children that they are donor offspring obligatory. The institutions are assumed to inform the prospective parents that informing the child is desirable.

Although in the political debate, the best interests of the child have been a major topic, there is no provision in the law that refers to such interests or to the right of the child to know its origins.[16]

Furthermore, there are no requirements regarding (written) consent and the like. This is partly regulated by other laws (for example, the law on patients' rights,[17] which requires the informed consent of all medical treatment, and the Embryo Law) and by professional standards.

There is no legal limit to the number of children per semen donor. The Health Council advice used to be 25 children at max (which is relatively high). In 2018, the Dutch Association for Obstetrics and Genealogy (NVOG) and Association for Clinical Embryology (KLEM) changed this to 12 families per sperm donor,[18] a view shared by the government.

In 2012 and 2019, the impact of the law on mandatory donor data registration was assessed. It turned out that the prescribed institution – the foundation donor data artificial fertilization (SDKB) – had set up a registration system that was open to the institutions applying assisted reproduction. The SDKB connects the data of the donor with the data given by the institution where the fertilization took place (with the person identifying data of the intended mother).[19] The evaluation of 2012 showed only a few institutions that did not always meet the registration requirement. By 2019, this had been improved. At that time, the investigators principally criticized the SDKB for not being sufficiently prepared for questions regarding donors and for not executing the law properly with respect to the transition from the old to the new situation in 2004. It turned out that all donors were asked again whether they wanted to be anonymous. The result is that some children whose mothers agreed on a non-anonymous donor ran into the fact that the donor had newly indicated that he wanted to be anonymous.[20]

Because the law is so recent, donor offspring who have the right to information do not exist yet. That the system works can be deduced from the facts that physicians have asked for medical records and an increasing number of parents and children for data on physical and social characteristics and received them.[21] It is unknown whether the data fulfilled their demands. With regard to the openness of parents on the procreation of the child, in 2012, the researchers concluded that most clinics bring it forward as important. They cautiously concluded – this part of the survey was not representative – that the prospective parents endorse and apply openness. The second evaluation makes clear that most clinics find it important to point out to expectant parents that telling the truth about parentage is crucial. The researchers of the first evaluation also looked at an unintended but expected side effect: the reduction in the number of donors. This effect indeed occurred.

IVF: Physicians taking the lead, hardly hindered by temporary decrees

In the Netherlands, the birth of Louise Brown in 1978 was noted with huge interest. Dutch doctors (although in the beginning only one or two) quickly saw opportunities and started with IVF.[22] The discussion after the birth of the first Dutch IVF baby in 1983 made clear that the technique had supporters and opponents.

Doctors performing it were enthusiastic and pointed at the great grief of childlessness.[23] Infertile women were very happy with a new chance to become mothers. When more hospitals were offering IVF, the discussion on whether IVF should be part of a health insurance package started. As usual in the Netherlands, the Health Council was asked for advice. Quickly the council issued an interim report (Gezondheidsraad, 1984). Remarkably, the Health Council almost self-evidently suggested that IVF does not raise ethical questions when used in infertile women in a stable heterosexual relationship. Another striking feature is that the Health Council addressed IVF and AI as comparable issues in this respect, although IVF is more invasive and technically more sophisticated. Both techniques were seen as acceptable ways of becoming pregnant, especially for heterosexual couples.[24]

Part of the feminist movement agreed and thought of the new technique as widening the options for women's self-determination. Another group of feminists, however, put the importance of this new option for realizing motherhood into perspective. They were suspicious about the medicalization of reproduction that would increase the involvement of men, and they feared this would entail a new form of repression of women (Kirejczyk et al., 2001). In particular, those concerned with women's health issues pointed at the dangers of hormone treatment for the women involved, the risks to the embryo, and the societal perils of embryo selection and enhancement. They started to insist on regulating the practice.

Relying, among other things, on the position of the Health Council, the minister of health issued a Temporary Decree on IVF (1985). The aim of the decree was the control of the impending proliferation of the IVF practice. Its essential element was only allowing IVF in institutions that were authorized to do so by the minister.[25] Through this, the Ministry could determine the total amount of IVF and impose quality requirements on the institutions involved.[26] The decree stimulated discussion of IVF because gynecological clinics and the newly founded patient organization for infertile couples, the Dutch Association for In Vitro Fertilization (NVRB, later renamed Freya), opposed the reduction of the number of clinics, the limitation of the persons who qualify for IVF, and the non-inclusion of IVF in health insurance packages. At that time, confessional political parties also became more and more interested in the topic.[27] Nevertheless, the Ministry of Health dawdled over proposing rules that would be more permanent.

In the second half of the 1980s, the number of IVF treatments increased enormously, from 400 in 1985 to 2,246 in 1988 (Kirejczyk, 1996). The Decree on IVF (1985) was a temporary one, and therefore clearer and more lasting rules became urgent. In 1988, the minister of health proposed to bring IVF permanently under the regime that makes ministerial authorization for the practice obligatory. With respect to content: The minister wanted to be very restrictive regarding research on embryos and was reluctant with respect to IVF for single women and lesbians.[28] This was in line with the view of the Christian Democratic party, the Council of Europe's concept-recommendation on ART, and the 1986 advice of the Dutch Health Council (Holtrust, 1993). The CDA, the only political party at the time that issued a viewpoint on the topic, took the position that political control of reproductive technologies was necessary (Wetenschappelijk Instituut voor het CDA, 1988). Respect for the intrinsic value of life was paramount, in the party's opinion. One of the proposed restrictions was that only a very limited number of embryos should be created, and they all should be implanted in the woman. Destruction of embryos and experiments with embryos should be criminalized, and assisted reproduction should only be allowed if there was a biological reason for childlessness (and therefore not for single and lesbian women).

The proposal of the minister of health was debated in 1989. The minister admitted that the practice of IVF treatments was booming and now estimated the annual demand at 4,500 treatments and the maximum number of IVF laboratories at 11.[29] The committee of the Second Chamber[30] agreed with the minister that the admissibility of IVF (and AID) as such was not the subject at stake. Furthermore, members of Parliament supported the minister's idea of putting the best interests of the child first.[31] The question of whether IVF should be refunded by health care insurance was avoided. The discussion focused on the question whether single and lesbian women were to be allowed access to IVF (the CDA and small religious parties were against and the other parties in favor) and whether research with embryos should be allowed (a similar political dividing line).[32] The new Planning Decree IVF was agreed on.

In 1989, the newly appointed Cabinet (a coalition of Christian Democrats and Social Democrats) announced legislation regarding IVF (and medical research with embryos). At that moment in time, 12 hospitals (eight academic and four general hospitals) were granted a license to carry out IVF. The government announced the proposal of a bill on fertilization techniques in order to regulate the practice.

However, the plan to propose a bill was never carried out by this Cabinet. In the mid-1990s, the 'purple' Cabinet (social democrats and the two liberal parties) started to write a new Planning Decree IVF. Research into the practice of IVF was carried out to give the new decree a better footing. Again, it became clear that the IVF practice had grown fast. The number of IVF treatments carried out in 1993 was twice the intended maximum. Furthermore, women in their 40s were offered IVF, although this was seen as undesirable; the indication for the treatment had been expanded (now also including male infertility); and one of the hospitals was carrying out IVF in combination with pre-implantation diagnosis.[33] Thus practice, once again, had taken its own path.

In 1998, the second 'Purple Cabinet' issued the new IVF Planning Decree. The leading role of the Dutch Association for Obstetrics and Genealogy in defining the direction of the policy to be followed is clearly visible therein.[34]

Meanwhile, public acceptance of homosexual relations in the 90s[35] had grown to such extent that equal access of homosexuals to IVF had become an issue. Access for lesbian couples to IVF treatment had never been explicitly denied by law but had been left for the hospitals to decide, resulting in some of the hospitals refusing such access to lesbian couples as well as single women. In 2000, the Equal Treatment Commission, at its own instigation, did research into hospitals' criteria for access and judged the policy of three of these hospitals refusing such treatments to lesbian couples to constitute direct discrimination on the ground of sexual orientation. The hospitals concerned justified their decisions by declaring that in the interests of the child, they did not want to use donor semen, a sine qua non for such couples. However, according to the Equal Treatment Commission, this reason could not be accepted as justifying discrimination. The commission also concluded about a hospital that refused single women that such a policy entailed unjustified indirect discrimination on the ground of marital status. The minister of health, wellbeing and sports reacted to the Equal Treatment Commission's report by writing: 'the interests of the (future) child has to be the starting point in deciding about each individual application, however, it does not justify the exclusion of lesbian or single women in general'.[36] The minister subsequently asked all hospitals to adapt their policy accordingly, promising further measures in case of non-implementation.

In 2016, the NVOG observed that doctors were more reluctant to assist homosexual couples, transgender, and single persons than heterosexual couples in reproduction involving donated gametes or embryos, notwithstanding their equal right to access (NVOG, 2016, p. 3). The association points to the protocol it formulated in 2010 to support doctors in their decision making (NVOG, 2010). It clarifies what could be a contraindication for giving assistance: Although a marginal assessment of the future parenting situation can be part of the procedure, this can only be a contra-indication if the doctor is convinced that the reproduction poses serious risks to the well-being of the child (NVOG, 2016, p. 7).

The rules for transactions with embryos are codified in the Embryo Law enacted in 2002.[37] The controversial part of this law involved research with embryos and will be addressed in the following.[38] With regard to transactions with gametes and embryos, the law provides first that the IVF institutions should establish a protocol concerning the control of it. Second, embryos and gametes not or no longer part of a project in which their genetic owners intended to reproduce themselves could be made available for another person's pregnancy or for scientific research. The Embryo Law stipulates who has a say over such decisions: in the case of embryos, both 'parents' for whose pregnancy the embryo initially is created (Zeegers, 2007). Furthermore, the law states that permission to use one's gametes or embryos must be in writing, that the donor must be well informed, and that the donation must be done without payment. With regard to these requirements, the NVOG formulated model regulations in consultation with the Ministry of Health, Welfare and Sports (Kwaliteitsinstituut voor de Gezondheidszorg CBO, 2003). These model regulations indicate, among others, the age limits of potential acceptors (maximum 45 years old) and donors of egg cells (between 18 and 40 years old) and that each procedure requires the permission of the hospital's medical ethics review committee.

The basic structure of the IVF regulations (embryo research excluded) is administrative authorization for clinics to carry out IVF (other clinics are prohibited to do so) under specific requirements (based on the NVOG model protocol). Much is left for the profession to decide. Because this law mostly contains many administrative obligations, the first and second evaluation of the Embryo Law were impact assessments addressing such obligations (Olsthoorn-Heim et al., 2006; Winter et al., 2012).

The most important estimated shortcoming is that some clinics did not design their own institutional protocol (as they should); they use the model protocol of the NVOG. The third evaluation is of a different type (Dondorp et al., 2021). The authors address the new technical possibilities that have developed in research with embryos and reflect on whether the existing rules should be reconsidered because of the promises that new technical possibilities entail for curing diseases and improving the wellbeing of less fertile couples (Dondorp et al., 2021, p. 191). We will come back to this under the fourth section.

A joint opinion on surrogacy

In the report of 1986, the Health Council discussed surrogacy, too.[39] The Council stated that surrogacy under certain conditions could be acceptable (especially in situations of a medical indication of the intended mother who lives in a situation that guarantees a good upbringing). The council stressed that surrogacy should be a free choice; however, commercialization, that is, women being paid for surrogacy, would be undesirable (Kirejczyk et al., 2001). The report addresses the following questions: Can a child have two mothers simultaneously? Is it lawful to become pregnant with the intention to give up the child? Are the arrangements between surrogate mothers and prospective parents binding? Is it allowed to ask for money for surrogacy? Opinions were divided, but the aversion against the possibility of commercial surrogacy in combination with IVF was almost general.

The Cabinet (the earlier mentioned coalition of CDA-PvdA) was even stronger in its rejection of surrogacy and declared surrogacy contracts void.

Remarkably, surrogacy, although it rarely occurred in practice, was the first aspect of ART to be regulated by law. In 1990, the government proposed a bill that aimed to discourage non-commercial surrogacy and to forestall commercial surrogacy.[40] The reasons given for this negative stance were the risks and emotional problems in the long term for the surrogate mother, increased risk of identity problems for the child, a disturbed process of bonding, the risk of disappointment for prospective parents, and difficulties in coming to a good relationship between child and parents. To discourage and prevent surrogacy, the government proposed to add two paragraphs to article 151 of the Penal Law. Together with an addition in the 1950s (article 151a, an article that concerns adoption), these additions were supposed to lead to the desired effect.

In the late 1950s, with the (then new) adoption law, paragraph 151a was added to the Penal Code. This paragraph mandates that placing children in another family would need the supervision of the Council of the Protection of the Child. Paragraph 151a is important for surrogacy because it creates obstacles to the recognition and adoption of a child by the prospective parents.[41] The new proposed paragraphs prohibited professional mediation for surrogacy and advertising therefor (151b) and the mediation of ceding a child (151c).[42]

These proposals were widely supported by the political parties. Nevertheless, they had different ideas concerning the underlying issues. Some parties were not against surrogacy per se but considered commercial surrogacy wrong (D66 and GL). Other parties felt, just like the government, that surrogacy as such is undesirable (VVD), and still other parties (the Protestant parties GPV and SGP) took the position that the government did not go far enough, that all forms of surrogacy should be prohibited. Both chambers of Parliament passed the bill.[43]

The debate on surrogacy has not ended with these Parliamentary decisions. At the end of the 1990s, one of the IVF clinics was permitted to carry out 'high-technological surrogacy'. The rationale for this kind of surrogacy is that this is the only way for women without a (functional) uterus to have their own genetic progeny (NVOG, 1999). In 1998, the new Planning Decree IVF permits surrogate motherhood under the conditions given by the NVOG (Timmermans, 2004). Since 2016, the NVOG has been asking for a new law on surrogacy in the Netherlands to prevent Dutch people going abroad.[44] Nowadays, the Dutch government intends to change the legislation on surrogacy, in response to the report of the State Commission Re-evaluation of Parenthood (2016) that was asked to formulate basic principles regarding the origin of legal parenthood and the creation of a legal possibility of surrogacy (and multiple parenthood). In its response to the report in 2019, the government states that the best interests of the child must come first and places great emphasis on creating the development of lineage identity.[45]

The basic structure of the paragraphs on surrogate motherhood is quite simple: It prohibits (professional) mediation and advertising for surrogacy without specific enforcement regulation. Therefore, police and prosecutorial authorities are the institutions in charge of enforcing compliance. Up to now, no arrests or prosecutions have taken place regarding article 151b and 151c.

That surrogacy takes place (although presumably in very small numbers) has become clear from a research report of the University of Utrecht (Boele-Woelki et al., 2011). In 2012, the Council of the Protection of the Child looked at 12 requests and in 2013 at 19 requests for adoption of a child born after surrogacy.[46] These requests concerned 'low-technological' surrogacy (surrogacy without the involvement of a doctor), as well as high-technological surrogacy and surrogacy abroad (Boele-Woelki et al., 2011). The researchers are convinced that surrogacy took place more often.

Nevertheless a political clash

The practice of creating embryos in IVF treatments brought with it new issues related to ART. As we have seen, the parliamentary discussion of research on embryos started in the late 1980s. In 1989, the government took the position that such research would only be allowed in exceptional cases and only if public health had a huge interest in it. Later on, in 1991, research that would be therapeutic for the embryo itself came to be distinguished from research in which the embryo would be lost, putting a ban on the latter. In 1993, a moratorium followed with the possibility to prohibit the latter kind of research by an Order in Council.

In 2002, the long-expected legislation on embryo research and the use of embryos otherwise as well as the use of human gametes followed. To an extent, these rules concern the donation of human gametes or embryos that have already been addressed under the second section. The rules concerning embryo research were more permissive than the CDA had proposed in 1989; for instance, the use of spare embryos for research is conditionally allowed. Unsurprisingly, in the parliamentary debates, there was opposition from the Christian Democrats and the other confessional political parties. However, the second 'Purple Cabinet' had already anticipated the most controversial issue in this respect by putting a moratorium on specially creating embryos for use in research.[47] In addition, the Embryo Law (2002) first stipulates that scientific research on human embryos would only be permissible when authorized by the Central Committee on Research Involving Human Subjects (CCMO). Second, the Embryo Law contains a ban on sex selection in embryos on non-medical grounds, earlier regulated by an Order in Council.[48] In 2020, the possibilities for sex selection on non-medical grounds were slightly widened, creating space for gender choice in cases where this would prevent offspring from carrying a serious sex-linked disorder.[49]

With respect to research therapeutic for the embryo, a distinction is made between research on the embryo in vivo and research on the embryo in vitro. The latter appeared to be controversial because of the involved selection of embryos, albeit selection on medical grounds, which the law has never explicitly forbidden. The Planning Decree Clinical Genetic Research and Counseling (2003) brought pre-implantation genetic diagnosis explicitly under the Specialist Medical Practice Act (WBMV), article 2. In this Decree, 'an increased risk for the potential parents in an individual case of giving birth to a child with a severe genetic condition' is the criterion formulated for PGD, which involves such embryo selection.[50] In May 2008, the secretary of state of health, welfare, and sports sought to widen the opportunities for PGD and make it available to parents with families where genetic mutations occur that are responsible for inherited breast cancer.[51] Her proposal led to fierce protests by a minister of the Christian Union (a religious party),[52] who, in addition to opposing her proposal, accused her of a breach of the Coalition Agreement. The CU had agreed to participate in the Cabinet (CDA, PvdA, and CU) on the condition that it would not enlarge the existing opportunities for abortion, euthanasia, and embryo research. The compromise that the secretary of state formulated averted a government crisis (Zeegers, 2011). First, 'a high individual risk of a severe genetic condition or disease' is the criterion for access to PGD laid down in the Regulation PGD, published in early 2009. Second, in deciding about access, medical professionals would have to take four indications into consideration: (a) the seriousness of the disease involved, (b) the treatability of the disease, (c) additional medical aspects, and (d) psychological and ethical aspects. Third, a National Indication Committee PGD, consisting of medical professionals, would be installed that would advise on requests for PGD in cases of genetic conditions for disease that previously had not been given access and for supervising the implementation of the guidelines for decision making, as described previously.[53] The Parliament accepted the inclusion under these conditions.

Human dignity and the principle of respect for life are the starting points of the Embryo Law. Therefore, the Embryo Law does not permit scientific research on human embryos unless deemed necessary by the Central Committee on Research Involving Human Subjects. In addition, it forbids, first, (temporarily) the creation of embryos specifically for research; second, development of the embryo in vitro after 14 days; and third, making changes in the germ line. However, according to Dutch law, the values announced as starting points for embryo research, with technology developing, have to be weighed anew each time against the interests connected to curing diseases and improving the wellbeing of less fertile couples (Dondorp et al., 2021, p. 191).

In line with this consequentialist reasoning, pre-implantation diagnostic (and selection) is not prohibited but conditional. The treatment is implemented for couples who have a high individual risk of giving birth to a child with a severe genetic condition or disease such as Huntington's disease or cystic fibrosis (Steinkamp et al., 2012). The Regulation PGD is the response to the parliamentary debate concerning the widening of access to PGD to include some inherited forms of cancer. This regulation consists of, first, guidelines for medical professionals' decision making on whether a client should be given access to PGD treatment and, second, the installment of a National Indication Committee PGD.

Steinkamp et al. (2012) assessed whether the professionals feel themselves sufficiently supported by the guidelines. The medical professionals answered that this is so to the extent that the indications in the guidelines offer four different angles from which each case can be approached in the decision-making process rather than four different, mutually exclusive criteria that each have to be decided on separately. With respect to the functioning of the National Indication Committee PGD, the medical professionals indicated they were satisfied and considered them expert and careful. However, Steinkamp et al. (2012) point to two critical notes: First, some medical professionals experienced its role as government interference in the doctor-patient relation. Second, some medical professionals experienced the course of events concerning new requests for access to PGD where they had to await the judgment of the National Indication Committee PGD as a doubling of decision making, as consultations between different disciplines and careful decision making on each case already take place at the PGD hospital itself.

Steinkamp et al. (2012) also call attention to the moral questions involved in PGD: Current developments in genomics make conceivable a quick diagnosis of more genetic conditions for diseases. What are the ethical implications, for instance, with regard to the decisions future parents have to take about testing their embryo?

Dondorp et al. (2021), in the third evaluation of the Embryo Law, point at a new technique that could be reason for reconsidering the ban on germline modification as well as the 14-day limit: the possibility of editing the human genome to prevent children with a severe genetic condition from being conceived (Dondorp et al., 2021, p. 56). The authors suggest that allowing the application of this technique in comparison might be more morally acceptable than the destruction of human embryos with serious genetic abnormality that is involved in pre-implantation genetic testing (PGT).

Infrastructure and use

Currently, the Netherlands has six clinics that collect sperm, three collecting eggs and one collecting embryos. Furthermore, there are 21 clinics that apply AI and 12 clinics that offer IVF (one of the latter offers PGT in addition).

About 350 men yearly donate sperm. Their sperm is kept icebound in one of the seven sperm banks available in the Netherlands. The demand for sperm is much higher than the useful sperm offered this way. About 900 new female clients a year ask for sperm treatment; waiting lists are resulting from this gap between supply and demand. Some sperm banks offer the possibility of using semen from foreign donors. The wait for semen from foreign donors is two-and-a half months against one to two years for semen from Dutch donors.[54]

Number of treatments

The number of treatments with donor sperm initially increased but now appears to have started a sharp decline. Something similar happened with egg donation treatments; treatments with embryos appear to be more stable.

As of 2019, 11,803 pregnancies are now registered with the SDKB (this also concerns treatments that took place before 2004): 11,689 as a result of sperm donation, 747 from egg donation, and 185 from embryo donation. More than 1,000 pregnancies are registered every year (Woestenburg et al., 2019, pp. 84–85).

Table 7.1 Numbers of treatments with donated gametes and embryos.[55]

	Semen	Eggs	Embryos
2010	644	52	6
2011	769	72	8
2012	881	62	17
2013	1003	95	19
2014	1126	65	31
2015	1030	63	28
2016	1180	63	29
2017	1290	53	27
2018	1222	44	30
2019	865	18	21

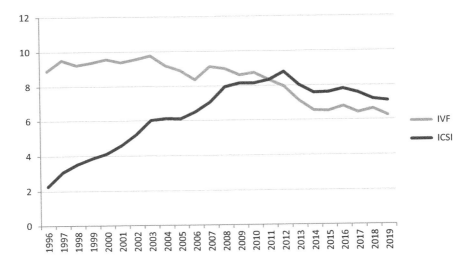

The total of IVF and intracytoplasmic sperm injection (ICSI) treatments between 1996 and 2008 rose from 11,154 to 16,927 and thereafter decreased to 13,341 in 2019. The proportion of IVF in this total – in 1996 starting out at 80% – has declined considerably. The proportion of ICSI in this total has risen and nowadays exceeds IVF treatment.

Figure 7.1 Numbers of IVF and ICSI treatments.[56]

Source: The graph is based on yearly reports: www.degynaecoloog.nl/nuttige-informatie/ivf-resultaten/

ART tourism from other countries to the Netherlands hardly seems to exist; at least, it is not a topic of debate. To some extent, Dutch citizens go to Belgian and Spanish hospitals for IVF, among other things because of the option to make use of gametes from anonymous donors.

Financing

IVF treatment is covered in health insurance, restricted to three efforts, for women no older than 42. Women younger than 38 are only allowed to have one embryo implanted on the first and second treatments; only in the case of their third treatment can two embryos be implanted. For women older than 38 years, the latter is allowed from the first treatment on.

As requesting payment for gametes is not allowed, sperm donors can get only refunds of the costs made, such as travel expenses. The clinic determines the age limit for sperm donors; there is no legal age limit. Egg cell donors, in addition to refunding of travel expenses and other costs, are allowed to receive an amount (680–900 euro) per treatment for compensation of the effort and any lost income.

ART regulation, the same but different

The debate on assisted reproduction started in the 1960s, a period in which much changed in the Netherlands. From a conventional quiet country, it turned into an experimental garden of all kinds of behavior (drugs, sex, and 'euthanasia'). Churches lost their grip on believers, and self-determination became a hotly debated topic. With respect to sex and reproduction, this in the first instance concerned the liberation of sexuality, resulting in the free sale of contraceptives repealing the crime of adultery, repealing a restrictive provision on homosexuality in the 1970s, and legislating abortion in the early 1980s. Assisted reproduction, although quite different in nature, strongly relates to this epoch of self-determination. If people have a say in not becoming parents, why not also in becoming one?

Assisted reproduction, like the issues mentioned previously, is a morality issue. In the Dutch political system, such issues are often characterized by potential value clashes between religious and secular political parties that make it hard to find compromises. Coalition governments that include religious parties put much emphasis on accommodating the potential conflicts such issues could engender. Delegation of considerations and 'decisions' to expert committees as well as focusing on procedures instead of substantial rules are well-known methods of depoliticization that are applied (Timmermans, 2004).

However, ART differs from these other moral issues in a couple of ways. First, because the way it reached the political agenda. The subject did not reach the political agenda because of the activities of single-issue movements.[57] AID had already been practiced for a few decennia in hospitals before the possible downsides of donor anonymity came to be debated in Parliament. The Christian Democrats was the first political party that through this and other issues expressed an interest in ART regulation. The party thought to protect the traditional family and the dignity of human life against secular views such as self-determination.

Second, assisted reproduction is different to the issues evolving from the liberation of sexuality as described previously because of its technological aspects. The latter aspects make decision making more complex and make it more tenable to leave regulation to a subsystem of medical professionals and advisory bodies.

Third, assisted reproduction differs from most topics mentioned previously because of the involvement of the medical profession. Not only do patients have an interest in the subject, but doctors and medical researchers have, too. Witness to this is the fact that physicians have taken the lead in making reproductive techniques available on such a scale despite the government's effort to restrict the quantity of IVF treatments.

The following norms and legislation developed around the application of the four reproductive techniques in Dutch medical practice. Once AID and IVF treatments were available, accessibility became an issue, and political authorities ended up hammering out equal access, for example, for heterosexual and homosexual partners, as the basic rule to follow in this regard. In all cases, donor registry became mandatory, as donor offspring have the right to know who their genetic parents are. With respect to surrogacy, a joint aversion to commercialization resulted in a legislative ban, but surrogacy as such is possible and became available even in its high-technological form. Whereas the law forbids selection of embryos on nonmedical grounds, it permits selection on medical grounds, as part of PGT, albeit under certain conditions.

How to characterize the political process regarding the norms and rules described previously? The religious-secular divide in the Dutch party system brings with it a large potential for conflict regarding morality issues, but, at the same time, Dutch governments are experienced in accommodating these. We observed examples of (political) actors coping with conflicts, even preventing them from manifesting, in the phase preceding as well the phase during the actual rule making.

In the phase preceding the actual rule making, the Health Council precooked decisions in its advice concerning reproductive technology. In addition, the government tried to delineate the boundaries within which this technology could develop without giving too much room for parliamentary debate, an example being its attempts to regulate IVF practice through Planning Decrees. The rather vague legal concept of 'personality right' in combination with the idea – widely shared among political parties – that the interests of the child should prevail, led to a majority of members of Parliament accepting mandatory donor registry. With respect to surrogacy, the lowest common denominator between parties, forbidding commercial surrogacy is the rule the 1990 legislation was based on. In the bill that led to the Embryo Law, government already anticipated societal support by formulating it as a compromise between those in favor of the use of embryos for research and those against it.

The rules resulting from the actual decision making are often procedural in addition to a few substantial bans: The legislature leaves the ultimate decision to the medical associations, such as NVOG, KLEM, or expert committees established by law, such as the CCMO. In some cases, the legislature, in addition to determining who can take the ultimate decision, also stipulates the values they should take into consideration, such as respect for human life and human dignity.

In sum, the political process regarding the norms and rules concerning assisted reproduction in the Netherlands fits with Dutch political culture. The Netherlands is a country of minorities and political fragmentation, the latter becoming even more relevant in recent decades. This has led to a political practice of consensus seeking through consultation but also, and even more relevant here, according a central role to expert advice. Whether it is the Health Council or groups of medical professionals, their contribution based on technocratic facts and practical experience is widely accepted as taking precedence over ideological differences. Therefore, according them the role of setting the parameters of legislation and/or taking the ultimate decision concerning ART rules is highly instrumental in keeping the practice developing without too much political contestation.[58]

Notes

1 Pre-implantation genetic diagnosis consists in examining an egg cell or an embryo in vitro for the purpose of diagnosing severe genetic conditions. Since 2017, this technique has been called pre-implantation genetic testing (PGT).
2 The CDA governed with either the right liberals (VVD) or the Social Democrats (PvdA) and other smaller parties.
3 Since 1994, coalitions between the former archenemies VVD and PvdA proved possible.
4 The government is legally obliged to seek their opinion, which usually carries considerable political weight.
5 The Health Council has a chairman, a vice-chairman, and some 130 members. Each member is recruited in a personal capacity and in relation to his or her special expertise in a certain field. Board members are appointed by the Crown. Their membership runs for four years and can be extended. The leadership of the Health Council has a policy, in principle, to prolong membership no more than twice.
6 Both Catholics and Protestants rejected AI (Takes, 2006).
7 Between the top year 1970 and 2003, the annual number of weddings declined by a third, and the number of children born out of wedlock increased by a factor of 14. In the 1960s, of first-born children, less than 1 in 30 was born out of wedlock. In 2003, this was 40% (the parents of these children often marry later on). The percentage of second and further children born out of wedlock was 23% in 2003 (Latten, 2004).
8 In the late 1980s, nearly a fifth of inseminations concerned these women (Kirejczyk et al., 2001).
9 Second Chamber of Parliament 1992/1993, 23 207, p 3.
10 ECLI:HR:1994:ZC1337.
11 There are no clear indications that the signing of the Convention on the Rights of the Child in December 1994 by the Netherlands – and in particular Article 7, which stipulates that children have, as far as possible, the right to know and be cared for by their parents, had an influence on this.
12 Two members of the Second Chamber voted against the bill; the First Chamber accepted the bill without voting [Second Chamber of Parliament 2000/01, 46 (2/6/2001), p 3548–49; First Chamber of Parliament 2001/02, 26 (4/23 2002, p 1322)].
13 In 2018, the Dutch Association of Obstetrics Gynecology and the Association for Clinical Embryology adopted a position setting out the requirements for donors (NVOG en KLEM, 2018). This concerns not only sperm donors but also donors of eggs and embryos. How to deal with these types of tissue is regulated in the Act on Safety and Quality of Human Materials 2003.
14 This age limit is under discussion because it is thought that younger children, too, should have this right.
15 In 2018, one-third of the intended mothers were lesbian, one-third single, and one-third heterosexual. The decline in the proportion of heterosexual couples is partly due to the fact that the use of new techniques makes these couples less dependent on donor sperm (Woestenburg et al., 2019, p. 109).

16 It is worth mentioning in this context that, since 2012, the guidance of children in their search for and contact with donors and half-siblings has been placed in the hands of an institute that specializes, among other things, in parentage issues (FIOM). They have already carried out about 300 projects. It is one of the signs that Article 7 of the Convention on the Rights of the Child is becoming increasingly important (Woestenburg et al., 2019).

17 Law on Medical Treatment Agreement (1994).

18 This is per clinic. It is clear from newspaper reports that some donors evade this by registering at multiple clinics. There is no check on this because there is no central register.

19 As of 2019, 4,292 donors were included in the system.

20 At the moment (2021), the courts are considering this situation.

21 Parents from 83 in 2011 to 450 in 2017; children from 5 in 2011 to 217 in 2017 (Woestenburg et al., 2019, p 87).

22 In 1982, the Dijkzigt Hospital in Rotterdam started with IVF and on May 15, 1983, the first IVF baby was born in the Netherlands.

23 Kirejczyk et al. (2001) state that there was a lot of media attention and that in the media, the feeling regarding infertility was an important element. IVF was seen as the solution to the needs of infertility, and they took the view that insurance companies not paying for the treatment would lead to a disadvantage for people without means, because then they were condemned to permanent childlessness.

24 In its report, the Council asked for legislation regarding property rights and the ways embryos and gametes should be treated (Gezondheidsraad, 1986).

25 They did so by placing IVF (temporarily) under Article 18 WZV (Law on Hospitals). This article makes it possible to prohibit certain operations and the purchase or use of certain equipment. This prohibition should be laid down in an Order in Council. Only hospitals which already carried out IVF were qualified.

26 The result is that carrying out IVF without ministerial authorization is forbidden and that the indication is clear (abnormalities of the fallopian tubes). Hospitals were obliged to collect systematic information on, among other things, the effectiveness and risks of IVF and to report this to the Ministry.

27 Besides the Christian political parties, there were other confessional organizations such as the Dutch Physicians' League who opposed IVF.

28 White Paper Artificial Fertilisation and Surrogacy.

29 Through collaboration with the Ministry of Education and Science, teaching hospitals were also governed by the regulation.

30 Before debate takes place in the Second Chamber, committees of Members of Parliament, consisting of all the parties in Parliament, discuss legislative proposals.

31 Feminists opposed the view that protection of the interests of future children was the central problem. They also saw women's interests. For example, the obligation for written consent of the husband (another CDA idea) gave the man control in a way that did not exist before. They supported the possibility of IVF (and AID) for single and lesbian women. Their argument relies on the prohibition of discrimination. Furthermore, they warned against the medicalization of reproduction by the new technologies and the low chances of success.

32 The number of reimbursed treatments was (and still is) limited to three, and no restrictions would be imposed on the type of indication (Regulation Subsidization Scheme of the Health Insurance Council In Vitro Fertilization 1989). Soon after the parliamentary agreement on the Planning Decree IVF, the commission that selects the treatments that will be refunded by health insurance companies decided to pay for IVF treatments carried out in institutions authorized by the decree.

33 PGD would be regulated in 2003.

34 For example, the Decree states that the application of in vitro fertilization takes place on the basis of the 'Indications for IVF' guideline of the NVOG, and IVF centers must participate in the uniform national IVF registration of the NVOG.

35 The European Value Studies show that in the early 1980s, the acceptance of homo-sexuality in the Netherlands had a score of 5.91 (on a scale of 1 to 10), which rose to 7.33 in the early 1990s.

36 Letter of Minister E. Borst-Eilers concerning her position on the judgment of the Equal Treatment Commission, CSZ/ZT/2076894, 28 June 2000.

37 Act of June 20, 2002, containing rules on operations with germ cells and embryos (Embryo Law).

38 Legally, an embryo in utero is considered born if his or her interests ask for it. If the fetus dies before birth, legally it is considered not to have lived. After birth, a human being becomes a holder of rights. At that time, the child has the right to a name (article 1:4 BW). With respect to the protection of the embryo, it is worth mentioning that in the Netherlands, abortion is legal until the third trimester if the woman is in a precari-ous position. What constitutes a precarious position is in practice left to the woman concerned. If the child cannot survive after birth, third-trimester abortion is possible. The doctor can invoke the defense of necessity.

39 In an interim report (1984), the Health Council did not object the use of donor eggs and took the position that surrogacy should not be introduced yet.

40 The government did not choose to ban (commercial) surrogacy because enforcement of the ban was considered very problematic and to be too great a breach of the privacy of parents. It was thought that the rules would have a preventive effect (Second Cham-ber of Parliament 1990–1991, 21 968 no. 3).

41 Discouraging is, among other things, that no separate scheme for the 'transfer' of the child is made. In the Netherlands, the woman from whom the child is born is the legal mother; the man to whom she is married (or has registered partnership) is the legal father. In cases of surrogacy, the surrogate mother (and possibly her partner too) have to cede the child. That is, they are deprived of parental authority by the court (in this procedure, the Council for the Protection of the Child also plays a role). And the prospective parents must be examined on being capable of raising a child (by the same Council). A slightly different course is taken if the prospective father is the genetic father of the child.

42 The status of surrogacy contracts is not clear. Generally these contracts consist of four provisions: The duty of the surrogate mother to be fertilized, the duty of the surrogate mother to cede the child after birth, the duty of the prospective parents to take the child after birth, and their duty to pay the agreed expenses. It is generally thought that the first three agreements cannot be enforced and that this does nullify the contract (Broekhuijsen-Molenaar, 1991; Schoots et al., 2004).

43 In the Second Chamber, the bill was accepted by CDA, VVD, PvdA, SGP, GPV, and Centrumdemocrats (other parties voted against); the First Chamber accepted the bill without voting [Second Chamber of Parliament 1992–93, 51 (2/3/1993), p 3729; First Chamber of Parliament, 37 (9/14/1993), p 1649].

44 In the Ukraine, for example, it is possible to make the 'wish-parents' the legal parents and therefore to avoid the involvement of the Council for the Protection of the child. Acting in this way is seen as *contra legem* in the Netherlands (van Vlijmen & van der Tol, 2012).

45 Kabinetsreactie op de aanbevelingen op het terrein van Draagmoederschap, meer-ouderschap en meerpersoonsgezag van de Staatscommissie Herijking ouderschap, 12 juli 2019 (State Commission Re-evaluation of Parenthood).

46 Circumstantial evidence is known through an interview with a judge. Research in 1995 showed that Dutch judges treated 30 cases of adoption after surrogacy in the early 1990s (*Trouw* 3/23/1995 www.trouw.nl/home/-discussie-nodig-over-draagmoederschap-~a3ff 7a96/).

47 The Cabinet, in elaborating on the bill, concluded this would not have enough soci-etal support from its consultation with scientific organizations, patient and women's organizations, and organizations with a religious background such as Pro Life and eccle-siastical organizations (Second Chamber of Parliament 2000/01, 27 423, nr. 3, p. 27).

However, all three evaluation reports have since advised lifting the ban on the creation of embryos for research purposes (Dondorp et al., 2021, p. 198).

48 In the Second Chamber, the bill was accepted with the votes of the Socialist Party (SP), PvdA, D66, and VVD in favor; confessional parties voted against. In the First Chamber, confessional parties voted against the bill, too [Second Chamber of Parliament 2001/02 10 (10/9/2001) p 428–29; First Chamber of Parliament 6/18 2002 (2001/02) 32 p 1536–37].

49 Act of 1 July 2020, amending the Embryo Law instead of Act in connection with the amendment of the ban on sex selection and use of gametes and embryos for quality assurance, *Staatsblad* 2020, 229.

50 Planningsbesluit klinisch genetisch onderzoek en erfelijkheidsadvisering (*Staatscourant* 23 januari 2003, 16, p. 11) and the Annex to Article 3 of the Planning Decree brings PGD under article 2 of the Specialist Medical Practice Act. PGD concerns research into the ovum or the embryo in vitro with respect to the diagnosis of constitutionally and hereditary disorders.

51 This was considered controversial because it concerns a hereditary disorder that is not fully penetrant, which means that not every person carrying the faulty gene will develop the condition involved (Zeegers, 2011).

52 The CU bases its politics on biblical principles, whereas the Christian Democratic Party sees the bible as a source of inspiration for individual members.

53 Regeling van de staatssecretaris van Volksgezondheid, Welzijn en Sport van 16 februari 2009, nr. CZ-TSZ-2912089, houdende regels ten aanzien van preïmplantatie genetische diagnostiek (PGD).

54 www.ad.nl/nieuws/het-is-angstig-stil-in-het-masturbatorium~ab8d8d4e/?referrer= www.google.com/

55 Ministerie Volksgezondheid, Welzijn en Sport, 'Jaarverslag 2019 Stichting donorgegevens kunstmatige bevruchting'.

56 The graph is based on yearly reports: www.degynaecoloog.nl/nuttige-informatie/ ivf-resultaten/

57 Zeegers's comparative chapter in this book addresses the role of parliamentary politics in ART regulation more generally.

58 At the same time, to the extent rules are formulated, the Dutch government wants them to be followed, as its assessments of the effects bear witness to.

References

Boele-Woelki, K., Curry-Sumner, I., Schrama, W., & Vonk, M. (2011). *Commercieel draagmoederschap en illegale opneming van kinderen*. Boom Juridische uitgevers.

Broekhuijsen-Molenaar, A. M. L. (1991). *Civielrechtelijke aspekten van kunstmatige inseminatie en draagmoederschap*. Kluwer.

Dondorp, W. J., Ploem, M. C., de Wert, G. M. W. R., de Vries, M. C., & Gevers, J. K. M. (2021). *Derde Evaluatie Embryowet*. ZonMw.

Embryo Law. (2002). *Act of June 20, 2002, containing rules on operations with germ cells and embryos*.

Gezondheidsraad. (1984). *Interim advies inzake in vitro fertilisatie*. Gezondheidsraad.

Gezondheidsraad. (1986). *Advies inzake kunstmatige voortplanting*. Gezondheidsraad.

Hoksbergen, R. C. A. (1985). *Een nieuwe kans, adoptie van Nederlandse en buitenlandse pleegkinderen*. Rijksuniversiteit Utrecht.

Holtrust, N. (1993). *Aan moeders knie: De juridische afstammingsrelatie tussen moeder en kind*. Ars Aequi Libri.

Kirejczyk, M. (1996). *Met technologie gezegend? Gender en de omstreden invoering van in vitro fertilisatie in de Nederlandse gezondheidszorg*. Uitgeverij Jan van Arkel.

Kirejczyk, M., van Berkel, D., & Swierstra, T. (2001). *Nieuwe voortplanting: Sociaal-historische en normatief politieke aspecten van de ontwikkeling van voortplantingstechnologie in Nederland*. Rathenau instituut.

Kwaliteitsinstituut voor de Gezondheidszorg CBO. (2003). *Modelreglement Embryowet*. Van Zuiden Communications.

Latten, J. (2004). *Trends in samenwonen en trouwen. De schone schijn van burgerlijke staat*. Central Bureau voor de Statistiek. www.cbs.nl/nr/rdonlyres/d479f5ba-87b2-4c6e-bccd-8306450af908/0/2004k4b15p046art.pdf

Lijphart, A. (1999). *Patterns of democracy. Government forms and performance in thirty-six countries*. Yale University Press.

NVOG. (1999). *Richtlijn hoogtechnologisch draagmoederschap*. NVOG.

NVOG. (2010). *Modelprotocol mogelijke morele contra-indicaties bij vruchtbaarheidsbehandelingen*. NVOG.

NVOG. (2016). *Standpunt 'Geassisteerde voortplanting met gedoneerde gameten en gedoneerde embryo's en draagmoederschap'*. NVOG.

NVOG en KLEM. (2018). *Landelijk standpunt spermadonatie. Specifieke eisen voor spermadonoren*. NVOG en KLEM.

Olsthoorn-Heim, E. T. M., de Wert, F. M. W. R., Winter, H. B., te Braake, A. M., Heineman, M. J., Middelkamp, A., & Nierse, C. J. (2006). *Evaluatie Embryowet*. ZonMw.

Schoots, M., van Arkel, J., & Dermoet, S. (2004). Wetsaanpassing in verband met draagmoederschap? *Tijdschrift voor Familie- en Jeugdrecht*, 26, 189–194.

Planningsbesluit klinisch genetisch onderzoek en erfelijkheidsadvisering. *Staatscourant 23* januari 2003.

Staatscommissie Herijking ouderschap. (2016). *Kind en ouders in de 21e eeuw*. Xerox/OBT, Den Haag.

Steinkamp, N., van Hoek, M., Boerboom, L., & van Leeuwen, E. (2012). *Evaluatie Regeling Preïmplantatie Genetische Diagnostiek (PGD). Besliskader – Behoefteraming – ethisch debat*. IQ Healthcare.

Takes, F. (2006). *Het recht om te weten. 'Het belang van het kind' in het debat over gametendonatie*. Universiteit van Nijmegen.

Timmermans, A. (2004). The Netherlands. Conflict and consensus on ART policy. In I. Bleiklie, M. L. Goggin, & C. Rothmayr (Eds.), *Comparative biomedical policy. Governing assisted reproductive technologies*. Routledge.

Vlijmen, S.C.A, van, & Vlijmen, S. C. A., & van der Tol, J. H. (2012). Draagmoederschap in opkomst: Specifieke wet- en regelgeving noodzakelijk? *Tijdschrift voor Familie- en Jeugdrecht*, 160–166.

Wetenschappelijk Instituut voor het CDA. (1988). *Zinvol leven. Een christen-democratische bijdrage aan de discussie over draagmoederschap, kunstmatige inseminatie, gift en in vitro fertilisatie*. Van Loghum Slaterus bv.

Weyers, H. (2015). Wet donorgegevens kunstmatige bevruchting: Administratieve helderheid gekoppeld aan een vaag doel. *Tijdschrift voor Familie- en Jeugdrecht*, 112–117.

Weyers, H. (2016). Mandatory sperm donor registration. Instrumental, symbolic or somewhere in between? A comparison of laws. *European Journal of Comparative Law and Governance*, (3) 24–39.

Winter, H. B., Dondorp, W. J., Woestenburg, N. O. M., Akerboom, C. P. M., Legemaate, J., & de Wert, G. M. W. R. (2012). *Evaluatie Embryowet en Wet donorgegevens kunstmatige bevruchting*. ZonMw.

Woestenburg, N. O., Frederiks, B. J. M., Dorscheidt, J. H. H. M., Floor, T., Bloemhoff, C. E., & Winter, H. B. (2019). *Tweede evaluatie Wet donorgegevens kunstmatige bevruchting*. ZonMw.

Zeegers, N. E. H. M. (2007). The working of power in communicative regulation. *Zeitschrift für Rechtssoziologie*, 28(1), 97–110.

Zeegers, N. E. H. M. (2011). The mobilizing force of legal rules. A case study in law and political science. In B. van Klink & S. Taekema (Eds.), *Law and method*. Mohr Siebeck.

8 IVF in Poland

From political debates to biomedical practices

Anna Krawczak and Magdalena Radkowska-Walkowicz

Introduction

For the last decade, the dispute on assisted reproductive technologies (ART)[1] in Poland has been particularly heated, and the procedure has remained in the centre of important political events. During the run-up to the presidential elections in 2015, ART was one of the main subjects broached by the candidates. This chapter will describe the current legal rules concerning embryo protection, gamete donation, PGD and access to ART and the contested issues around these topics. Subsequently, it presents an analysis of the politico-historical Polish debate on in-vitro fertilization (IVF) and assisted reproductive medicine in order to provide context for understanding the current dispute surrounding the procedure. The position of the Catholic Church has played a key role in mounting controversy on IVF. We will confront this position with the attitude of Polish society towards IVF. Finally, we will analyse statistical data together with issues concerning the financing and availability of IVF as they are linked to the dispute and the law.

This chapter is based on many years of anthropological research on IVF in Poland. This research has examined IVF as a biomedical category that interferes in the private lives of many people, as well as a political phenomenon (Krawczak, 2016; Radkowska-Walkowicz, 2012, 2013, 2014, 2018). Between 2011 and 2014, we carried out our research as part of the project: *The Family and Reproduction in the Context of Development of Genetics and New Medical Technologies*, while between 2013 and 2018, it was part of the project: *New Reproductive Technologies – The Childhood Studies Perspective*.[2] In both projects, we carried out discourse analysis as well as classical ethnographic research such as in-depth interviews and participant observation. When analysing the discourse, we mainly focused on the study of mainstream media as well as high-volume Catholic press, where the subject of IVF is frequently discussed. We also analysed parliamentary debates, texts released by the Catholic Church and statements made by Catholic Church authorities as well as internet forums focused on reproductive technologies and infertility. We conducted about 145 interviews: 70 with people suffering from infertility, 45 (including 5 group interviews) with children born through IVF and 30 with doctors involved in ART treatment (gynaecologists, embryologists, and psychologists). Moreover, one of our co-authors, Anna Krawczak, has been a longtime patient-activist in the

DOI: 10.4324/9781003223726-8

Association for Infertility Treatment and Adoption Support, "Our Stork", and has acted as chairperson of the organization for many years; she is also a member of the European Society of Human Reproduction and Embryology (ESHRE).

In this chapter, we will attempt to describe the landscape of Polish IVF, with a focus on public discourse. While in other texts we delved into the private experiences of those suffering from infertility (Krawczak, 2016; Radkowska-Walkowicz, 2013, 2018), we present in this chapter the context necessary to understand the situation of particular individuals who struggle with their infertility or with the criticism of a technology without which they would not have been born.

The Act on Infertility Treatment (embryo protection, same-sex couples, gamete and embryo donations, PGD)

The Act on Infertility Treatment, passed in July 2015, was the first Polish piece of legislation regulating the principles of infertility treatment. By adopting the law, Poland became the last EU country to fulfil obligations imposed on the Member States by the Tissue Directive 2004/23/WE[3] along with subsequent implementing directives. The solutions introduced by the Act were divided into four important areas, which to date remain points of dispute for the participants in the Polish debate on IVF. We include arguments that the restrictions of the act are excessive developed by patient groups, feminists, left-wing parties and some politicians from the centre. We have also included arguments for tightening the current law proposed by conservative politicians and representatives of the Catholic Church. However, one should note the distinctions within these groups; for instance, some centrist conservatives do not agree with a total ban on IVF but would like only to limit the number of fertilized eggs and ban freezing embryos (Klawiter, 2017; Polska Agencja Prasowa, 2016). On the other hand, some centrist liberals do not agree with the postulate to destroy surplus embryos or to provide access to IVF for same-sex couples and/or single women (Polska Agencja Prasowa, 2015).

Embryo protection

The law prohibits embryo destruction. Thus, every embryo capable of proper development must be transferred into a uterus. In order to prevent the creation of surplus embryos on a scale that would make transferring them impossible, only six oocytes can be fertilized unless other IVF attempts were unsuccessful. The act also creates a ban on handing embryos over for scientific research. For conservative groups represented by the parties and think tanks that adhere to Catholic doctrine (i.e. the Law and Justice party, the Kukiz15' party, the Solidarna Polska party, the Porozumienie party and think tanks such as the Institute for Legal Culture Ordo Iuris), the current protection of embryos is not sufficient. In terms of political power, the parties mentioned previously (Law and Justice, Solidarna Polska and Porozumienie) currently form the government by reaching parliamentary majority. These parties are alarmed that the legal definition of an "embryo capable of proper development" is not clear and state that protection should apply to any embryo regardless of its embryological evaluation. Conservative groups demand a ban on both the creation of surplus embryos as well as on embryo freezing, although their ultimate postulate would be a total ban on ART due to their discordance with the Catholic doctrine. At the same time, feminist movements, patient groups and ART medical professionals consider the current law too restrictive and believe that handing over embryos for scientific research and destroying embryos should be legalized together with the possibility of fertilizing more than six oocytes in one cycle of IVF. It does not mean, however, that those three groups are consistent in their postulates or that they have real political influence on legislation comparable with the position of the conservative groups described previously. Hence, the non-governmental stakeholders (patients' groups, feminists and ART doctors) present common demands in terms of equal access to ART (in vitro reimbursement) (Kongres Kobiet, 2009; Polskie Towarzystwo Medycyny Rozrodu, 2015), but at the same time, they vary in their attitudes on such issues as embryo destruction or passing embryos on for scientific purposes (only patients' groups publicly articulate this postulate), fertilizing more than six oocytes per cycle (only patients' groups and feminist groups raise this issue; the Polish Society of Human Reproduction and Embryology has never issued an official statement regarding the liberalization of the Law on Infertility) and non-anonymous gamete donations (only patients' groups demand this legal solution).

Single parenthood and same-sex couples

According to the law, access to ART methods is restricted only to heterosexual couples, thus excluding single women and same-sex couples. Following this restriction, all embryos of single women or same-sex couples created before the act came into force cannot be transferred if a prospective mother does not indicate the legal father of the child to be born. This is due to a law that states that each child born through ART must have a legally indicated father, which is impossible in the case of single women and single-sex couples who use heterologous donation. In order to prevent the law from being circumvented by single women or lesbians, who could go to a clinic with a man who is not their partner, the legislation stipulated that every future father who is not genetically linked to the offspring must certify to the head of the Civil Registry Office that he will undertake all paternal duties including alimony (with inability to deny paternity regardless of the results of DNA tests). As a result of this law, forced embryo donation was created in Poland as all embryos of single women created before the act came into life can be currently donated willingly and anonymously to a heterosexual couple or can undergo anonymous and mandatory donation to a heterosexual couple 20 years after being deposited in a cryobank. The third option is to take the frozen embryos out of Poland to a foreign clinic at the expense of the patient. However, this last option may be unaffordable for many single women or lesbian couples who have their embryos frozen. Conservative groups have not raised any objections in this case, as they believe that the current law excluding single women and same-sex couples is appropriate. Meanwhile, feminist groups, ART medical professionals, some left-wing parties and some of the patients' groups are demanding equal access to ART for single women and same-sex couples.

Heterologous donation

According to the law, the donation of oocytes, sperm and embryos is legal, completely anonymous and reserved for heterosexuals only. The recipients must remain in a marriage or common-law marriage, but in the latter case, the partner of the future mother must confirm to the head of the Civil Registry Office that he will act as the child's legal father and will undertake all his legal obligations. This law is accepted by doctors, as they believe that maintaining the anonymity of the donor lies in the interest of the entire family. Opponents, in this case patient groups, are asking for fully transparent gamete and embryo donation due to the rights of children as stated in the Convention on the Rights of a Child. In 2012, the Association for Infertility Treatment and Adoption Support, "Our Stork", launched a social campaign focused on the issue of non-anonymous donations, entitled "Telling and Talking" [Powiedzieć i Rozmawiać]. Despite moderate media interest, the main idea of the campaign remained politically ignored. Furthermore, most ART doctors that we interviewed acknowledged the existence of the campaign but were opposed to the idea of legal changes such as releasing the donor's personal information (Montuschi, 2009).

Preimplantation genetic diagnosis

Preimplantation genetic diagnosis (PGD) is legal under the new law, although acceptable only for couples undergoing ART with medical (genetic) indications to perform PGD. Therefore, the rights to access PGD procedures for patients who are fertile but carry genetic diseases are still pending: the law allows IVF treatment only for those with clinically proven infertility, as stated in art. 5, par. 6, st. 2:

> 2. The treatment of infertility through the procedure of in vitro fertilization can be performed after exhausting other methods of treatment conducted by a period of no less than 12 months. The procedure of in vitro fertilization can be done without exhausting other treatments and in less than 12 months from the beginning of infertility treatment if in accordance with current medical knowledge, medical treatment is not possible to get pregnant as a result of these methods.
>
> (Kancelaria Sejmu, 2015)

All embryos with confirmed genetic or morphological malformations are considered incapable of proper development and may be destroyed. Thus, for the conservative groups mentioned earlier (the ruling party, coalition parties and think tanks that adhere to Catholic doctrine), much like for conservative Christians in other countries, the issue of PGD is important and closely linked to the use of metaphors concerning negative Nazi eugenics (Doolin & Motion, 2010). These groups believe that PGD should be banned, because each embryo has the right to live. Opponents, mainly doctors and patient groups, argue that the right to PGD should be extended to anyone who has indications for its use regardless of the state of their fertility. The ban on positive eugenics put in place by the act has not been questioned in public debate, irrespective of worldviews.

Surrogacy

Currently, surrogacy is indirectly prohibited in Poland in other legal acts which state that all surrogacy agreements are null and void (art. 58 par. 1 st. 1 Civil Code) and the mother of a child is always the woman giving birth (art. 61[9] Family and Custody Code). The introduction of the Infertility Act did not bring any changes here. Currently the legalization of surrogacy is more a debate among specialists, that is, in medical and academic circles.

Polish debate before 2005

To clarify the Polish law and the discussion on it, we now focus on the debate on IVF in Poland. The history of Polish IVF, like the history of IVF in general, is both a political and a medical history. Just as with many other medical innovations, IVF is not a neutral technology and can be linked to many bioethical, economic and political disputes. Yet in Poland, the extent to which IVF has become entangled in current political debates, including electoral campaigns, seems exceptional. The history of Polish IVF is a kind of microhistory, which reveals various tensions and power plays that have surfaced in Polish history since 1989. By examining the discussions surrounding the subject of IVF, one can easily draft a map of political disputes in Poland. Just as in the case of abortion, the dispute over IVF

> represents a coded discourse that reflects fundamental concerns, including the shape of the state itself, the state's obligation to society (and vice versa), the rule of law, and . . . the scope of the protection of civil rights and fundamental freedoms.
>
> (Gal & Kligman, 2000, p. 10; Zielińska, 2000, p. 24)

The IVF debate is a playing field where political actors are busy negotiating the national "moral code" (Mayer, 1999, p. 3). This debate also centres on national identity and gender norms, something that Michel Herzfeld has called cultural intimacy (1997), as well as on the conditions for participating in an "imagined community that is the nation" (Anderson, 1983).

History of IVF in Poland

When Louise Brown, the world's first baby conceived through IVF, was born in Oldham, Great Britain, in 1978, alongside accolades praising the scientific breakthrough, voices of criticism could also be heard.[4] The media in Poland at the time likewise released a mixture of approval and criticism. In 1978, in "Tygodnik Powszechny", Józefa Hennellowa, a well-known Polish Catholic columnist, warned against excessive enthusiasm:

> Now this barrier of nature's threat has been crossed: man has interfered with the very beginning of human existence. Instead of a real being and its imponderable scientific and psychological intimacy – strange hands and laboratory equipment, an artificially prepared environment, a number of procedures that are shocking for a human embryo. How will the new human cope with that?
>
> (1978, p. 1)

Nine years later, on November 12, 1987, after 39 unsuccessful IVF attempts, the first Polish test-tube child was born thanks to Professor Marian Szamatowicz and his team at the Department of Gynaecology at the Medical University of Białystok. Until November 2012, the girl remained anonymous, like thousands of other Polish children conceived through IVF. The mainstream press, when reporting on the first Polish IVF procedure, described it as an important and electrifying event, with rare critical commentary. Criticism of IVF was found in the Catholic press and in the public addresses of representatives of the Church. The division that is so clearly visible today could already be sensed at that time. On the one hand, there are people who placed great hopes on IVF.[5] On the other, meanwhile, there is the very critical stance of the Catholic Church. Journalist Iwona Konarska described this tension as follows:

> The media went crazy. . . . Białystok was deluged with letters. One priest would rail from the pulpit about the inhumane practices of the clinic, which, according to him, were even more harmful than drug addiction and drunkenness, and the women would talk of their dreams in which they were cuddling babies. They were begging, writing that their husbands wanted to leave them, and that their hands were reaching out for other people's infants.
>
> (Konarska, 2004)

In the first years of IVF in Poland, the mainstream media were – in comparison to the 2000s – rather reserved in their moral assessment of the procedure. The only exception was in the form of reports about new, controversial achievements in the field of reproductive medicine (like ICSI technology or surrogate motherhood). Despite the mainstream (namely non-Catholic) press being relatively friendly (or silent) regarding IVF, one could observe a gradual increase in the political tension surrounding the procedure around the beginning of the 1990s. The issue of evaluating IVF turned into a political matter. As such, at present, a politician's attitude towards IVF gives them a particular position in the political game, just as do their attitudes towards the nation's history or taxes. Various players in this game are, in a way, forced to take a stand concerning IVF. The discussion on IVF accompanied changes in the political system, and through this discussion, the government had to redefine and interpret its relations with the Catholic Church.[6] Ideological issues concerning individual worldviews and moral values, including those connected with sexuality and reproductive health, were placed at the centre of the dispute concerning the shape of the state and its degree of secularity.

In the 1990s, opponents of IVF pursued a strategy whereby the procedure was attributed to the socialist regime. This is well depicted by a disagreement concerning IVF in Warsaw's Children's Memorial Health Institute hospital (CZD) where the first test-tube baby was born in 1988. Soon after, the hospital's director shut down the IVF programme, claiming that the technology is an "invention of the PZPR" [the Communist party which governed the Polish People's Republic from 1948 to 1989] and was invented in the Soviet Union (Konarska, 1991).

IVF and the Catholic Church

Today IVF is no longer a symbol of the Communist faith in science but is instead perceived by its opponents (often associated with Catholic Church) as a "Nazi" technology, a eugenics-related experiment that also represents Western "culture/ the civilisation of death". This transition from "Communist" to "Nazi" can be observed in the document entitled "Eugenika – w imię postępu" (Braun, 2010) bought and broadcast by Polish Public Television several times between 2016 and 2019.[7] The term "Culture [the Civilisation] of death" was coined by Pope John Paul II, an unquestionable authority for nearly all political fractions in Poland:

> While it is true that the taking of life not yet born or in its final stages is sometimes marked by a mistaken sense of altruism and human compassion, it cannot be denied that such a culture of death, taken as a whole, betrays a completely individualistic concept of freedom, which ends up by becoming the freedom of "the strong" against the weak who have no choice but to submit.[8]
>
> (John Paul II, 1995, passus 19)

The very same reference to Nazi ideology, and the concept of the civilization of death, is also used as a frequently cited retort to a liberal attitude towards abortion, IVF and an individual's general attitude towards "protection at conception", which is thought to be characteristic of secular, Western European countries.

The Catholic Church in Poland has had an unfavourable stance on the procedure from the very beginning, but it has remained restrained in its criticism until recent years. Some conflicts in this matter arose among smaller, local communities, as pointed out by Marian Szamatowicz when he began his work on IVF. Szamatowicz himself came into conflict with Church authorities in Białystok: "The archbishop insisted that we stop all work on the method. It was said during a sermon in church: there are many calamities – alcoholism, drug addiction but also something worse. In a clinic in Białystok doctors are murdering people" (Szamatowicz, 2009, p. 94).

At the end of 2007, Ewa Kopacz, the minister of health at the time, said she would attempt to reimburse IVF procedures from the state budget. These words marked the beginning of an ongoing, turbulent debate. This debate that has undoubtedly been affected by the development and availability of Internet access on the one hand and on the other by the polarization in Polish political life and generally in Polish society (Applebaum, 2018). The minister's proclamation struck a chord with political forces affiliated with the Catholic Church.

Therefore, the Polish debate on IVF is, to a large extent, a debate concerning the place and the role of the Catholic Church in Poland. This includes preserving its "monopoly on morality" (Inglis, 1998). The debate is also a result of the struggle for the support of the Catholic Church for a particular political party. The Church's official teachings serve as the main foundation for legitimizing views opposing IVF. The issue of protecting human embryos, also in the context of IVF, is discussed in many Catholic publications, for instance, in the documents of the Congregation for the Doctrine of Faith, but most of all in the instructions: *Donum vitae* (*Instruction on respect for human life in its origin and on the dignity of procreation replies to certain questions of the day*) and more recently *Dignitas personae: On Certain Bioethical Questions* and the encyclical *Evangelium vitae*, as well as the *Catechism of the Catholic Church* (Szymański, 2009). These texts have tremendous influence on passing judgements concerning IVF in the rhetoric of its opponents. The *Donum vitae* reads:

> The human being is to be respected and treated as a person from the moment of conception; and therefore from that same moment his rights as a person must be recognized, among which in the first place is the inviolable right of every innocent human being to life. . . . since the embryo must be treated as a person, it must also be defended in its integrity, tended and cared for, to the extent possible, in the same way as any other human being as far as medical assistance is concerned.[9]

It is also for that reason that the Catholic Church has expressed its negative opinion concerning embryo cryopreservation:

> *The freezing of embryos*, even when carried out in order to preserve the life of an embryo – cryopreservation – *constitutes an offence against the respect due to human beings* by exposing them to grave risks of death or harm to their physical integrity and depriving them, at least temporarily, of maternal shelter and gestation, thus placing them in a situation in which further offences and manipulation are possible.

Moreover, the document states that life ought to be created only within a marriage: "The child has the right to be conceived, carried in the womb, brought into the world and brought up within marriage", which unequivocally means that IVF and most forms of heterologous fertilization are considered wrong. Further, "even in a situation in which every precaution were taken to avoid the death of human embryos, homologous IVF and ET [embryo transfer] dissociates from the conjugal act the actions which are directed to human fertilization", thus also making these procedures contrary to the teachings of the Church. Masturbation, which is part of IVF, also turns out to be problematic: "Masturbation, through which the sperm is normally obtained, is another sign of this dissociation: even when it is done for the purpose of procreation, the act remains deprived of its unitive meaning".[10] A statement issued by the Team of Experts on Bioethics with the Episcopal Conference of Poland in understanding with the Presidium of the Episcopal Conference of Poland is representative of the opinions of Polish bishops as well as many Catholic journalists:

> Human dignity is encroached upon in non-organic fertilization procedures since conception occurs not during the act of love, but in the course of experimental technical procedures. This carries the signs of "human production" . . . we justify opposition to IVF also basing upon natural law, or the data of universal knowledge, commonly recognized norms, to which all people, regardless of perspective, are obligated. . . . The killing, selection and freezing of human embryos is morally unacceptable. They are human beings, who deserve full legal protection, especially the protection of the right to life.
>
> (Konferencja Episkopatu Polski, 2010)

Stigmatization

The main actors in the debate on IVF in Poland are representatives of the Catholic Church as well as like-minded columnists and politicians. A smaller role is played by scientists, doctors and bioethicists, while the voices of infertile patients and people born through IVF are rarely encountered in the media. (Maciejewska-Mroczek & Radkowska-Walkowicz, 2017). "We are spoken about, but we are not spoken with", one twenty-some-year-old born using IVF told us.

One woman whose child was born after IVF told us during an individual interview:

> The Church has taken over the entire arena, assuming that either you are pro-life or against. One is not a murderer or anything, you are simply undergoing a medical procedure, trusting that the doctor is neither a quack nor a fraud but that they have graduated med school and know what they are doing, performing a medical procedure that I, as an adult, either accept or I don't. I want to sign all the appropriate documents and don't wish to have a religious discussion. . . . Yes, there is no place for women in the Church and most certainly not for women who have made a choice.

Often arguments raised by IVF opponents in public debate not only stigmatize infertile couples and doctors specializing in ART but also people born through IVF (Radkowska-Walkowicz, 2017), who are represented by IVF opponents as monsters, suffering from serious health, psychological and social problems (Radkowska-Walkowicz, 2012).

Our interviewees often addressed negative opinions concerning IVF. In July 2015, Magda Kołodziej, the first child born through IVF in Poland, wrote a letter to one of the newspapers:

> Something inside me burst. I can no longer sit still and listen to all these lies. I can no longer allow for my family and myself to be disrespected. Do all these God-fearing defenders of the unborn know how they are hurting us, children conceived in vitro, our parents, and finally, our own kids? I am not broken, I do not have a crease on my forehead, I don't suffer from a smaller head circumference, and in addition, I have two wonderful daughters born naturally.
>
> (Polska Newsweek, 2015)

Many of those involved in the public discussion do not seem to care that children do not function in a media vacuum and that they also hear tales of "living at the expense of their brothers and sisters", another argument made by IVF opponents. They also hear stories of dishonourable births and about the mental and physical defects that supposedly affect them. We spoke to a teenager who compared the process of stigmatizing IVF children with anti-Semitism: "The society makes us different, just because we were conceived through IVF. Just like Jews in the past". Agnieszka is also certain that the rhetoric on IVF is stigmatizing:

> It's not like if you sling mud around, accusing people of murder, then you yell about the civilization of death, Frankenstein's babies, that you're not in fact stigmatizing IVF children. We hear all of it, we read about it, all this mudslinging doesn't go unnoticed. . . . I see a lot of bluster and members of parliament – usually male – who are exploiting the situation, joyfully scream-ing on TV. For them the problem is virtual but in reality this problem is a person – with arms, legs and a name.
>
> (Danielewski & Wybieralski, 2012)

The new abortion debate

The debate on abortion and regulations concerning the conditions for terminat-ing a pregnancy represents an important context for the debate on IVF in Poland. Throughout the last few years, the IVF debate became "the new abortion debate" (Chełstowska, 2011, p. 104). The effective comparison of IVF to abortion is the main strategy of IVF opponents, and language is the main weapon used in this battle. The success of "pro-life" rhetoric in Poland is above all an effect of reshap-ing language, where the term "termination of pregnancy" was replaced by "mur-der", "foetus" was replaced by "unborn" and "conceived child", while "pregnant women" became "mothers". Notably, this new language was incorporated into offi-cial state documents (Chełstowska, 2011, p. 102). Rhetoric against IVF is based on the same rules: IVF became the "production of people", the freezing of embryos became "freezing children" and embryo selection became "eugenics" (Radkowska-Walkowicz, 2014).

In both the IVF and abortion debates, the arguments and emotions are similar, just as are their protagonists and antagonists: they use the same overly emotional references to fundamental issues, such as life and death. As far as the two subjects are concerned, the topics of the "holocaust of the unborn", disregard for human dignity and a wounded woman's body are all referenced. The Family Planning, Human Embryo Protection and Conditions of Permissibility of Abortion Act, which has been in force since 1993, is very restrictive and has been criticized by many interest groups in recent years. Nonetheless, groups connected to the ruling party[11] demanded that the law be tightened further, and since January 2021, a pregnancy may be terminated in only two cases: if it threatens the life or health of the mother or if there is justified suspicion the pregnancy is a result of an unlawful act, such as rape or incest. This change means a practical ban on abortion in Poland, which has sparked huge protests across the country.

Unlike abortion, IVF was not regulated by law for many years. This only changed with an act that came into force in 2015[12] (more subsequently); however, this did not affect the dynamics or the quality of the debate on IVF in Poland.

Social attitudes

In a country where more than 90% of Poles declare themselves Catholics (a little more than half of Poles admit that they lead religious lives in accordance with the teachings of the Catholic Church), it would seem that such criticism of IVF by the Catholic Church and ruling party politicians should result in low support for IVF by the general public (Hall, 2012). However, according to polls conducted since the 1990s by CBOS (the Public Opinion Research Center), over 75% of Poles accept the use of IVF by married couples, and about 50% accept it for common-law relationships as well as for single women (Centrum Badania Opinii Społecznej, 2015). This is probably due to the family-oriented nature of Polish society, where the family constitutes the most important point of reference and child-rearing is perceived as the most basic form of self-fulfilment and the pursuit of happiness (Radkowska-Walkowicz, 2013). The Church's opinion on ART is partially ignored within Polish society also due to its moral liberalization. In line with the general European trend, Poles have an open attitude to, among others, sexual issues such as birth control. High selectiveness in the moral sphere is a significant element of Polish religiousness (Grotowska, 1999). In Poland, as in many other countries, the privatization of religiousness is quite apparent as it becomes more independent from the institution (Borowik, 1997). It is worth noting, however, that the process does not follow a linear path, and some issues concerned with "traditional" religiousness may actually be bolstered. At the same time, although there is strong identification with Catholicism, Polish society is of the opinion that the Church "has too much power" in social life (Maciejewska-Mroczek & Radkowska-Walkowicz, 2018).

According to the CBOS report, attitudes towards faith and Church teachings affect the degree of acceptance of IVF:

> Nearly every other Pole (46%) states they are a person of faith, following the teachings of the Church. An almost identically sized group (47%) is made up of people of faith who consider themselves to be believers on their own terms. Only some consider themselves agnostic: they cannot unequivocally declare whether they are religious (3%) or whether they have no faith at all (overall 4%). The attitude towards IVF is relatively least unambiguous among respondents belonging to the first category. . . . But also in this group there is a prevalence towards support for the method by married couples experiencing fertility problems. . . . the acceptance of this method by people who claim to follow Church teaching is not a result of ignorance of its opinion on the matter.
>
> (Centrum Badania Opinii Społecznej, 2010, p. 3)

One can therefore speak of a deliberate lack of acceptance and refusal to accept the negative narratives that the hierarchs of the Catholic Church have spun around IVF. Nevertheless, attention should be paid to the recent strong position of nationalist-Catholic discourse in Poland. An element of this process is to strengthen the conviction that moral laws derived from the language of the Catholic religion are an element of Polishness, and as such, they can protect us against the threat of so-called Western civilization.

Controversies surrounding the act on infertility

The current Polish law is a compromise between the demands of various politically significant players (doctors, conservative and centrist politicians, media, patient communities and women's pressure groups) and the pragmatic necessity to adapt Polish law to EU requirements. Consequently, the law is too conservative for patients and feminist groups and too progressive for the Catholic Church; conservatives consistently raise demands for its tightening, ranging from introducing significant restrictions such as a ban on freezing embryos and fertilizing only one egg cell to banning IVF altogether.[13]

At present, the Polish law discriminates against single women and same-sex couples, and – probably without such intention on the part of the legislature – it has led to the violation of the principle of *lex retro non agit* (Latin: the law does not operate retroactively). This was due to the legislature's adoption of only a three-month period of *vacatio legis*, which in practice created a situation where all embryos of single women and same-sex couples created before November 2015 have symbolically become state property and can no longer be used by the people whose gametes have been used to create said embryos.

These people and couples were allowed only three months to collect their embryos and transfer them before the window of opportunity was closed permanently. It should be noted that for many such people, embryo collection was not possible at the time for pragmatic reasons: they could have been pregnant at the time, their current state of health could not allow for an embryo transfer or for other reasons they were not ready to become pregnant at the time even though they planned a pregnancy in the future. The embryos of such patients are currently deposited in cryobanks. They cannot be destroyed (the act prohibits the destruction of embryos), nor can they be taken away by the genetic mother because, as already mentioned, one condition for the transfer of an embryo is to indicate the man who will agree to act as father (including taking on the legal obligation of alimony and parental authority). They were thus not only literally, but also symbolically, frozen. Women who are owners of such embryos may decide to give them up for an anonymous heterosexual couple or get in touch with a foreign clinic which would perform the transfer (costs of embryo transport and transfer have to be borne by the patient), or they may refuse to make any decision at all. In the latter case, 20 years after the embryos were registered in a cryobank,[14] they will be handed over by the clinic to a heterosexual couple. Similar regulations concern all other couples who have surplus embryos but for a number of reasons cannot or do not want to use them all for their own treatment. Many patients who are members of the patients' forum run by the Our Stork Association (currently over 100,000 registered users who are affected by the problem of infertility) have stated that they will wait for a change in the law and that until the act is in force, they do not want to make any binding decisions. Some couples have decided to donate their embryos, while the smallest group has or is planning to take their frozen embryos to foreign clinics in order to have them legally destroyed, donated to scientific research or given up for an open embryo donation. The Czech Republic is selected most frequently by Polish couples seeking to have their embryos destroyed, while couples who have decided to give up their embryos in an open donation most often travel to Great Britain.

In light of these issues, it is also interesting to look at the statutory order of the anonymity of donation, which in Polish practice exposes the blurry borders of the biomedical paradigm adopted by the legislature.

On the one hand, there is a requirement for the clinical confirmation of the legitimacy of the use of gametes or donor embryos and the stipulation that the donor is selected solely by the doctor. On the other hand, the doctor should pick a donor based on the compliance of blood type with the recipients as well as phenotypic likeness. It seems that the intention of this law is not only to turn donation into a purely biomedical procedure and to reject a social perspective that is well indicated in source literature and usually favours non-anonymous donation (Dennison, 2008; Freeman, 2015; Frith, 2001). Most of all, it supports striving for social neutralization of donation by removing its possible distinguishing features: blurring the trace of the "other blood" and physical differences between parents and children. Embryos are therefore property of the state, which controls the morality of its citizens and aims to provide two heterosexual parents for every child born as a result of ART, but also – in the case of heterologous donations – they are property of a society that embraces principles of the naturalization of kinship.

Infrastructure and financial support

Number of treatments

The main source of information on the number of infertility treatment centres and their activities are reports from the Fertility and Infertility Section of the Polish Society of Gynecologists and Obstetricians, submitted voluntarily by ART clinics as part of the European IVF Monitoring project run by the European Society of Human Reproduction and Embryology. Additionally, there are two other sources: data from the so-called Reimbursement program ("Program – Treatment of infertility through IVF 2013–2016") and data from patient monitoring of infertility treatment centres; however, these data are only collected periodically. (see Table 8.1. in Appendix).

Table 8.1 Overview of treatment numbers in Poland.

Type of procedure	Number of initiated cycles	Number of oocyte retrievals	Number of transfers	Number of pregnancies (pregnancies with unknown outcome)	Number of deliveries*	Effectiveness (in conversion: procedure/ transfer/ clinical pregnancy)
IVF	884	865	710	256 (46)	177	36%
IVM (in vitro maturation)	NA	56	41	14	9	34%
ICSI	12,525	12,411	10,661	4,109 (870)	2,727	38,5%
FER (frozen embryo replacement, both IVF and ICSI)	NA	NA	5961	1737 (428)	1026	29%
PGD	259	251	133	57 (2)	50	43%
Egg donation (both fresh and frozen oocytes)	NA	NA	892	386 (58)	273	43%
Embryo donation	NA	NA	298	109 (20)	81	36,5%
IUI-H (intrauterine insemination with husband's or partner's semen)	12447	NA	NA	1537 (305, pregnancy losses – 177)	1055	12,3%
IUI-D (intrauterine insemination with donor semen)	2145	NA	NA	405 (66, pregnancy losses – 45)	294	19%

Hence, in Poland, there is not (and never has been) a system that would require all ART clinics to report their results and then subject them to external verification. Thus, all data regarding the effectiveness of ART clinics, and even the number of these facilities, come from the actual centres providing ART services, so the credibility of data in the report by EIM Polska should be treated with caution.

According to EIM reports in Poland, there are currently at least 35 ART clinics offering homo- and heterologous insemination, IVF, IVM and ICSI/IMSI fertilization (including preimplantation PGD), as well as treatments using donor cells and embryo donation procedures. The latest data from 2013 (Table 8.1) provide the following values for the number of procedures performed and their effectiveness:

The data in Table 8.1 come from 2013, before the Act on Infertility Treatment entered into force and introduced a limit on the number of fertilized oocytes, a ban on ART treatments by single women, the prohibition of intra-family gamete donation and many other changes which were discussed in the previous section concerning the Act on Infertility Treatment. These changes may influence the results of procedures currently performed in Poland. This is indirectly demonstrated by the difference between the reported results of IVF and ICSI procedures in 2013 (IVF – 36%, ICSI – 38.5%) and the effectiveness of these procedures in 2017 provided by the Ministry of Health on the basis of the results of the refunding program (32% in total for IVF and ICSI procedures).[15] The refunding program was adopted in 2013, before the Act on Fertility was passed, but its regulations placed a rule on all participating centres. This rule, which became binding law two years later, was an order to fertilize a maximum of six oocytes at the same time (unless the woman is over 35 years of age or her previous IVF attempts were unsuccessful) and – resulting from the recommendation of the Polish Society of Reproductive Medicine and Embryology – an order to transfer one embryo, or two embryos in special cases (Kuczyński et al., 2012). This policy is aimed at limiting the number of multiple pregnancies and resulting complications but, above all, at establishing a political compromise concerning the fate of surplus embryos, the number of which was first limited by the Reimbursement Program and, later, in the act.

Financial support

ART methods – apart from temporary or local exceptions – are not covered by private health insurance in Poland or by the universal system of health insurance (National Health Fund, NFZ). The first historical exclusion of IVF from the list of procedures reimbursed by the state was a decision made in 1992 by the then-minister of health, Władysław Sidorowicz, who decided that ART procedures are not medical methods and should not be covered by public funding (Radkowska-Walkowicz, 2013). Since that time and until July 2013, the costs of all ART procedures were fully covered by patients. 2012 saw the first changes in the state's approach to funding ART procedures. The local government in one Polish city, Częstochowa, passed an act on the partial reimbursement of IVF procedures for its residents. Even though the qualifying criteria for the local reimbursement program were very restrictive (only married couples residing in Częstochowa and women aged 20–37 years old, which led to only 12 couples being able to take advantage of the program in its first year [Romanek, 2013]) and the actual amount reimbursed was relatively low (app. 650 EUR with the average IVF costs being 2800–3500 EUR), the program gained a lot of attention in the media and revived the hopes of infertile couples for reimbursement on a national scale (Wołczyński & Krawczak, 2012). Currently, in 2021, the cost of the procedure remains at similar level (2800–3500 EUR plus the cost of examinations and medication, adding up to 3500–4650 EUR depending on the given procedure and clinical indications), while the average gross salary is 5411 Polish zlotys (around 1200 EUR). Therefore, the perspective of paying for IVF out of one's own pocket is unattainable for many Polish patients.

The success of the Częstochowa program probably had political impact on the government's decision to create a national IVF reimbursement program, which took place in July 2013. Between 2013 and 2016, the national IVF reimbursement program included over 22,600 couples and resulted in the births of at least 5300 children, with some of the women still pregnant or planning to be via transfers of frozen embryos obtained through the program (Polska Agencja Prasowa & Rynek Zdrowia, 2016). The conditions for admission to the national reimbursement program were more liberal than in Częstochowa, as it applied to couples regardless of their marital status (including common-law relationships), the maximum age for women was 40 (no age limit for men), the couple had to document infertility lasting at least 12 months (unless the reason for infertility was indisputable, for instance fallopian tube obstruction) and each couple was entitled to a full refund of three cycles of IVF (along with cryopreservation of possible surplus embryos and paid cryotransfers). At the same time, the guidelines for the program limited the number of fertilized oocytes to six, and the refunding did not cover couples using procedures that used donor gametes and embryos. Single women and same-sex couples did not have access to the program; however, they were able to use the procedures in private ART centres. Additionally, the costs of hormonal medication used in IVF were covered by co-financing up to 70% of its value starting from 01.07.2014, irrespectively of the use of the refunding program (Ministerstwo Zdrowia, 2014).

In the fall of 2015, the right-wing Law and Justice party (*Prawo i Sprawiedliwość*) became the governing party in Poland, and one of the first decisions made by the new health minister, Konstanty Radziwiłł, was to axe the IVF reimbursement program (Dziennik.pl, 2015), effectively terminating it in July 2016. As the IVF reimbursement program was being shut down, the Ministry announced it was preparing to introduce a new fertility support program, called the "Comprehensive Reproductive Health Protection Program in Poland". Its role was to improve the availability of infertility diagnostics by creating 16 public reference facilities, but it would not provide reimbursement for ART procedures. Only diagnostics and less invasive methods such as cycle observation, ovulation induction, laparoscopy and so on were covered. In reality, the program was not addressed to couples with confirmed infertility but to those who suspected fertility issues and wanted to investigate the problem. Despite ministerial assurances that the program would kick off in 2015 and those public funds would be used to supply hospitals, organize training and run public service announcements, the first patients of the reproductive health program were admitted only in December 2017, three years after it was announced. Until now, recruitment has only been carried out by one clinic instead of the planned 16. Only couples who have not previously been diagnosed or treated for infertility were invited to participate in the program.

At present, that is, in 2021, no national co-financing system for using advanced methods of infertility treatment exists in Poland, so patients have to fully pay for IVF therapy. Nonetheless, the reimbursement of hormonal medication has been maintained. Some cities are offering IVF refunding programs for their inhabitants, designed similarly to the Częstochowa program; however, only residents of a specific city (among others, Gdańsk, Warsaw, Łódź, Poznań) can benefit from them, and the procedure is only partially co-financed, usually in the amount of 3000 PLN (Miłkowska, 2017). Thus, people living in small towns and villages, or in cities where the local government has not decided to finance IVF treatment, still depend on their own financial resources when considering the decision to undergo infertility treatment.

Summary

Although ART has been successfully performed in Poland for over 30 years, it is still discussed and questioned as a method of infertility treatment. What is more, many myths surround ART, two of which are key in the Polish discourses on IVF: the myth of a technology that creates baby monsters, victims of a modern-day Frankenstein that are sick and unhappy, and the myth of a neutral medical technology, the use of which causes no social consequences.[16] IVF in Poland is seen above all as a political and ideological phenomenon,[17] but Polish reproductive medicine is doing well in the area of ART, at least regarding the growing number of ART centres and their quality of services. Polish infertility treatment clinics achieve similar results to clinics in other European countries and offer the majority of ART techniques currently available. Although the law regarding IVF addresses most postulates of the communities associated with reproductive medicine, it remains – much like the Polish debate on IVF – imperfect, exclusionary and politically charged. For a great number of infertile people in Poland, ART services are unaffordable. For those living in same-sex couples or who are single, these procedures are inaccessible. Finally, for all people undergoing IVF, this process is likely to be socially stigmatizing and connected with moral choices in terms of forced surplus embryo donations.

Appendix

Table 8.2 Data collection of ART in Poland.

Source	Data verifi- cation	Type of data	Data collection period	Who collects the data?	Who do the data concern?
EIM Polska report	No	Number of ART clinics, number and type of ART procedures, number of embryos transferred, post-IVF complication, success rate (clinical pregnancies, births)*	Since 1999 until now	Polish Society of Gyneco- logists and Obstetri- cians, Fertility and Infertility Section	ART clinics, which voluntarily submitted reports (no reporting obligation). The last report from 2013 includes 34 facilities
Program – infertility treatment using IVF between 2013 and 2016	Yes	Number and type of refunded ART procedures, number of transferred embryos, post-IVF complications, success rate (clinical pregnancies, live births)**	Between 2013 and 2016	Ministry of Health	All ART clinics that participated in the program (compulsory reporting): 26 clinics (between July 2013 and December 2013); 31 clinics (between 2014 and 2016)
Patient moni- toring of infertility treatment clinics	Partial	Number of ART clinics, description of their offer and operations; qualitative data verified by auditors based on observations and interviews with staff and patients	Between 2014 and 2015	Association for Adoption Support and Treatment of Infertility NASZ BOCIAN	Thirty-five ART clinics that agreed to participate in the monitoring process, with 44 confirmed ART clinics operating in 2014

Source: (Janicka et al. 2021)

* Births refer to the WHO ICMART definition and concern live births as well as premature births; data provided by patients voluntarily.

** Data concerning live births were provided by patients voluntarily.

Notes

1 In this chapter, we use the term ART whenever we refer to the discourse on assisted reproductive technology in general. We use the term IVF in reference to the particular Polish public debate where the in vitro fertilization procedure itself (not ART as such) engages the attention, interests and doubts of politicians, media, clergy, NGO representatives and so on.

2 The project was supported by the National Centre of Science in Poland under grant no. 2012/07/E/HS3/01024, 2013–2018.

3 Directive 2004/23/EC of the European Parliament and of the Council of 31 March 2004 on setting standards of quality and safety for the donation, procurement, testing, processing, preservation, storage and distribution of human tissues and cells.

4 On the ambivalent attitude to IVF at the beginning of its history from a worldwide perspective, see Turney (1998).

5 For IVF as a "hope technology", see Franklin (1997).

6 For an analysis of 1989 as a key moment in reproductive legislation in Poland, particularly concerning abortion and birth control, see Mishtal (2009) and Radkowska-Walkowicz (2014).

7 Since 2016, Polish Public Television's (TVP) management has been appointed by the ruling Law and Justice (Prawo i Sprawiedliwość) party. More about Polish anti-IVF discourse: Radkowska-Walkowicz (2012, 2014) and Korolczuk (2016).

8 All quotations from *Evangelium Vitae* follow the translation on the Vatican's official website: http://w2.vatican.va/content/john-paul-ii/en/encyclicals/documents/hf_jp-ii_enc_25031995_evangelium-vitae.html [access: 02.08.2019].

9 All quotations from *Donum vitae* according to translation on Vatican's official website: www.vatican.va/roman_curia/congregations/cfaith/documents/rc_con_cfaith_doc_19870222_respect-for-human-life_en.html.

10 According to the position of the Pontifical Council for the Pastoral Care of Health Care Workers, artificial insemination using the husband's sperm is only allowed on the condition that the sperm used for fertilization was obtained through intercourse (using a special, perforated condom). Only then is the low tubal oocyte transfer (LTOT) method allowed by moving the woman's gamete from the ovary to the fallopian tube or the uterus where it can be fertilized. It also allows for the gamete intra-fallopian transfer (GIFT) method, that is, moving both gametes to the fallopian tube. Nonetheless, media publications by Church hierarchs or journalists who support them make no mention of whether these medical technologies are accepted by the Church.

11 In 2015, the elections in Poland were won by a right-wing, nationalist party, Prawo i Sprawiedliwość (PiS, in English: Law and Justice), which has close ties to the Catholic Church. The current Polish president, Andrzej Duda, also comes from its ranks.

12 Act from 25.06.2015 on infertility treatment, Journal of Laws 2015 item 1087.

13 Since November 2015 (the date of the Act on Infertility introduction), there have been several parliamentary attempts to legally limit ART. That is, three attempts were made through the amendment to the Act on Infertility entitled "the Bill on the protection of the life and health of unborn children conceived through IVF, amending the Act of June 25, 2015, on Infertility, the Act of June 6, 1997 – Criminal Code and the Act of February 25, 1964 – The Family and Custody Code", Druk nr 525: 18th December 2016, 22nd of August 2017, 6th November 2018. One attempt through parliamentary petition in the introduction to the law on the "Clause of conscience" regarding pharmacists (pharmacists would be able to refuse to sell drugs for ovarian stimulation in IVF procedure): "Petition regarding the amendment to the Act of 7 January 1993 or the Law on Family Planning, Human Embryo Protection and Conditions of Permissibility of Abortion Act, of the Act of 6 June 1997 – Penal Code and the Act of 23 April 1964 – Civil Code", petition no. BKSP-145–122/16, 19th August 2016. Another attempt concerned the amendment to the Act on Family Planning and was raised by Polish pro-life movements with the inclusion of the articles that concern ART.

14 The duration of embryo freezing counts, according to the Act, not from the moment of their actual creation and freezing but from the moment cryobanks were established by law. This means that an embryo created in the 1990s was only formally registered in November 2015, and the 20-year count started at that moment.
15 Results submitted by the facilities that participate in the government program, source: www.nasz-bocian.pl/node/55452 [access: 27.01.2018].
16 For more on the biomedical discourses that co-exist in Poland and on those related to Catholic worldviews, see Maciejewska-Mroczek and Radkowska-Walkowicz (2018).
17 For more on the relation between nationalism and IVF discourse in Poland, see Radkowska-Walkowicz (2014).

References

Anderson, B. (1983). *Imagined communities. Reflection on the origin and spread of nationalism.* Verso.

Applebaum, A. (2018). A warning from Europe: The worst is yet to come. *The Atlantic.* www.theatlantic.com/magazine/archive/2018/10/poland-polarization/568324/

Borowik, I. (1997). *Procesy instytucjonalizacji i prywatyzacji religii w powojennej Polsce.* Wydawnictwo UJ.

Braun, G. (2010). *Eugenika – w imię postępu.* Telewizja Polska, Film Open Group.

Centrum Badania Opinii Społecznej. (2010). *Etyczne aspekty zapłodnienia in vitro.* www.cbos.pl/SPISKOM.POL/2010/K_096_10.PDF

Centrum Badania Opinii Społecznej. (2015). *Opinie o dopuszczalności zapłodnienia in vitro. Komunikat z badań.* http://cbos.pl/SPISKOM.POL/2015/K_096_15.PDF

Chełstowska, A. (2011). Stigmatisation and commercialisation of abortion services in Poland: Turning sin into gold. *Reproductive Health Matters, 19*(37), 98–106. https://doi.org/10.1016/S0968-8080(11)37548-9

Danielewski, M., & Wybieralski, M. (2012, July 30). Niepokalanie poczęta. Agnieszka, najstarsze w Polsce dziecko z in vitro. *Gazeta Wyborcza.* www.wysokieobcasy.pl/wysokie-obcasy/1,53662,12200284,Niepokalanie_poczeta__Agnieszka__najstarsze_w_Polsce.html?disableRedirects=true

Dennison, M. (2008). Revealing your sources: The case for non-anonymous gamete donation. *Journal of Law and Health, 21*(1), 1–27.

Doolin, B., & Motion, J. (2010). Christian lay understandings of preimplantation genetic diagnosis. *Public Understanding of Science, 19*(6), 669–685. https://doi.org/10.1177/0963662509354537

Dziennik.pl. (2015, December 1). *Minister Radziwiłł wygasza program in vitro. Podał termin końca refundacji.* https://zdrowie.dziennik.pl/aktualnosci/artykuly/507101,minister-zdrowia-konstanty-radziwill-wygasza-program-in-vitro-podal-termin-konca-refundacji.html

Franklin, S. (1997). *Embodied progress. A cultural account of reproduction.* Routledge.

Freeman, T. (2015). Gamete donation, information sharing and the best interests of the child: An overview of the psychosocial evidence. *Monash Bioethics Review, 33,* 45–63. https://doi.org/10.1007/s40592-015-0018-y

Frith, L. (2001). Gamete donation and anonymity. The ethical and legal debate. *Human Reproduction, 16*(5), 818–824. https://doi.org/10.1093/humrep/16.5.818

Gal, S., & Kligman, G. (2000). Introduction. In S. Gal & G. Kligman (Eds.), *Reproducing gender: Politics, publics, and everyday life after socialism* (pp. 3–19). Princeton University Press.

Grotowska, S. (1999). *Religijność subiektywna. Studium socjologiczne na podstawie wywiadów narracyjnych*. Nomos.

Hall, D. (2012). Questioning secularization? Church and religion in Poland. In D. Pollack, O. Müller, & G. Pickel (Eds.), *The social significance of religion in the Enlarged Europe. secularization, individualization and pluralization* (pp. 121–141). Ashgate.

Hennelowa, J. (1978, August 6). Niepokoje nad „dobrą nowiną". *Tygodnik Powszechny*, 1–3.

Herzfeld, M. (1997). *Cultural intimacy: Social poetics in the nation-state*. Routledge.

Inglis, T. (1998). *Moral monopoly. The rise and fall of the catholic church in modern Ireland*. University College Dublin.

Janicka, A., Spaczynski, R. Z., Koziol, K., Radwan, M., & Kurzawa, R. (2021). Assisted reproductive medicine in Poland, 2013–2016: Polish Society of Reproductive Medicine and Embryology (PTMRiE) and Fertility and Sterility Special Interest Group of the Polish Society of Gynaecologists and Obstetricians (SPiN PTGiP) report. *Ginekologia Polska*, 92(1), 7–15. https://doi.org/10.5603/GP.a2020.0142

John Paul II. (1995). *Encyclical Evangelium Vitae: To the bishops, priests and deacons, men and women religious lay faithful and all people of good will on the value and inviolability of human life*. Libreria Editrice Vaticana. http://w2.vatican.va/content/john-paul-ii/en/encyclicals/documents/hf_jp-ii_enc_25031995_evangelium-vitae.html

Kancelaria Sejmu. (2015). *Ustawa z dnia 25 czerwca 2015 r. O leczeniu niepłodności*. http://prawo.sejm.gov.pl/isap.nsf/DocDetails.xsp?id=WDU20150001087

Klawiter, J. (2017). *Ustawa o zmianie niektórych ustaw w związku z ochroną zdrowia i życia dzieci poczętych*. https://orka.sejm.gov.pl/Druki8ka.nsf/Projekty/8-020-1141-2018/$file/8-020-1141-2018.pdf

Konarska, I. (1991, July 6). Szatańskie probówki. *Polityka*, 10.

Konarska, I. (2004). Szczęście z in vitro. *Przegląd*. www.przeglad-godnik.pl/pl/artykul/szczescie-vitro

Konferencja Episkopatu Polski. (2010). *Oświadczenie Zespołu Ekspertów Konferencji Episkopatu Polski ds. Bioetycznych w porozumieniu z Prezydium Konferencji Episkopatu Polski*.

Kongres Kobiet. (2009). *Postulaty z I Kongresu Kobiet "Kobiety dla Polski, Polska dla kobiet"*. https://www.kongreskobiet.pl/cele-i-postulaty

Korolczuk, E. (2016). 'The purest citizens' and 'IVF children'. Reproductive citizenship in contemporary Poland. *Reproductive Biomedicine & Society Online*, 3, 126–133. https://doi.org/10.1016/j.rbms.2016.12.006

Krawczak, A. (2016). *In vitro. Bez strachu, bez ideologii*. Muza.

Kuczyński, W., Kurzawa, R., Oszukowski, P., Pawelczyk, L., Poręba, R., Radowicki, S., Szamatowicz, M., & Wołczyński, S. (2012). Rekomendacje dotyczące diagnostyki i leczenia niepłodności – skrót. Polish gynecological society and polish society for reproductive medicine recommendations for the diagnosis and treatment of infertility. *Ginekologia Polska*, 83(2).

Maciejewska-Mroczek, E., & Radkowska-Walkowicz, M. (2017). Do 'in vitro children' exist? The 'ontological choreography' between public debates and private experiences in Poland. *Children's Geographies*, 17(1), 36–48. https://doi.org/10.1080/14733285.2017.1380781

Maciejewska-Mroczek, E., & Radkowska-Walkowicz, M. (2018). Between monster child and innocent baby. Managing fear and hope in Polish debates on in vitro fertilisation. In J. Ahlbeck, P. Lappalainen, K. Launis, & K. Tuohela (Eds.), *Childhood, literature and science. Fragile subjects* (pp. 184–195). Routledge.

Mayer, T. (1999). Gender ironies of nationalism. Setting the stage. In T. Mayer (Ed.), *Gender ironies of nationalism. Sexing the nation* (pp. 1–24). Routledge.

Miłkowska, K. (2017, June 1). Oto 7 miast, które dofinansowują in vitro – gdzie i na jakich warunkach? *Chcemy Być Rodzicami.* www.chcemybycrodzicami.pl/oto-6-miast-ktore-dofinansowuja-in-vitro-gdzie-i-na-jakich-warunkach/

Ministerstwo Zdrowia. (2014). *OGŁOSZENIE w sprawie podziału środków finansowych pomiędzy realizatorów programu zdrowotnego pn. Program – Leczenie Niepłodności Metodą Zapłodnienia Pozaustrojowego na lata 2013–2016.* http://www2.mz.gov.pl/wwwmz/index?m r=m15&ms=739&ml=pl&mi=739&mx=0&mt=&my=739&ma=032743

Mishtal, J. (2009). Matters of "Conscience": The politics of reproductive healthcare in Poland. *Medical Anthropology Quarterly, 23*(2), 161–183.

Montuschi, O. (2009). „*Powiedzieć i Rozmawiać" Jak rozmawiać o poczęciu dzięki dawstwu z dziećmi w wieku 0–7 lat Poradnik dla rodziców.* www.nasz-bocian.pl/sites/default/files/2020-02/powiedziec%20i%20rozmawiac%200-7.pdf

Polska Agencja Prasowa. (2015, August 4). Kidawa-Błońska zaskoczona stanowiskiem Episkopatu ws. In vitro: 'Ja uważam, że to jest dobre, a nie złe'. *WPolityce.Pl.* https://wpolityce.pl/polityka/261385-kidawa-blonska-zaskoczona-stanowiskiem-episkopatu-ws-in-vitro-ja-uwazam-ze-to-jest-dobre-a-nie-zle

Polska Agencja Prasowa. (2016, October 6). *Kilku posłów Kukiz'15 wycofało swoje poparcie. Projektu ws. In vitro został wycofany.* https://wiadomosci.dziennik.pl/polityka/arty kuly/532616,kilku-poslow-kukiz15-wycofalo-swoje-poparcie-projektu-ws-in-vitro-zostal-wycofany.html

Polska Agencja Prasowa, & Rynek Zdrowia. (2016, June 30). In vitro: To już koniec rządowego programu. *Rynek Zdrowia.* www.rynekzdrowia.pl/Polityka-zdrowotna/In-vitro-to-juz-koniec-rzadowego-programu,163358,14.html

Polska Newsweek. (2015, July 10). Magdalena Kołodziej, pierwsze w Polsce dziecko z in vitro: Wstyd mi za Polskę. *Polska Newsweek.* www.newsweek.pl/polska/in-vitro-pierwsza-polka-z-in-vitro-magdalena-kolodziej/q1zj044

Polskie Towarzystwo Medycyny Rozrodu. (2015, July 7). *List otwarty Polskiego Towarzystwa Medycyny Rozrodu.* http://ptmrie.org.pl/pliki/akty-prawne-i-rekomendacje/stanowiska/list-otwarty-ptmr-do-senatorow-rp.pdf

Radkowska-Walkowicz, M. (2012). The creation of "monsters": The discourse of opposition to in vitro fertilization in Poland. *Reproductive Health Matters, 20*(40), 30–37. https://doi.org/10.1016/S0968-8080(12)40647-4

Radkowska-Walkowicz, M. (2013). *Doświadczenie in vitro. Niepłodność i nowe technologie reprodukcyjne w perspektywie antropologicznej.* Warsaw University Press.

Radkowska-Walkowicz, M. (2014). Frozen children and despairing embryos in the "new" post-communist state: The debate on IVF in the context of Poland's transition. *European Journal of Women's Studies, 21*(4), 399–414. https://doi.org/10.1177/1350506814542881

Radkowska-Walkowicz, M. (2017). "Jak zaczęła się twoja historia". Nowe technologie reprodukcyjne i nowe formy stygmatyzacji. *Lud, 101,* 149–169. https://doi.org/10.12775/lud101.2017.04

Radkowska-Walkowicz, M. (2018). How the political becomes private: In vitro fertilization and the Catholic Church in Poland. *Journal of Religion and Health, 57*(3), 979–993. https://doi.org/10.1007/s10943-017-0480-3

Romanek, B. (2013, March 20). Częstochowa: In vitro – rusza druga edycja tego programu zdrowotnego. *Częstochowa – Nasze Miasto.* https://czestochowa.naszemiasto.pl/czestochowa-in-vitro-rusza-druga-edycja-tego-programu/ar/c8-1781190

Szamatowicz, M. (2009, March 14). Samo życie. *Polityka,* 94–95.

Szymański, Ł. (2009). *In vitro.* Wydawnictwo Petrus.

Turney, J. (1998). *Frankenstein's footsteps: Science, genetics, and popular culture.* Yale University Press.

Wołczyński, S., & Krawczak, A. (2012). *Program Polityki Zdrowotnej „Leczenie niepłodności metodą IVF dla mieszkańców Częstochowy w latach 2012–2014.* Rada Miasta Częstochowy.

Zielińska, E. (2000). Between ideology, politics and common sense: The discourse about reproductive rights in Poland. In S. Gal & G. Kligman (Eds.), *Reproducing gender. Politics, publics, and everyday life after socialism* (pp. 23–58). Princeton University Press.

9 From safeguarding the best interest of the child to equal treatment

Legislating assisted reproductive techniques in Sweden

Anna Singer

Introduction

Sweden was the first country in the world to introduce legislation on assisted reproduction in 1984 through the Insemination Act (*Lagen om insemination*), in effect on 1 March 1985.[1] The In Vitro Fertilization Act (*Lagen om befruktning utanför kroppen*) followed in 1988.[2] Without amendment, both laws were incorporated into the Genetic Integrity Act (*Lagen om genetisk integritet m.m.*) of 2006.[3] Reports prepared by the Insemination Committee (*Inseminationskommittén*) laid the foundation for the views on assisted reproduction and what interest should be protected by the laws. The reasoning behind these laws has to a great extent influenced the development of the following legislation concerning the use of different methods of assisted reproductive technologies (ART).[4] The development can be characterized as cautious, as new methods have been allowed only after thorough investigation of possible risks and consequences for the resulting child. Hence, egg donation was allowed as late as in 2003. Following that amendment to the law, the development has proceeded in a somewhat higher pace, reflecting a more open view towards assisted reproduction. In 2005, lesbian couples were given access to ART as long as the fertilized egg came from the woman giving birth. From April 2016, single women were given access to in vitro fertilization (IVF) and donor insemination, and in 2019, embryo donation became legal.

When first regulated in 1985, ART using donated gametes was considered to raise problems of a legal, ethical and psychological nature. It was deemed necessary to guarantee that the best interests of the child would always remain in focus, and this goal is still valid today. However, the definition of what the best interest of the child is has changed. The starting point was to give the child two parents of different sexes, what can be described as a traditional family. Another requirement long upheld was a genetic link to one of the legal parents and access to information about the donor. Furthermore, the number of clinics that could provide treatment with donated cells was limited in order to, among other things, ensure that treatment would be given under ethically acceptable conditions.

DOI: 10.4324/9781003223726-9

Step by step, these requirements have been abolished. The one requirement that has not changed over time is the protection of a child's right to access information about the donor. The latest change in the law entered into effect as of 1 January 2019. It is now possible to use donated reproductive cells from two different donors and to donate embryos. A genetic link between the child and one of the future parents is no longer considered necessary to protect the best interest of the child.[5] The number of clinics that can provide treatment with donated cells has also increased in order to make ART more accessible to those who want to become parents.

Since the beginning of the 1980s, ART have been the subject of ongoing legislative attention in Sweden. With the introduction of new techniques, the foundational laws of 1985 and 1988 have slowly been reformed. There has been very limited political debate concerning the legislation on assisted reproduction until lately, possibly as a result of the moderate reform speed but also due to the fact that the use of ART has for a long time and to a large extent been perceived as a medical matter and not a question of public policy. Along with recent changes in the law, evidence of changing views on ART can, however, be seen in the discussion concerning donor insemination for single women in 2016[6] and more recent calls for allowing surrogacy arrangements.[7] The focus has shifted from a doubtful attitude towards ART to an emphasis on the right to become a parent and the right to equal treatment. The previous ambition to give the child a traditional family has been replaced by the acknowledgment of different family forms. The regulation has largely been the result of rather consensual politics, with single parliamentarians, in many cases from the conservative side of the Parliament, as opposing voices. The fact that methods not allowed in Sweden are offered and available elsewhere to residents in Sweden has been a driving force behind legislative action in Sweden during the last decade. Apart from what methods should be allowed, central questions of the debate have been how to regulate the establishment of legal parenthood following assisted reproduction with donated gametes and how to secure a child's right to knowledge about genetic origin.

In the following, the motives behind the Swedish legislation regarding ART are presented and explored.[8] The description is chronological, starting with background on the first legislation in 1984. All subsequent changes of the laws have been preceded by thorough investigations by government-appointed committees, which in some cases include parliamentarians from all political parties and in other cases include one special examiner supported by different experts from academia, government agencies and organizations. The reports from the committees, covering, among other things, a review of the use of different methods, results and suggestions of possible law reforms, have been widely circulated to different authorities, universities and non-governmental organizations. The reports and the responses they have evoked have been the basis for the ensuing government bills, thus providing informative background to the laws.

The first legislation – regulating a medical matter

Donor insemination

Legislative background

In Sweden, as in many other countries, donor insemination has been practiced since the 1920s. During the period 1945–48, there were 56 donor inseminations done in Sweden, resulting in seven pregnancies.[9] Demand for insemination treatment increased after the 1940s, both in Sweden and abroad. It has been estimated that in 1974, about 100 children were born in Sweden using donor insemination, and at the beginning of the 1980s, the number of children born using donor insemination was at least 230.[10]

The question of regulating donor insemination was raised already in a proposal of a Children and Parents Code in 1946. In a government report, medical and legal experts noticed that donor insemination was practiced but concluded that legislation was not called for. According to the experts, any disputed matters could be resolved in practice without the support of specific legal provisions.[11]

However, the then operating Medical Board, a state agency responsible for monitoring and guiding health care in Sweden (later transformed to the National Board of Health and Welfare, *Socialstyrelsen*), was of the opposite opinion and believed that donor insemination ought to be regulated. In 1947, a special commission was appointed and delivered a government report with a proposal for regulation. According to this proposal, donor insemination should be offered only to married women with the consent of her husband.[12] The proposal did not result in legislation. While the reasons for this are not fully clear, it has been suggested that the government considered the number of inseminations with donor too small to motivate regulation. It could also have been opposition from different interest groups, such as the Church.[13] Although the Church had not been especially significant in the discussions concerning the regulation of ART, a common view from the bishops of the Church of Sweden was quoted by the commission, which stated that insemination using sperm and eggs from the couple within the marriage was acceptable. Donor insemination, on the other hand, was criticized and considered to violate the core of paternity.[14] The fact that Swedish children were available for adoption could also have been a reason for not regulating donor insemination.[15]

However, in the early 1980s, renewed calls came for legislation regarding various forms of ART, in particular from the medical profession, mainly due to an increase in the use of donor insemination. The then-existing regulation regarding paternity determination was considered insufficient to safeguard the interests of the child.

After an initiative from the Swedish Society of Medicine (*Svenska Läkaresällskapet*), the government in 1981 appointed a special examiner. The committee formed – the Insemination Committee – was given the task of mapping the scope and forms of donor insemination in Sweden. Based on the results of this survey, the committee was to consider whether legislation was required, both in terms of paternity determination and the forms of treatment as such, and to propose the necessary regulation.[16] The starting point for the committee's work was that insemination was to be permitted only as long as it was consistent with the child's best interest. This included having two parents. It was also deemed necessary that the doctor, before treatment, should examine whether the parents' medical, social and psychological circumstances were such that donor insemination was advisable. In short, the resulting child should be able to grow up under "good conditions".

During the mandate of the Insemination Committee, the deficiencies in the protection of the child's legal status became clear in a case decided by the Supreme Court in 1983.[17] The case concerned the revocation of legal paternity. In the case, a former husband requested to have his paternal rights and obligations terminated following divorce from the child's mother, since the child was born after insemination with an anonymous donor. The court found that the man was not the child's biological father and the fact that he had consented to the insemination was not an obstacle to have paternity revoked. His request was granted, and the child was left without a legal father.

The then-existing regulation meant that a man who had once been declared a child's legal father through the pater est rule or through paternity confirmation could always have his legal status as a child's father revoked with reference to the lack of genetic relationship if the child had been conceived through donor insemination. If paternity was revoked, it was the donor who should be declared the legal father according to the then-applicable rules. Since the donors were generally anonymous, it became in reality impossible to establish legal paternity for children conceived through donor insemination if a previously established paternity was revoked. New rules for the establishment of legal paternity after donor insemination were deemed necessary in order to satisfy the child's need, and right, to a legal father.

Therefore, a basic question for the committee's investigation was how the child could be secured a legal father. Several possible alternatives were discussed. A ban on donor insemination was not seen as a realistic solution considering the extent of the use of donor insemination. It was furthermore assumed that a ban would not be respected; the risk of continued donor insemination in violation of the law was high, since it is a method that can be performed independently of assistance from health facilities. In addition, the practice of donor insemination was considered a valuable option for spouses or cohabiting couples that could not have children.[18] In addition, the best interests of the child did not call for a ban on the method as such.[19] Another possible solution considered for establishing paternity after donor insemination was adoption. However, this would require fundamental changes in the legal regulation of adoption, including an option to adopt a child that is not yet conceived and a possibility to cancel an adoption before the child was conceived. Adoption was therefore not considered a realistic alternative to protect children conceived through donor insemination.[20]

1984 Insemination Act

The solution ultimately proposed by the Insemination Committee came, after some changes, to form the basis of the Insemination Act that entered into effect on 1 March 1985. The law made it possible for married or cohabiting couples to receive donor insemination. Insemination was for a long time perceived as a method to help couples that were involuntarily childless due to infertility or hereditary disease, not as an alternative to fertilization "the natural way". Hence, single women did not have access to donor insemination. It was also pointed out that an underlying value was that a child ought to have both a mother and a father to enable positive development and that society should not encourage or be part of a child having only one parent from the onset of life.[21] The committee found it "reasonable that the legislation, in a realistic manner is in accord with society's view with regard to the family formation pattern".[22]

The Insemination Act also stipulated that donor insemination within the healthcare system could only be done at a publicly financed hospital under the supervision of a specialist in gynecology and obstetrics and with the permission of the National Board of Health and Welfare.[23] The purpose of establishing these requirements was to guarantee that the treatment would be given under ethically acceptable conditions. In addition, the centering of treatment at certain hospitals was assumed to facilitate research and follow-up of the activities, not least regarding the living conditions of the children born through the use of ART. In the law, it was stated that before treatment, the doctor should examine the future parents' medical, social and psychological circumstances in order to establish that the child would grow up under "good conditions". Even if this is an impossible task, the requirement underlined the responsibility of society when contributing to the conception of a child.

In addition, a new rule was introduced in the Children and Parent Code for determining legal paternity after insemination. The law stated that the man who consents to the insemination of his spouse or cohabiting partner was to be deemed the father of the child if it was likely that the child was conceived through the insemination.

To serve as the basis for legal paternity, the man's consent did not require insemination according to the Swedish regulation. Paternity could be established regardless of whether the treatment was given within the Swedish health care system, abroad or through an at-home-insemination. If there was, for some reason, no valid consent from the husband or cohabitant of the woman (a situation that should not arise if the insemination is done according to the Insemination Act and later the Genetic Integrity Act, that is at a Swedish health facility) the donor could be given the opportunity to confirm paternity as the biological father if the mother agreed.[24] It was not possible to establish the donor as the father through court decision since the child had not been conceived through intercourse. This changed in 2005, when genetic relationship was established as the principal ground for paternity.[25] However, a donor within the framework of the Genetic Integrity Act cannot be declared the child's father by court.

It is clear that the ambition of the legislature in 1985 was to ensure that a child conceived thorough ART, as far as possible, should have a legal father, even if this meant that the child did not have access to information about his or her genetic origin. This view changed with the reform of the rules for establishing legal parentage in force from 1 January 2019. The law now states that consent to assisted reproduction with donated sperm is valid only if the treatment is given in Sweden and according to the Genetic Integrity Act or at a competent health care facility abroad and the child conceived through the treatment has a right to information about the identity of the donor. Access to information about genetic origin is now in effect considered more important than having a legal father.[26]

The most controversial aspect of the Insemination Act was, however, the prohibition of the use of anonymous donors. The child was considered to have an indispensable right to have access to information about the donor's identity.

The child's right to information about the donor

The Insemination Committee proposals were in general unanimously accepted, with one exception – the child's right to have access to information about his or her genetic origin. The committee declared that a "self-evident prerequisite for permitting the undertaking of [donor insemination] should be – as in the case of adoption – that the needs and interests of the prospective child be fulfilled and safeguarded in a satisfactory way".[27] The best interest of the child included, according to the committee, a right for the child to have access to information about the donor's identity. Relying on the experiences of adopted children, who according to the Swedish regulation always have had access to information about their biological parents through the Swedish population register, the committee found no reason to treat children through donor insemination differently. The requirement that all donor insemination be carried out within publicly funded hospitals was to safeguard the child's right to this information. Information about the donor should be kept in a special journal at the hospital where the treatment was received, and the child would be entitled to access the information as soon he or she had reached sufficient maturity.[28] To withhold information about the child's origin from the child would be a departure from the fairness principle, since most children have knowledge about their origin.[29] The result was inclusion into the law a rule which gave the "mature enough" child the right to access hospital records showing the donor's identity. The social authorities were obliged to assist the child in the search for information. The committee acknowledged that many parents would probably not inform the child of how he or she was conceived but hoped that openness about this process would eventually prevail. The committee considered a registration of information about the insemination in the population register, but the minister of justice did not find this "functional".[30]

Not allowing anonymous donors was a suggestion that evoked protests from, in particular, the medical professions involved in ART.[31] They feared that the availability of sperm donors would cease if donors were not guaranteed anonymity.[32] Another argument against the right to information was that the situation of the sperm donor was not taken into consideration. However, with reference to the principle of best interest of the child, the subsequent law gave the "mature enough" child the right to obtain information about the donor, that is, the genetic father.[33]

After the introduction of regulation in 1985, the number of inseminations initially indeed decreased. One reason for this decline was that new donors who agreed to be non-anonymous had to be recruited. The fact that the child had a right to knowledge about the donor's identity might also have deterred intended parents from seeking the assistance of the Swedish health care. However, over time, the number of treatments steadily increased until 1995, when they decreased again. Of major importance for this more recent decline was the increased use of microinjections, providing improved means of helping men with impaired fertility to have children, thereby decreasing the need for donor insemination. In recent years, the number of donor inseminations has again increased slightly, which can at least partly be explained by the fact that this treatment was made available to lesbian couples in 2005 and to single women in 2016. In 2015, there were 959 donor inseminations performed and around 150 children born as a result.[34]

Statistics from the National Board of Health and Welfare do not fully reflect the number of children born in Sweden after donor insemination, since the statistics only cover treatment by Swedish health facilities. Many parents, both couples and singles, go to other countries for treatment. There are several reasons behind such a decision. Long queues at clinics offering donor insemination suggest that many intended parents are deterred by long waiting periods for treatment, especially if treatment can be obtained without delay at clinics abroad. The fact that children conceived through donor insemination at a Swedish health facility have the right to access information about the donor may also be a reason some are turning to clinics in other countries where anonymous donors are used.

It should be pointed out that infertility treatment in Sweden is, and has always been, included in the national health insurance and thus available for a small fee for Swedish residents. The first three treatment cycles are usually available for the regular patient fee, usually between 10 and 30 Euros, varying somewhat between the different Country Councils that are responsible for providing health care in Sweden. Further treatment must be paid for by the intended parent(s).

Until 2018, the legislation concerning donor insemination regarding the conditions for use of the method and the establishment of paternity had remained mainly unchanged after the introduction of the law in 1985. Protecting the child's right to knowledge has been an important goal for the ensuing legislation concerning the use of other methods of assisted reproduction with donated cells, culminating in new regulation entering into force 1 January 2019. The new regulation will be described in "And Now – Parenthood for the Involuntarily Childless".

In vitro fertilization

After presenting their first report in 1983, the Insemination Committee continued its work with a review of ethical, judicial, medical and psycho-social aspects of fertilization outside the body – in vitro fertilization – and surrogate motherhood.

In the mid-1980s, these methods of assisted reproduction had not yet become widespread in their use, neither in Sweden nor elsewhere. However, the technology was in rapid development. As was the case with donor insemination, these methods made it possible to create relationships between children and parents not based on genetics, something that was considered problematic by the committee.

In its second report, "Children Through Fertilization Outside the Body" in 1985, the committee addressed IVF treatment, egg donation and surrogacy.[35] The report laid the foundations for the In Vitro Fertilization Act in 1988.[36]

It is noticeable that the committee in its second report expressed a rather cautious attitude towards ART that was not clearly pronounced in the first report. The committee now declared, "a limit should be set to how far to go regarding manipulations to remedy childlessness".[37]

The committee found the manipulation through insemination when using sperm from the woman's husband or cohabiting man insignificant, since it consists only of the transfer of sperm from man to woman in an artificial way for conception. Donor insemination involved a higher degree of manipulation. However, according to the committee, donor insemination did not depart from the natural life process in the sense that a man's sperm is transferred to a woman.[38]

A further increase in the degree of manipulation existed when using fertilization outside the body, IVF. The committee found this procedure completely against the natural life process. Additionally, it increases the possibilities for manipulation within the very conditions of life. The committee formulated its starting point for assessing which forms of assisted reproduction could be considered acceptable as follows:[39]

> We want to make it clear at the outset that, in our opinion, it can never be a human right to have children. Nature's incompleteness must sometimes be accepted. No human being can be treated solely as a means of satisfying others, but each individual has his own human worth. The goal of using artificial fertilization methods must be in the best interest of the future child.

The committee thus formulated an approach that since has echoed in several different contexts when the desirability of different methods of assisted reproduction has been assessed. However, despite the rather restrictive view on IVF, the committee suggested allowing treatment for couples using their own reproductive cells. The fact that the genetic parents of the child would also be the legal parents seemingly could compensate for the ethical objections to the use of the method.

The committee considered other forms of ART undesirable and hence concluded they should not be allowed. IVF with donated sperm was not allowed since the combination of sperm donation and IVF was considered too big a deviation from the "natural order" of things. Egg donation entailed an even greater deviation.

> The Committee declared that "[e]gg donation is a complicated method of fertilisation which goes completely against the natural process of life. We cannot

disregard that the method can involve risks of physical and mental strain for the pregnant woman and the developing child. The investigation regarding egg donation as having so many features of technical construction for solving the problem of childlessness that the method is ethically indefensible. In the Committee's view egg donation should be prohibited in Sweden".[40]

The resulting In Vitro Fertilization Act thus made IVF treatment for married or cohabiting couples with the use of the couples' own reproductive cells possible. Egg donation was not allowed, nor surrogacy arrangements. IVF treatment could only be given at publicly funded hospitals.[41] The same investigation of the couples' medical, social and psychological circumstances as should be done prior to donor insemination was prescribed when using IVF in order to establish that the child would grow up under "good conditions". The purpose of establishing these requirements was also in this situation to guarantee that the treatment would be given under ethically acceptable circumstances. In addition, the concentration of treatment to certain hospitals was assumed to facilitate research and follow-up of the activities. Minor changes were also done in the Children and Parent Code making it possible to establish paternity after IVF based on the man's consent to treatment.

The first legislation – a hesitant acceptance of ART

The impression is that the Insemination Committee in the reports from 1983 and 1985 wanted to prohibit everything that could be forbidden, thus demonstrating a slightly doubtful view on the use of ART. This cautious approach might partly explain the lack of political debate on the matter.[42] The thorough examination of the questions and the extensive reports on the subject also contributed to the acceptance of the proposals. It was considered better to regulate what could not be forbidden.

The fact that assisted reproduction for a long time was defined as a medical matter, and thus in the hands of medical professionals, might also have contributed to the limited political discussion. As the Insemination Committee put it:

> The Committee finds [donor insemination] to be a method in certain cases to help families who cannot have children due to the man's infertility.[43]
>
> IVF is a method of remedying involuntary childlessness. The Committee's understanding is that the method should be used only where there are medical obstacles against fertilization in the natural way.[44]

The medical profession was on the whole positive towards the regulation of donor insemination and IVF. The only real debate or controversy around the first laws on assisted reproduction was the abolition of donor anonymity, a proposal that followed from the strong emphasis that the 1981 Insemination Committee put on the legal protection of the rights of children. The special examiner Tor Sverne was at the time Parliamentary Ombudsman, and he had at the end of the 1970s chaired the highly acclaimed Commission on Children's rights with the task to investigate how the legal position of children in Sweden could be strengthened. He was a strong children's rights advocate and had a very high position in the legal profession in Sweden. This might partly explain why his suggestion that children should have the right to access information about the donor prevailed over the rather negative response from the medical profession.

The next step – equal treatment of all women

Egg donation and IVF with donated sperm

Already five years after the introduction of the In Vitro Fertilization Act in 1988, the Parliamentary Committee on Health and Welfare (*Riksdagens socialutskott*) declared that a new investigation on egg donation was justified.[45] As a consequence, the Ministry of Health and Social Affairs gave the Swedish National Council on Medical Ethics (*Statens medicinsk-etiska råd*) (Ethics Council) the assignment to review a number of questions about fertilization outside the body, including egg donation and sperm donation in combination with IVF.[46]

The Ethics Council published its conclusions in 1995.[47] The Council suggested allowing IVF with egg donation and sperm from the woman's spouse or partner for women of childbearing age. Similarly, in the opinion of the Council, IVF with donated sperm should be allowed using the woman's own egg. However, the Council opposed egg donation in combination with sperm donation, since the result would be that the child would not have any genetic link to the legal parents.

The report from the Ethics Council was referred by the Ministry of Health and Social Affairs to many public and private authorities and organizations in Sweden for their opinion. During this procedure, many of those involved pointed out the need for further investigation into the risks of ART.[48] Consequently, the National Board of Health and Welfare carried out an investigation of the risks with ART, in particular IVF, in cooperation with the Swedish Pediatric Society (*Svenska barnläkarföreningen*) and the Swedish Association for Obstetrics and Gynecology (*Svensk Förening för Obstetrik och Gynekologi*). The need to rule out problems with the use of the IVF technique as such motivated the delay in acting on the suggestions from the Ethics Council from 1995. The risks for the child in connection with IVF treatment were mainly the result of the implantation of more than one egg. The risks were minimized if only one fertilized egg was transferred to the woman and the guidelines were changed accordingly.[49] Critique against this came from the medical profession, since it most likely would reduce the probability of success of the treatment.[50]

The Ministry of Health and Social Affairs published a government report in 2000 following the investigation by the National Board of Health and Welfare and the report from the Ethics Council.[51] The Ministry suggested a few amendments to the law, including allowing for IVF with donated egg or sperm, although not in combination.

The Ministry report was favorably received by many different institutions and organizations during the referral. One argument in favor of the proposal was the equal treatment of men and women. In 2003, an amendment of the In Vitro Fertilization Act was made, making IVF treatment with donated sperm or eggs possible.[52] Allowing for the use of IVF with donated sperm was a reform that did not cause any controversy or even discussion. Apparently no reason was found to differentiate between donor insemination and IVF with donated sperm as long as the egg came from the woman giving birth.

The law also stipulated that IVF treatment involving donated gametes could only be offered at academic research hospitals. The government was of the opinion that use of IVF in new situations should be closely controlled and evaluated. This could be achieved if the treatment was centered at certain hospitals where there were also medical specialties other than gynecology and obstetrics available.[53]

IVF treatment with both egg and sperm from donors was still not permitted. This limitation was motivated by the argument that a child should have a genetic link to at least one of the legal parents. The perspective of the child was emphasized in the legislative process. The government agreed with the recommendations of the Ethics Council and shared the view of the Church of Sweden that it was reasonable to apply the precautionary principle when introducing new methods. In the assessment of different methods to treat involuntary childlessness, it was vital to guarantee the child's interest since the child had nothing to say about the procedure of conception.[54]

At the time of this proposal, the principle of non-anonymous donors was well established in Sweden compared to when the principle was first introduced in 1985. A child conceived through IVF treatment with a donated egg was entitled to information about his or her origin in the same way as children born after donor insemination. In this context, the matter of surrogacy was brought to attention once again. However, no suggestion to regulate this was put forward, since this method for alleviating childlessness was not considered ethically justifiable.[55]

When egg donation was introduced, there were no rules regarding determination of maternity. The lack of a rule was considered a possible source of uncertainty in the situation where children were conceived through IVF treatment with donated eggs. The legal presumption was that the woman giving birth was the child's legal mother, but it was not clear if this would also hold in the case of a non-genetically related birth mother. Consequently, amendments to the Children and Parents Code stated that the woman who gives birth to a child conceived by IVF treatment with a donated egg is considered the child's legal mother. Furthermore, it followed that the consenting husband or cohabitee to the woman receiving the treatment is considered the child's legal father if, considering all the circumstances, it is probable that the child has been conceived through the treatment.[56] This rule was the same as that applicable after donor insemination.

The number of children born after IVF treatment with donated sperm is approximately at the same level as children born after IVF treatment with donated eggs. In 2005, 186 treatments with donated eggs resulted in 59 pregnancies and 44 births. In 2009, 321 egg donations resulted in 111 pregnancies and 87 births.[57] In 2018, the number of children born through egg donation was 96.[58]

Lesbian couples' access to ART

In the beginning of the 1980s, the Investigation of Homosexuals' Situation in Society considered, among other questions, if homosexual couples should be allowed to adopt children. Equal treatment of same-sex couples was a question that had then been on the political agenda in Sweden for quite some time. However, the conclusion was not to introduce such a possibility.[59] The Partnership Committee reached the same decision in 1993.[60] The main reason for this was that there was no agreement between researchers on the consequences for children who grow up in same-sex families. Furthermore, joint parenthood for couples of the same sex was assumed to most likely be in contradiction with then-current values of society.[61]

In 1999, a Parliamentary committee, the Committee on Children in Homosexual Families, received the task to investigate and analyze the conditions for children in same-sex families. In their report from 2001, the committee concluded that the legal differences in the then-existing legislation regarding possibilities for homosexual and heterosexual couples to adopt were no longer substantively justified.[62] Research concerning children with homosexual parents showed that there were no grounds to believe that same-sex registered partners or cohabitees were unable to offer children a good environment to grow up in or to offer them the care and need they were entitled to. Based on this, the conclusion was that there were no reasons that could justify prohibiting lesbian couples' access to ART.[63] The committee proposed that both adoption and donor insemination be allowed for same-sex couples.

In 2003, same-sex couples received the right to apply for adoption under the same conditions as different-sex couples.[64] In 2005, new rules came into effect through amendments, giving lesbian couples the right to donor insemination and IVF treatment at public hospitals under the same conditions as heterosexual couples.[65] Since sperm donation was not allowed in combination with egg donation, it meant that the birth mother in these cases was always the genetic mother of the child.

A guiding principle for regulation concerning the use of ART was from the onset to give the child two parents who can provide the child with economic, social and legal stability.[66] The rules concerning the establishment of parenthood thus needed reform in order to allow two women to become parents together. The result was that the woman consenting to the insemination of her partner, wife or cohabitee is considered the child's parent if the child is conceived through treatment at a Swedish hospital. Parenthood – the legal term for the consenting woman is in this case parent – is established by confirmation or court decision. However, for a child conceived through treatment abroad or through an "at-home-insemination", the donor, if he can be identified, should be established as the legal father. The wife of the birth mother had to adopt the child in order for the child to be their common child.[67]

The law for the establishment of parenthood for the child's second parent was changed from 1 January 2022. Legal status for the wife of the birth mother is now established in the same way as for a man married to the birth mother.[68]

Until 1 January 2019, there was a difference between consenting men and women in the way parental status was established. A man consenting to the treatment of his wife or cohabitee would always be the child's legal father regardless of where the treatment was given. A consenting woman would only be considered a parent if the treatment was received at a Swedish hospital. In all other cases, paternity should, if possible, be established. Adoption was the only way to joint parenthood in these cases. The reasons for this difference were "the actual circumstances" of the situation when a child is born to two women and the assumption that many donors to lesbian couples could have an interest in becoming the child's legal father.[69]

The driving force behind the introduction of donor insemination for lesbian couples was the ambition to abolish unequal treatment between homo- and heterosexual couples. This law proposal did not encounter any serious resistance or debate in the Parliament.[70] Again, the explanation could be the thorough investigations that proceeded the government proposal. Nevertheless, it is noticeable that this extension of the use of donor insemination to a certain degree goes against the declaration of the Insemination Committee 20 years earlier that it can never be a human right to have children and that nature's incompleteness sometimes must be accepted. The right to equal treatment as an argument carried great weight and would continue to do so for the following developments, not the least for the claims to give single women access to donor insemination.

Single women's right to access donor insemination and IVF treatment

Giving single women access to ART on under the same conditions as couples was a question that had been discussed in the Parliament already in connection with the debate in 1984 concerning the government bill on insemination.[71] The Parliamentary Committee on Justice then referred to the opinion of the Parliamentary Committee on Health and Welfare, which stated that it is not a human right to have access to donor insemination. Society should not provide this treatment if it could not be assumed that the child would have good conditions for positive development. The Committee on Justice saw no disagreement about the desirability for a child to have a mother and a father. To deprive the child altogether of a paternal figure was not acceptable at the time. The child's best interest must prevail over the equality of different groups of women.[72] The Committee on Justice concurred with the Committee on Health and Welfare that psychiatrists and child psychologists had underlined the importance of a mother and a father for a child's development. The Committee on Justice could not stand behind an arrangement that from the beginning would deprive a child of a legal father.[73]

The parliamentary discussion concerning the right of single women continued thereafter, with increasing intensity. In the fall of 2005, a Parliament member from the Left party submitted a motion asking the government to present a law proposal giving single women access to donor insemination.[74] The motion was denied with, among other things, reference to the statements concerning the right of the child to two parents made in the then-recently accepted law on joint parenthood for lesbian couples.[75] The following year, there were more motions in the Parliament from representatives from five out of six parties, with the exception of the Christian Democratic Party, urging for regulation of insemination for single women. The motions were again denied, but the Parliamentary Committee on Health and Welfare called for the government to closely follow the question and act if and when it became motivated.[76] In 2008, motions in the Parliament from six out of seven parties called for single women's access to donor insemination. The Committee on Health and Welfare did not support the motions, this time with reference to a government investigation in the matter from a child rights perspective.[77] In 2011, the Committee on Health and Welfare did not support motions concerning single mothers, again with a reference to ongoing investigations into the matter done by the government.[78]

There have been several arguments against giving single women access to donor insemination. One is the right of the child to two parents, another the fact that the Swedish legislation puts an obligation on society through the social welfare authorities to try to have paternity to all children born by unmarried mothers established. A right for single women to have donor insemination would be in contradiction to this obligation. The child's right to know and be cared for by his or her parents according to article 7 in the UN convention the Rights of the Child has also been referred to in these discussions as an argument against donor insemination for single women.

Finally, in 2013, the government appointed a special investigator – the Committee on Increased Possibilities to Address Involuntary Childlessness – to examine several questions concerning assisted reproduction.[79] The committee was, among other tasks, asked to submit suggestions that would enable single women to access ART to the same extent as married and cohabiting couples.[80] The result was the interim report *Assisted Fertilization for Single Women* in 2014,[81] which led to a government bill in 2015.[82] The conclusion was that a general ban for single women's access to ART was no longer justified.[83] The Parliament accepted the proposed legislation in January 2016, and the law came into force 1 April 2016. The law had wide support in Parliament; all political parties endorsed it except the Christian Democrats and the Sweden Democrats, both on the conservative end of the political scale.

An explanation expressed in the preparatory work for the development of the legislation was the change in society: the prevalent values and the attitude towards the traditional family had shifted. Family forms had changed, and single parenthood was no longer socially stigmatized. In addition, it was pointed out that many women go abroad to have donor insemination. It was also pointed out that there are no indications in research that a child with a single parent has a less favorable upbringing than a child with two legal parents.

When the law came into force, IVF was only permitted with the use of an egg from the single woman due to the requirement of a genetic tie to at least one of the parents. This changed from 1 January 2019 through the amendments to the Genetic Integrity Act accepted by the Parliament in June 2018. A genetic tie to one of the parents is no longer a requirement.[84]

The following applies regarding determination of parenthood where a woman has undergone assisted fertilization while single. The basic premise is that there is no need to determine paternity or parenthood if the mother has undergone insemination or IVF under the Genetic Integrity Act. She will be the child's only parent if she was single at the time of treatment in accordance with Chapter 1, Section 5, of the Act and it is likely, in view of all of the circumstances, that the child was conceived through the treatment. However, if any of the conditions are not fulfilled, paternity shall be determined in accordance with general rules. This means that the sperm donor is given the opportunity to confirm paternity on a voluntary basis subject to the consent of the mother of the child or if the child, if he or she has reached the age of majority, approves of the confirmation.[85]

Reflections on the second phase of legislation – equal treatment

Central principles throughout the process of developing legislation on ART in Sweden are equal access to health care on equal conditions, autonomy and the right to self-determination, non-discrimination, informed consent, the principle of the child's best interest and the principle of caution.[86] The first legislation on ART in place in 1985 and 1988 highlighted and protected the interests of the child and the principle of caution. This was done by giving the child a right to access identifying information about the donor, by limiting the treatment to certain clinics and by control of the future parent's abilities to give the child a good upbringing. Later on, equal treatment as an argument for the expansion of the use of ART gained momentum. Equal treatment as an argument was visible already in the discussion concerning egg donation but increased in weight in a society where equal treatment of men and women has long been a prominent political goal. However, it has also been the argument that has caused public and parliamentary debate, albeit limited. Proponents of a more traditional view of the family unit refer to the child's right to a mother and a father when opposing the extension of the use of different methods of assisted reproduction. This argument has not carried much weight in view of the fact that around 25% of children in Sweden grow up in one-parent families.

And now – parenthood for the involuntarily childless

The 2019 reform of the Genetic Integrity Act – background

After presenting the report on access to ART for single women in 2014, the Committee on Increased Possibilities to Address Involuntary Childlessness continued its work. Major questions that remained for consideration were the use of combined donated reproductive cells from man and woman, embryo donation and surrogacy arrangements. The establishment of legal parenthood following ART with donated cells also needed consideration.

The committee published the final report, *Different Ways to Parenthood*, in February 2016.[87] It suggested allowing for IVF with a combination of donated egg and sperm and embryo donation by couples themselves going through fertility treatment. In addition, it was suggested that treatment should be available at more health facilities than before. The committee did not propose that surrogacy arrangements should be allowed. The proposal from the committee also included recommendations concerning the establishment of legal parenthood for children conceived through different methods for assisted reproduction. Around 100 different authorities, courts, universities and organizations received the report for comments. Following the referral of the committee report, the government in March 2018 presented a bill to the Parliament with amendments that closely followed the recommendations of the committee. The bill was accepted by the Parliament in June 2018 and the amendments entered into effect on 1 January 2019.

The new amendments to the Genetic Integrity Act and the Children and Parent Code confirm that ART are no longer seen as means to alleviate medical obstacles to parenthood "the natural way" but rather as a means to make it possible for those who want to become parents to do so. This attitude towards the use of ART is first visible with the permission for lesbian couples to access donor insemination in 2005 and later on when single women received the same right in 2015. The new amendments expand the use of ART with donated gametes, indicating that genetic kinship is of little importance for the relationship between children and parents. Against this background, it is interesting to notice that reforms of the rules concerning legal parenthood in order to strengthen the child's right to access knowledge of genetic origin have resulted in an emphasis on genetic kinship that is difficult to reconcile with the emphasis on social parenthood. This will be elaborated on in the following.

Combined donation and embryo donation

Combined donation

One of the questions the committee had to consider was whether there is reason to mandate a genetic tie between a child and the prospective parents.[88] Ever since the first introduction of legislation in 1985, ART has only been allowed using the couple's own gametes or with donated egg or donated sperm, not both.[89] A genetic link with one of the prospective parents has been considered necessary in order to protect the best interest of the child. This position was further strengthened by the opinion of the Ethics Council in a report in 1995, when the majority of the council stated that ART with donated gametes from two donors should not be permitted. The reasons were, according to the council, that the acceptance of a method resulting in no genetic links between the child and the parents could be perceived as too far reaching a way to compensate for the shortcomings of nature through technical solutions.[90] At the referral of the report, a majority of the commentators agreed with the majority of the Ethics Council. However, there were quite a few that concurred with the suggestion of the council minority that egg and sperm donation combined should be accepted, arguing that combined donations was comparable to adoption and that pregnancy, birth and the first hours following birth are important for the attachment between mother and child. The subsequent government bill in 2001 concerning egg donation nevertheless maintained the ban on combined donations. The reasons stated were the risk of a technical view on procreation and the risk of an objectification of reproductive cells, something that could lead to an undesirable technified view of human beings.[91]

After 2001, several motions in the Parliament called for permitting ART with donated egg and sperm. For a long time, the motions were rejected by the Parliamentary Committee on Health and Welfare and subsequently by the Parliament.[92] The government finally in 2013 appointed the Committee on Increased Possibilities to Address Involuntary Childlessness with the task to investigate, among other questions, the use of combined donation of reproductive cells.

In its final report in 2016, the committee suggested that the use of combined donation of reproductive cells should be permitted and hence that the requirement of genetic link between parent and child be abolished. The committee had done a thorough investigation on the possible effects on the children resulting from the use of only donated gametes and concluded that available knowledge did not indicate any risks for children conceived through this method.[93]

The use of combined donation of cells is only to be permitted if there is a need for the treatment and when the risks to the parties involved, especially to the child, can be regarded as acceptable. The treatment should also be medically justified.

Embryo donation

After reaching the decision to allow for combined donation, the question of embryo donation was brought to the fore. The committee found no reason to object to this type of ART but set up certain conditions. Couples or single women who have gone through IVF treatment themselves can donate fertilized eggs. A requirement for donation of fertilized eggs is that they have been created from the egg or sperm from the donor couple. If the donor is a single woman, the embryo must come from her own eggs. The reason for this requirement is that it would not be appropriate if the child could have genetic siblings in an unlimited number of families.[94] Another requirement for donation is that the donor couple or the woman be the parent(s) of at least one child. Situations where the donor remains childless while the recipient of the embryo will have a child from the donated embryo can be prevented with this requirement.[95] In all other respects, the current rules that apply to donation for fertilization outside the body shall apply equally here.[96]

In an attempt to simplify the process for involuntarily childless individuals or couples to become parents, the previous limitation of the number of clinics providing ART with donated gametes has been abolished.[97] Such a treatment can now be provided by clinics other than university hospitals after receiving approval from the Health and Social Care Inspectorate (*Inspektionen för vård och omsorg*).

The child's right to knowledge about genetic origin

The amendments to the regulation concerning ART also address the donor child's right to information. On request, children conceived through donated reproductive cells can give consent in writing to disclose information about them to other people conceived through reproductive cells from the same donor or donors. Similarly, a donor-child should be able to access details and information about other donor-siblings. On request, the social welfare committee is obliged to assist a person who is not certain but has reasons to suppose that he or she has been conceived through a treatment using donated cells in finding out whether any further details are noted in a separate record.[98] There is also a provision in the Children and Parents Code stating that the parents to a child conceived through assisted reproduction with donated gametes are obliged to inform the child about this.[99]

Surrogacy arrangements – still not permitted

As with questions concerning single women's access to ART and embryo donation, the question about surrogacy arrangements has been on the political agenda for some time. Surrogacy arrangements were discussed already by the Insemination Committee in their first report in 1983 on insemination and further elaborated in the report on IVF in 1985. The Insemination Committee declared that surrogate motherhood was, in their opinion, a most dubious phenomenon, mainly with regard to its character of bargaining over children. If surrogacy arrangements were to be allowed, several legislative changes to the then-current legal system were necessary in order to create guarantees for the prospective child. Some of these amendments would be in conflict with the legal perception of parenthood. Even though surrogacy arrangements could be helpful to some couples, the Insemination Committee did not find reason to consider such changes.[100] At the time, there was general political and societal consensus regarding this view. The question of surrogacy arrangements was again discussed in the Ministry report in 2000 on treatment of involuntary childlessness.[101] The conclusion was again that surrogacy arrangements should not be permitted. Several reasons were stated for this conclusion, such as the difficulties of legally regulating questions of parenthood and to protect the surrogate mother's legal position. It was also declared that it was contrary to human dignity to use another human being in order to solve the involuntary childlessness of couples and furthermore that surrogacy arrangements were not desirable from the child's perspective.[102]

During the last decade, several Parliament members have made motions in the Parliament suggesting that an investigation of surrogacy arrangements should be done. The arguments have been that since it is a complicated question, more knowledge is needed and that it is not self evident what is ethically acceptable. The calls for an investigation have been supported by the fact that during the last years, many Swedish couples have made surrogacy arrangements abroad and that children conceived in this way are placed in a very insecure legal position concerning legal parentage. Calls for an investigation were, however, for a long time rejected by the Parliament.[103]

The Committee on Increased Possibilities to Address Involuntary Childlessness was finally given the assignment to take a stand on the issue of whether surrogate motherhood should be allowed in Sweden, assuming that, if allowed, it should be altruistic. Independently of the question of allowing surrogacy arrangements according to Swedish law, the committee should also consider if there is a need for special rules for the establishment of legal parenthood to children born through surrogate motherhood abroad.[104]

The committee found that commercial surrogacy arrangements should not be permitted in the Swedish health system and that society should counter that type of arrangements. The committee was also of the opinion that altruistic surrogacy should not be allowed despite acknowledging that there would be advantages to allowing it within the Swedish system. Allowing altruistic surrogacy arrangements would enable involuntarily childless people to become parents, and the Swedish legislation could provide security and better guarantees for the involved parties than what is the case in many of the countries where it is possible to have children through surrogate arrangements. The child's right to knowledge about origin and parents could also be safeguarded. The committee, however, concluded that the disadvantages were greater that the advantages. The committee found that there are serious gaps in knowledge regarding the consequences for a child born in a surrogacy arrangement, as well as concerning the surrogate mother's own children. There could also be a risk of pressure and commercialization. A third disadvantage was attributed to the application of the mater est rule and the possibilities of the surrogate mother to change her mind once the child is born.[105]

The government accepted the recommendations of the committee, and no changes to the law were proposed. The same rules as before apply. There is no explicit ban on surrogacy arrangements as such, but contracts concerning surrogacy arrangements are not legally recognized in Sweden. The woman giving birth is the legal mother, and paternity is established according to the general rules, which makes it possible for the genetic father to be identified as the child's legal father. His wife or cohabitee will then have to adopt the child in order for them to reach joint legal parenthood.

Despite declaring that there was no reason to legislate in order to protect children born abroad through surrogacy arrangements, the committee nevertheless suggested changes in the law regulating the establishment of paternity for children born abroad. The Social Welfare Committee in every municipality is obliged to assist in the establishment of paternity to children born by an unmarried mother if the child has residence in Sweden, that is, if the mother is residing in Sweden. No such obligation has existed when the child is born abroad, even if the father is Swedish. Through changes in the Law on International Paternity Issues, Swedish authorities, the Social Welfare Committee and courts can now, after 1 January 2019, under certain conditions, establish paternity for a Swedish man who is the genetic father of a child born abroad through a surrogacy arrangement, even when the child remains abroad.[106] Once paternity is established, the child can acquire a Swedish passport and hence enter Sweden. The regulation can be criticized for making an unjustified difference between genetic fathers and genetic mothers. It is, however, a reflection of the current regulation of the establishment of paternity in Swedish law.

Legal parenthood after assisted reproduction with donor

In order to protect the right of the child to access knowledge of his or her genetic origin, the rules for establishing paternity after donor insemination outside of the Swedish health care system have been altered. Paternity to children conceived before 1 January 2019 is established according to the old rules. This means that the husband or cohabitee of the woman giving birth is considered the legal father of the child conceived through ART with donated sperm if he has given his consent to the treatment. His paternity is established through the pater est rule, voluntary confirmation or court decision. If he has consented to the treatment, he cannot have his paternity revoked.

According to the new law, this rule will be applicable only when the donor insemination has taken place in Sweden and according to the Genetic Integrity Act or at a competent health care facility abroad, and the child conceived through the treatment has a right to information about the identity of the donor. In other cases, if the child is conceived through treatment abroad without the right to knowledge about the donor or through at-home insemination, the child's genetic father, that is, the donor, is considered the father and should if possible be legally identified as such.[107] The only way for a consenting man or woman to become the child's second parent is through adoption.[108] The same rules now apply to couples of the same or different sexes who become parents through ART abroad.

If paternity has been established in non-conformity with the rules, as could be the case when paternity is established through the pater est rule, the paternity can without limitations in time be revoked by the legal father; the child; or, if the child is underage, the child's custodian. The somewhat surprising conclusion is that if the child cannot have access to the donor's identity, there should be no legal father![109]

Concluding remarks

The initiative towards legislation concerning ART in Sweden came from the medical profession. This also meant that for a long time, the question of ART was perceived as a medical matter, and the discussion concerning the different methods was concentrated to the medical sphere. Even though there were different opinions on the formulation of the first regulation, the Insemination Committee managed to set the framework guarding the interests of the child in a way that for a long time guided the following development. The initially relatively limited public and parliamentary discussion concerning ART in Sweden can also be understood in light of the process preceding any new legislation. The legislative process in Sweden traditionally takes a long time because of the wide and extensive consultation procedures applied. In all instances when new methods are subject to regulation, the government has appointed a Parliamentary committee or commission. The committees have regularly been given the task to thoroughly investigate a question, organize hearings and collect available research concerning the matter at hand. Resulting reports are sent to different organizations and authorities for comments that are then considered, although not always followed, when formulating the government bills. The bills are then submitted to the Parliamentary Committees; in the case of ART, usually to the Parliamentary Committee for Health and Welfare, where parliamentarians from all parties discuss the proposals. When a government bill finally reaches the Parliament for decision, there is usually firm parliamentary support for the bill.

The discussion on what methods that can be allowed within the Swedish health care system has thus been rather limited and for a long time carried out within the medical framework. The legislation can be characterized as restrictive to the use of ART with donated gametes and has from the first legislation in 1985 underlined that the best interest of the child should be the guiding principle. This has been interpreted as the protection of the rights of the child to two legal parents, one genetic parent and a right to access information about genetic origin. During the following decades, the emphasis has shifted to a more open view on the right to become parents and equal treatment of women and men regardless of family forms. One by one, the original requirements set up to protect the best interest of the child have been abandoned, and today the best interest of the child is basically defined as the right to information about the donor.

Though the regulation of ART in Sweden has undergone substantial reforms in recent decades, it is noticeable that these changes have not evoked much public controversy or criticism. One possible explanation for this lack of public debate may be that some matters of family life are not generally discussed widely in Swedish society but rather are often treated as highly personal matters. For many individuals and couples, the fact that ART is a medical matter may have further reinforced the impulse to keep such discussions relatively private. In addition, in matters of public policy over the last century, a bedrock principle of Swedish law and society has been that the government should not propose rapid or radical law reforms that are not accepted by a broad consensus among the people as a whole. From this perspective, the slow and steadfast nature of the legislative process in Sweden may be respected and accepted as a necessity, particularly when it promotes a sense of socio-political fairness and stability while the government adjusts to and accommodates evolutions in public opinion.

Nevertheless, a final explanation of the lack of public discourse over ART reforms may be that many Swedish individuals and couples dissatisfied with regulation have respected the political process by choosing to travel quietly and privately abroad for ART that is not available at home, whatever legal risks or difficulties that may have entailed. The willingness of Swedish citizens and residents to travel for ART while waiting for reform may be seen as a "middle way" – generally trusting that the government and legislature will eventually come to the right political decisions over time, while those who have the will or means to travel may be able to privately mitigate the costs of waiting through the legislative process to form their families through ART until such reforms come to pass.

Swedish abbreviations

Prop. Government bill (*proposition*)
SOU Swedish Government Official Report Series (*Statens offentliga utredningar*)
NJA Periodical containing cases reported from the Swedish Supreme Court (*Nytt juridiskt arkiv*)
Ds Ministry Publication Series (*Departementsserien*)
Bet. Parliamentary Committee Report
Dir. Committee directives

Notes

1 Government Bill, Prop. 1984/85:2 on artificial insemination (*om artificiella inseminationer*).
2 Government Bill, Prop. 1987/88:160 on in-vitro-fertilization (*om befruktning utanför kroppen*).
3 Government Bill, Prop. 2005/06:64 Genetic integrity etc. (*Genetisk integritet m.m.*).
4 Assisted reproductive technology.
5 Government Bill, Prop. 2017/18:155 Modern rules on assisted fertilization and parenthood (*Modernare regler om assisterad befruktning och föräldraskap*).
6 Government Bill, Prop. 2014/15:127 Assisted fertilization for single women (*Assisterad befruktning för ensamstående kvinnor*).
7 See, among other, Swedish Government Official Report, SOU 2014:29 Assisted fertilization for single women (*Assisterad befruktning för ensamstående kvinnor*); Swedish Government Official Report, SOU 2016:11 Different ways to parenthood (*Olika vägar till föräldraskap*) and Parliamentary Committee on Health and Welfare, bet. 2017/18:SoU20 Modern rules on assisted fertilization and parenthood (*Modernare regler om assisterad befruktning och föräldraskap*).
8 I thank LL.M. Mohima Munin for valuable help assembling background material for this chapter.
9 Swedish Government Official Report, SOU 1953:9 Proposal to legislation about insemination p. 15. (*Förslag till lagstiftning om insemination*) During the same period, 95 inseminations with sperm from the husband (AIH) was done, resulting in 16 pregnancies.
10 See Swedish Government Official Report, SOU 1983:42 Children conceived by artificial insemination, main report of the Insemination Investigation (*Barn genom insemination, Huvudbetänkande av inseminationsutredningen*) p. 50.
11 Swedish Government Official Report, SOU 1946:49 Inheritance Code expert's proposal to the Children and Parent Code (*Ärvdabalkssakkunnigas förslag till föräldrabalk*) p. 64.
12 Swedish Government Official Report, SOU 1953:9, pp. 63–64.
13 Swedish Government Official Report, SOU 1983:42, p. 34.
14 Swedish Government Official Report, SOU 1953:9, pp. 56–57.
15 Swedish Government Official Report, SOU 1983:42, p. 34.
16 Swedish Government Official Report, SOU 1983:42, p. 25.
17 Supreme Court Case NJA 1983, p. 320.

182   *Anna Singer*

18 See e.g. Swedish Government Official Report, SOU 1983:42, p. 68.
19 Swedish Government Official Report, SOU 1983:42, p. 58; Government Bill, prop. 1984/85:2, p. 7.
20 Swedish Government Official Report, SOU 1983:42, p. 74.
21 Swedish Government Official Report, SOU 1983:42, pp. 68–70.
22 Swedish Government Official Report, SOU 1983:42, p. 205. (Author's translation.)
23 Follows from the Genetic Integrity Act ch. 6.
24 Since 2016, single women can receive donor insemination. In such a case, no consent from a second parent is necessary. See section "Single women's right to access donor insemination and IVF-treatment".
25 Government Bill, prop.2004/05:137 Assisted reproduction and parenthood (*Assisterad befruktning och föräldraskap*).
26 Recent changes of the rules concerning the establishment of paternity are described in section "Legal parenthood after assisted reproduction with donor".
27 Swedish Government Official Report, SOU 1983:42, p. 204. (Author's translation.)
28 Swedish Government Official Report, SOU 1983:42, p. 45.
29 Swedish Government Official Report, SOU 1983:42, pp. 116–124.
30 Government Bill, Prop. 1984/85:2, p. 17.
31 Assisted reproduction in the Nordic Countries. A comparative study of policies and regulation. TemaNord 2006:505, pp. 20–22.
32 Swedish Government Official Report, SOU 1983:42, pp. 120–121.
33 Government Bill, Prop. 1984/85:2, pp. 15–17.
34 Q-IVF Nationellt kvalitetsregister för assisterad befruktning. Årsrapport 2017, pp. 10–11.
35 Swedish Government Official Report, SOU 1985:5 Fertilization outside of the body. (*Befruktning utanför kroppen*).
36 Government Bill, Prop. 1987/88:160.
37 Swedish Government Official Report, SOU 1985:5, p. 66.
38 Swedish Government Official Report, SOU 1985:5 i.a., p. 47.
39 Swedish Government Official Report, SOU 1985:5, pp. 38–39. (Author's translation.)
40 Swedish Government Official Report, SOU 1985:5, p. 66.
41 In 2015, this was done at 16 clinics in Sweden. Q-IVF Nationellt kvalitetsregister Årsrapport 2017. Available at www.qivf.se.
42 Parliamentary Committee Report, Bet. 1987/88:SoU26 on in-vitro-fertilization (*Social-utskottet, om befruktning utanför kroppen m.m.*).
43 Swedish Government Official Report, SOU 1983:42, p. 205.
44 Swedish Government Official Report, SOU 1985:5, p. 65.
45 Bet. 1993/94:SoU2, pp. 9–10. Some ethical issues (*Vissa etiska frågor*).
46 Regeringsbeslut 1994–06–23 nr 34.
47 SMER, Assisted fertilization. Comments on certain issues related to fertilization outside of the body. (*Assisterad befruktning. Synpunkter på vissa frågor i samband med befruktning utanför kroppen*).
48 Ministry Publication Series, Ds 2000:51 Treatment of involuntary childlessness (*Behandling av ofrivillig barnlöshet*) p. 17.
49 Government Bill, Prop. 2001/02:89, pp. 30–31.
50 Government Bill, Prop. 2001/02:89, p. 27.
51 Ministry Publication Series, Ds 2000:51, pp. 31–36.
52 Government Bill, Prop. 2001/02:89 Treatment of involuntary childlessness (*Behandling av ofrivillig barnlöshet*).
53 Government Bill, Prop. 2001/02:89, p. 50. In 2015, this was done at seven clinics in Sweden. Q-IVF Nationellt kvalitetsregister Årsrapport 2017. Available at www.qivf.se.
54 Government Bill, Prop. 2001/02:89, p. 23.

55 Government Bill, Prop. 2001/02:89, p. 55.
56 Government Bill, Prop. 2001/02:89, pp. 57–59.
57 Socialstyrelsen, (2012) Officiell statistik. Graviditet, förlossningar och nyfödda barn. Assisterad befruktning 1991–2009.
58 Q-IVFFertility treatments in Sweden. National report 2020, p. 24.
59 Swedish Government Official Report, SOU 1984:63 Homosexuals and society (*Homosexuella och samhället*); Government Bill, Prop. 1986/87:124 on the situation for homosexuals in society (*om de homosexuellas situation i samhället*).
60 Swedish Government Official Report, SOU 1993:98 Partnership (*Partnerskap*).
61 SOU 1993:98, p. 106.
62 Swedish Government Official Report, SOU 2001:10 Children in homosexual families. (*Barn i homosexuella familjer*) p. 18.
63 Swedish Government Official Report, SOU 2001:10, pp. 332–344.
64 Government Bill, Prop. 2001/02:123. Partnership and adoption. (*Partnerskap och adoption*). This required until 1 September 2018 that the couple be married or registered partners. Government Bill, Prop. 2017/18:121 Modern adoption rules (*Modernare adoptionsregler*).
65 Government Bill, Prop. 2004/05:137 Assisted reproduction and parenthood (*Assisterad befruktning och föräldraskap*).
66 Government Bill, Prop 2004/05:137, pp. 41–42.
67 The previous Registered Partnership Act from 1994 was abolished in 2009, making marriage gender neutral, Prop. 2008/09:80 Marriage matters. (*Äktenskapsfrågor*).
68 Government Bill, Prop. 2020/21:176 Modern rules for confirmation of parenthood, paternity examination and to achieve a gender neutral parenthood presumption (*Modernare regler för bekräftelse av föräldraskap, faderskapsundersökningar och för att åstadkomma könsneutral föräldraskapspresumtion*), pp. 23–33.
69 Government Bill, Prop. 2004/05:137, p. 44.
70 Parliamentary Committee Report, Bet. 2004/05:LU25 Assisted fertilization and parenthood (*Assisterad befruktning och föräldraskap*).
71 Government Bill, Prop. 1984/85:2.
72 Parliamentary Committee Report, LU 1985/86:10 on artificial insemination (*om artificiella inseminationer*).
73 Parliamentary Committee Report, LU 1985/86:10, p. 10.
74 Parliamentary motion, Motion 2005/06:L262 Assisted fertilization and egg donation (*Assisterad befrukting och äggdonation*).
75 Parliamentary committee report, Bet. 2005/06:LU9 Guardianship and Parenthood. (*Förmynderskap och föräldraskap*).
76 Parliamentary Committee Report, Bet. 2006/07:SoU8.
77 Parliamentary Committee Report, Bet. 2008/09:SoU13.
78 Parliamentary Committee Report, Bet. 2010/11:SoU9.
79 *Utredningen om utökade möjligheter till behandling av ofrivillig barnlöshet.* Parliamentary Committee Report, Bet. 2011/12:SoU26.
80 Government directives, Dir. 2013:70 Increased possibilities to address involuntary childlessness (*Utökade möjligheter till behandling av ofrivillig barnlöshet*).
81 Swedish Government Official Report, SOU 2014:29 Assisted fertilization for single women (*Assisterad befruktning för ensamstående kvinnor*).
82 Government Bill, Prop. 2014/15:127.
83 Government Bill, Prop 2014/15: 127, p. 12.
84 Government Bill, Prop. 2017/18:155.
85 Government Bill, Prop 2014/15:127, pp. 18–19.
86 Swedish Government Official Report, SOU 2016:11, pp. 233–234.
87 Swedish Government Official Report, SOU 2016:11. Summary in English, pp. 47–72.

88 Government directives, Dir. 2013:70.
89 Government Bill, Prop. 1984/85:2.
90 SMER, Assisterad befruktning. Synpunkter på visa frågor i samband med befruktning utanför kroppen, 1995. Supra note 48.
91 Ministry Publication Series, Ds 2000:51 2000:51 Treatment of involuntary childlessness. (*Behandling av ofrivillig barnlöshet*); Government Bill, Prop. 2001/02:89, p. 52.
92 See e.g. Parliamentary Committee Reports, bet. 2004/05:SoU 10; 2005/06:LU9; 2006/07:SoU8; 2008/09:SoU13; 2009/10:SoU11; 2011/12:SoU26; 2013/14:SoU10 and bet. 2014/15:SoU7.
93 Swedish Government Official Report, SOU2016:11, pp. 287–358. (in English pp. 49–50)
94 Government Bill, Prop. 2017/18:155, p. 31.
95 Government Bill, Prop. 2017/18:155, p. 32.
96 Swedish Government Official Report, SOU 2016:11, pp. 52–54.
97 Government Bill, Prop. 2017/18:155.
98 Genetic Integrity Act, ch. 6 s. 5 a and 5 b; Government Bill, Prop. 2017/18:155, pp. 36–38.
99 Children and Parents Code ch. 1 s. 15.
100 Swedish Government Official Report, SOU 1985:2, p. 50.
101 Ministry Publication Series, Ds 2000:51.
102 Government Bill, Prop. 2001/02:89, p. 55.
103 See i.a. Parliamentary Committee Reports, bet. 2004/05:SoU10; 2005/06:SoU16; 2008/09:SoU13; 2009/10:SoU11 and 2010/11:SoU9.
104 Government Directives, Dir. 2013:70.
105 Swedish Government Official Report, SOU 2016:11, pp. 57–59.
106 Law on International Paternity Issues s. 3 a and 5. Government Bill, Prop. 2017/18:155, pp. 44–49.
107 This was confirmed by the Svea Court of Appeal in 2016 in two cases where the children were conceived though an at-home insemination, cases T 7894–15 and T 7895–15.
108 Swedish Government Official Report, SOU 2016:11, pp. 569–579: prop. 2017/18:155.
109 This might, however, change. In 2020, yet another committee was appointed, Dir. 2020:132 A parental regulation for everyone (*En föräldraskapsrättslig reglering för alla*), with the task, among others, to decide whether the scope for revoking parenthood should be limited. The committee report is due in June 2022.

References

Government Bills

Prop. 1984/85:2 on artificial insemination (*om artificiella inseminationer*).
Prop. 1986/87:124 on the situation for homosexuals in society (*om de homosexuellas situation i samhället*).
Prop. 1987/88:160 on in-vitro-fertilization (*om befruktning utanför kroppen*).
Prop. 2001/02:89 Treatment of involuntary childlessness (*Behandling av ofrivillig barnlöshet*).
Prop. 2001/02:123. Partnership and adoption (*Partnerskap och adoption*).
Prop. 2004/05:137 Assisted reproduction and parenthood (*Assisterad befruktning och föräldraskap*).
Prop. 2005/06:64 Genetic integrity etc. (*Genetisk integritet m.m.*).
Prop. 2008/09:80 Marriage matters (*Äktenskapsfrågor*).
Prop. 2014/15:127 Assisted fertilization for single women (*Assisterad befruktning för ensamstående kvinnor*).
Prop. 2017/18:121 Modern adoption rules (*Modernare adoptionsregler*).

Prop. 2017/18:155 Modern rules concerning assisted fertilization and parenthood (*Modernare regler om assisterad befruktning och föräldraskap*).

Prop. 2020/21:176 Modern rules for confirmation of parenthood, paternity examination and to achieve a gender neutral parenthood presumption (*Modernare regler för bekräftelse av föräldraskap, faderskapsundersökningar och för att åstadkomma könsneutral föräldraskapspresumtion*).

Parliamentary committee reports

Bet. 1987/88:SoU26. on in-vitro-fertilization (*om befruktning utanför kroppen m.m.*)

Bet. 1993/94:SoU2 Some ethical issues (*Vissa etiska frågor*)

Bet. 2004/05:LU25 Assisted fertilization and parenthood (*Assisterad befruktning och föräldraskap*)

Bet. 2004/05:SoU10 Health care issues (*Hälso- och sjukvårdsfrågor*)

Bet. 2005/06:LU9 Parliamentary committee report 2005/06:LU9 Guardianship and Parenthood (*Förmynderskap och föräldraskap*).

Bet. 2005/06:SoU16 Genetic integrity etc. (*Genetisk integritet m.m.*)

Bet. 2006/07:SoU8 Health care issues (*Hälso- och sjukvårdsfrågor*)

Bet. 2008/09:SoU13 Health care issues (*Hälso- och sjukvårdsfrågor*)

Bet. 2009/10:SoU11 Health care issues (*Hälso- och sjukvårdsfrågor*)

Bet. 2010/11:SoU9 Health care and dental care issues (*Hälso- och sjukvårdsfrågor och tandvårdsfrågor*)

Bet. 2011/12:SoU26 Assisted fertilization (*Assisterad befruktning*)

Bet. 2013/14:SoU10 Health care issues (*Hälso- och sjukvårdsfrågor*)

Bet. 2014/15:SoU7 Health care issues (*Hälso- och sjukvårdsfrågor*)

Bet. 2017/18:SoU20 Modern rules on assisted fertilization and parenthood (*Modernare regler om assisterad befruktning och föräldraskap*)

Bet. LU 1985/86:10 on artificial insemination (*om artificiella inseminationer*)

Parliamentary motions

Motion 2005/06:L262 Assisted fertilization and egg donation (*Assisterad befruktning och äggdonation*)

Swedish Government Official Report series

SOU 1946:49 Inheritance Code Expert's proposal to the Children and Parent Code (*Ärvdabalkskakkunnigas förslag till föräldrabalk*).

SOU 1953:9 Proposal to legislation about insemination (*Förslag till lagstiftning om insemination*).

SOU 1983:42 Children conceived by artificial insemination, main report of the Insemination Investigation (*Barn genom insemination, Huvudbetänkande av inseminationsutredningen*).

SOU 1984:63 Homosexuals and society (*Homosexuella och samhället*).

SOU 1985:5 Fertilization outside of the body (*Befruktning utanför kroppen*).

SOU 1993:98 Partnership (*Partnerskap*).

SOU 2001:10 Children in homosexual families (*Barn i homosexuella familjer*).

SOU 2014:29 Assisted fertilization for single women (*Assisterad befruktning för ensamstående kvinnor*).

SOU 2016:11 Different ways to parenthood (*Olika vägar till föräldraskap*).

Ministry publication series

Ds 2000:51 Treatment of involuntary childlessness (*Behandling av ofrivillig barnlöshet*).

Government directives

Dir. 2013:70 Increased possibilities to address involuntary childlessness (*Utökade möjligheter till behandling av ofrivillig barnlöshet*).

Court case

Supreme Court Case NJA 1983 p. 320.
Svea Court of Appeal cases T 7894–15 and T 7895–15.

Authorities publications

Assisted reproduction in the Nordic Countries. A comparative study of policies and regulation. TemaNord 2006:505

National Board of Health and Welfare (*Socialstyrelsen*) Code of statutes SOSFS 1997:20 M

National Board of Health and Welfare (*Socialstyrelsen*) Code of statutes SOSFS 2012:20 M

National Board of Health and Welfare. (2012). Official Statistics. Pregnancies, birth and newly born. Assisted fertilization 1991–2009. (*Officiell statistik. Graviditet, förlossningar och nyfödda barn. Assisterad befruktning 1991–2009*).

National Board of Health and Welfare. Assisted fertilization. Statistics Health and disease 2003:3. (*Epidemiologiskt centrum, Assisterad befruktning. Statistik Hälsa och sjukdomar 2003:3*).

Q-IVF Nationellt kvalitetsregister för assisterad befruktning. Årsrapport 2017.

SMER, Assisted fertilization. Comments on certain issues related to fertilization outside of the body. (*Assisterad befruktning. Synpunkter på vissa frågor i samband med befruktning utanför kroppen*).

10 Expectations regarding the convergence of domestic laws on ART

Heleen Weyers[1]

Introduction

In the previous chapters, we presented the regulation of assisted reproductive technologies (ART) in eight European countries and the path that has been taken to get there. In essence, this legislation concerns the regulation of physicians' behavior: which techniques they are allowed to use under which circumstances. Whereas in the early years of the developments in many countries, physicians were mainly the ones who decided which techniques they would use and how to apply them, nowadays in all the countries of the European Union, governments have taken part of the control.

In the country reports, at least two trends can be seen. First, all countries in which heterologous insemination is allowed started with anonymous donation. At the end of the 1980s, countries started to ban anonymous donation of gametes. The first country that prohibited clinics from carrying out insemination with the semen of an anonymous donor explicitly in a law was Sweden (1988), followed by Austria (1992), the Netherlands (2004) and Germany (2017). The Czech Republic, Denmark, Italy and Poland don't prohibit anonymous donation.[2] Second, in the beginning, only heterosexual married couples received ART treatment. This started to change in the 1990s by also allowing cohabiting heterosexual couples access. Nowadays, in five countries of our sample, lesbian couples also have formal access: the Netherlands (2000), Sweden (2005), Denmark (2006), Austria (2015) and Germany.[3]

In this chapter, I seek to answer the question of whether we can expect convergence of formal domestic laws regarding two topics of ART regulation: non-anonymous donation and access for lesbian couples to ART in our eight countries (and in the European Union in general). To answer the questions, I will test two propositions: first, the proposition that European law leads to convergence of domestic law (Koffeman, 2015; McGleenan, 1999) and, second, Kurzer's (2001) proposition that changes in the values of citizens in European countries lead to convergence of domestic law.[4]

After going into the two propositions, I will discuss value change as a driving force of the convergence of domestic law; thereafter, the role of the European

DOI: 10.4324/9781003223726-10

Court of Human Rights (ECtHR) on convergence will be discussed, and in the last section, I will answer the research question.

Two propositions regarding convergence of domestic laws

European law leads to convergence of domestic laws

That convergence of domestic laws regarding ART is to be expected is argued by McGleenan (1999). His argument is that the jurisprudence developed by the European Court of Justice (ECJ) in relation to Articles 59 and 60 of the Treaty of Rome (nowadays Articles 56 and 57 of the Treaty of the Functioning of the European Union – TFEU)[5] generates a structural downward pressure in a way that means ultimately, any regulation in Europe in relation to reproductive technology will gravitate towards the most liberal laws available.

To illustrate this, McGleenan uses the example of the British case of Mrs. Blood, who wanted to use the sperm of her deceased husband. She asked permission to take the sperm to Belgium to get pregnant. By applying British law, the Human Fertilization and Embryology Authority (HFEA) refused to give this permission.[6] Mrs. Blood appealed, referring to the Treaty of Rome, in particular Article 59. She thought she could do so because in an Italian case, the ECJ had ruled that

> The freedom to provide services includes the freedom, for the recipients of services, to go to another member state in order to receive a service there, without being obstructed by restrictions, even in relation to payments, and that tourists, persons receiving medical services and persons traveling for the purpose of education or business, are to be regarded as recipients of services.
>
> (McGleenan, 1999, p. 278)

That ART might be seen as a service could be deduced from a ruling of the ECJ in 1991 regarding abortion. The ECJ concluded that abortion "is a medical activity which is normally provided for remuneration and may be carried out as part of professional activity and can be seen as a service" (McGleenan, 1999, p. 278). And, indeed, the Court of Appeal decided that the HFEA had given inadequate consideration to the effect of Article 59 on the right of Mrs. Blood to freedom of movement in order to obtain a service.

Thus, domestic law in the countries of the European Union cannot stop people crossing borders to receive ART services which are prohibited in the country of origin, and according to McGleenan, this will automatically lead to changes in domestic laws to adapt to the new situation.

Koffeman (2015), who researched reproductive law in three countries (Germany, Ireland and the Netherlands), saw various kinds of reaction to cross-bordering for ART that prove McGleenan right, this time as a result of the European Convention for the Protection of Human Rights (ECHR) and the rulings of ECtHR.

Different from the TFEU, some articles of the ECHR which are important with respect to ART – and morality issues in general – leave states discretion for national differences. These articles are expressly formulated in relatively vague rights and freedoms. In this way, these rights and freedoms can be limited by countries, subject to the conditions set out in the articles. The main issue here is whether the restriction imposed by the contracting state is necessary in the interest of one of the objectives listed in the articles. The question of whether the restriction is sufficiently justified is ultimately answered by the ECtHR. In these answers, the ECtHR often uses the "doctrine of margin of appreciation".[7] If the court grants the margin of appreciation, it holds back. This means that the converging effect of the ECHR/ECtHR is less sure than that of the TFEU.[8]

Koffeman develops one argument against the necessary convergence of ART regulation: outsourcing the law. Outsourcing, according to Koffeman (2015), is not so much expressly voiced at the national level but is an implication of an approach taken by the ECtHR in the case *A, B and C v. Ireland* (2010). In this case, the court ruled that the prohibition of abortion for health and well-being reasons did not exceed the margin of appreciation accorded in that respect to Ireland. The fact that Irish women could lawfully travel abroad for an abortion with access to appropriate information and medical care in Ireland was considered sufficient by the ECtHR as a minimum level of protection under the convention.[9]

With respect to ART, the ruling in *S.H. and Others v. Austria* (2011) is an example.

> the Court also observes that there is no prohibition under Austrian law on going abroad to seek treatment of infertility that uses artificial procreation techniques not allowed in Austria and that in the event of a successful treatment the Civil Code contains clear rules on paternity and maternity that respect the wishes of the parents. (see, mutatis mutandis, A, B and C v. Ireland, § 239)[10]

In the fourth section of this chapter, the positions of the ECtHR on donor anonymity and access for lesbian couples to ART will be discussed to see whether we can expect a convergence of formal regulation in our eight countries.

Changes in values lead to convergence of domestic law

McGleenan's arguments suggest that states are forced by EU law to adopt ART regulation that they reject. Kurzer (2001), who researched policies regarding abortion, alcohol and drugs, argues that open borders indeed lead to harmonization of domestic rules, but her overall conclusion differs from McGleenan's. She concludes that

> national peculiarities are shrinking and . . . a modest rate of cultural convergence has occurred. Dutch drug policy is becoming more punitive, Nordic

anti-drinking measures are liberalizing, and Irish attitudes towards abortion are softening.

(Kurzer, 2001, p. 2)

In Kurzer's opinion, the TFEU does not impose convergence; she considers national citizens the agents of change. Their thinking, for example, in Ireland on abortion, had altered, and the removal of borders created an opportunity to act according to their preferences. Until the completion of the European Union, authorities could ignore the emergence of new desires and habits among their populations. Cross-border movement drew attention to domestic rules, and the tensions and contradictions between law and societal norms became more overt (Kurzer, 2001, pp. 177–178). Kurzer's argument can be reformulated as: Changes in values are driving forces of convergence in formal domestic laws. The basic idea behind values as a driving force is the relation between the values of inhabitants of a country and its regulations. For example, if Polish people value the traditional family very much, one would not expect Polish law to abolish donor anonymity, and if the Dutch are very tolerant regarding homosexuality, one would expect Dutch law to allow lesbian couples access to ART. Therefore, if values regarding families, child rearing and homosexuality in European countries are moving in the same direction, one would expect domestic law to do the same.[11] The influence of changes in values on convergence of domestic laws will be discussed in the next section.

Values as a driving force

Changes in views on donor anonymity and access for lesbian couples take place in the context of a much broader change in family formations in Europe in general, which in their turn are part of even broader social changes such as individualiza-tion,[12] secularization,[13] changes in economic and employment structures[14] and the expansion of the welfare state (Tomka, 2013, p. 71).

With respect to households, we see a decline in size caused by a lower number of children and a higher number of people living alone. Not only has the size of households and their composition changed, a fundamental change regarding personal relations in families has taken place, too. Families became more egalitarian, and the autonomy of their members increased (Tomka, 2013, p. 71). Increasing equality was, among other things, caused by a rise in female employment. The autonomy of family members was stimulated by a changing attitude to children which can be characterized as increasing respect for children's personality and autonomy (Tomka, 2013, pp. 71–74). After the 1960s, we saw a pluralization of family forms. Not only did the number of divorces rise significantly, there was also a significant proliferation in cohabitation and extramarital birth.

According to Astor and Dompnier (2017), the countries in this book can be divided into three groups with respect to family values.[15] According to these authors, Denmark, the Netherlands and Sweden belong to one group ("liberal conception of family")[16] and Italy and Poland to another group ("compulsory coercive conception of family"[17]). Austria, the Czech Republic and Germany show split conceptions influenced by, among other factors, age and religious affiliation. For example, the older one becomes, the less liberal one is, and the sentiment of duty generally increases with age (Astor & Dompnier, 2017, pp. 17–20).

With this background information, I will now focus on two values which relate to lifting donor anonymity (opinions regarding important qualities in child rearing) and one that relates to access to ART for lesbian couples (opinions regarding acceptance of homosexuality).

Changing views on child rearing

It is said that the child, or at least what is meant by that nowadays, is a product of the 19th century. According to Ariès (1965), for example, children hardly formed a separate social category before that time (adult in pocket format). This idea changed after the appearance of Rousseau's *Emile* in 1762. The conviction took shape that children differ essentially from adults. Pedagogy and education became important themes, and the role of the state in the latter became ever greater.

In the 19th century, government interventions were aimed at protecting the child. In the 70s of the 20th century, the focus shifted from protection to liberation/emancipation. Children were entitled to more and more rights. An important example of this development is the United Nations Convention on the Rights of the Child.

The European Values Study (EVS) can inform us on changes in the qualities seen as important in rearing children. Halman et al. (2012) note that

> Because society continuously changes, upbringing does too. In many European countries, child rearing used to be predominantly about teaching discipline, obedience, good manners and respect for adults. However, in the modern, individualized society, upbringing is much more about personal attention for the child's emotional and personal development. Parents in post-modern societies emphasize qualities such as responsibility, respect, creativity, and independency because those are the virtues that support individual freedom and self-actualization.
>
> (Halman et al., 2012, p. 29)

Granting the right to know one's origins can be seen as an example of emancipation, an example of attention for the individual freedom and self-actualization of the child. Therefore, one would expect a country in which inhabitants consider self-actualization of the child important (a country in which obedience is less subscribed to and independence emphasized, to pick out two of the virtues mentioned in the quote) to ban anonymous donation and vice versa. In the following, I will present data from the EVS to show changes in time regarding the importance of obedience and independence, and I will link these changes to the presence of laws banning donor anonymity.

Table 10.1 shows that in most countries, a decline has occurred in the importance of obedience (the Czech Republic is an exception, an increase from 21% in 1990 to 35% in 2018) and an increase in the importance of independence.

Obedience as a quality important in the upbringing of children seems to be a value that is not seen as very important (the mean in 2018 is 17%; the highest percentage in 2018 is scored by the Czech Republic: 35%).[18] The greatest change happened in Poland: In 1990, 42% considered obedience an important quality, and in 2018, only 20% did so.

Many more inhabitants think of independence as an important quality for children (mean in 2018 is 63%; lowest percentage Poland: 29%). The range is also considerably larger: obedience between 7% – Sweden – and 35% – the Czech Republic (28%); independence between 29% – Poland – and 79% – Denmark (50%). Some countries show big changes regarding the importance of independence: Sweden with an increase of 50% in four decades, the Czech Republic 25% in three decades and the Netherlands 30% in four decades.

These data show the trend towards the autonomous child Halman et al. (2012) mentioned, but some countries (namely Austria, Denmark, Germany and Sweden) have progressed more in this direction (that is, they have lower scores on obedience and higher scores on independence) than others.[19]

If the postulated relation between values and domestic laws exists, one would expect these four countries to have banned donor anonymity in their domestic laws. And one would not expect Italy, Poland and to a lesser extent the Netherlands to have done so.[20] Therefore, five of seven countries (the Czech Republic is left out) fit the expectation, and two do not (Denmark, which did not prohibit anonymous donation, and the Netherlands, which did).

If we add other European countries[23] to the comparison, we see more or less the same relation between values regarding child rearing and laws prohibiting doctors to make use of anonymous donors.

Six[24] of the seven countries which lifted donor anonymity have a relatively low score on obedience and a relatively high score on independence.[25] Four of the six countries which did not enact such a law have relatively high scores on obedience and relatively low scores on independence.[26] Thus, a relation between values of child rearing and (not) lifting donor anonymity exists.

Changes in attitudes towards homosexuality

Regarding homosexuality, we also see a first wave of emancipation at the end of the 19th century. This change consists of identifying homosexuality as a physical illness or mental disorder rather than a morally reprehensible act (but sexual contacts between homosexuals remained illegal in many countries). The next step in normalization was the elimination of homosexuality from the Diagnostic and Statistical Manual of Mental Disorders and elimination from the internationally used list of diseases. Since then, emancipation of homosexuals has meant realizing equal rights. This includes same-sex marriage and/or civil union, the possibility of adoption for same-sex couples and access to ART.

Table 10.1 Changes in values regarding child rearing in percentages.

	Obedience[21]					Independence[22]				
	1981	1990	1999	2008	2018	1981	1990	1999	2008	2018
Austria*		26	17	14	15		65	70	65	69
Czech R		21	17	26	35		52	69	65	73
Denmark	14	20	14	14	10	55	81	81	79	78
Finland*		26	30	21	21		58	58	52	48
France	18	53	36	28	25	16	27	29	27	38
Germany*		23	12	12	11		72	70	71	76
Italy	27	34	28	32	22	22	31	41	39	43
Netherlands*	23	34	26	30	19	27	49	53	49	57
Norway*	26	31		21	14	53	86		86	87
Spain	30	43	49	29	42					47
Poland		42	32	32	20		12	22	40	29
Sweden*		20		15	7	18	36	69	65	68
Switzerland*		20		15	10		42		64	67

* Prohibition of using anonymous donors

Regarding the acceptance of homosexuality, two questions are asked in the EVS. One refers to the acceptance of homosexuals as neighbors, the other to the acceptance of homosexuality in general.

Table 10.2 shows a clear trend towards more acceptance of homosexuality between 1990 and 2018. In 2018, homosexuality is the least accepted in Poland (30% of the population would not want to have homosexual neighbors, and 59% considers homosexuality not justified). The Czech Republic follows at a distance

Table 10.2 Changes in values regarding homosexuality in percentages, five countries added.

	Objecting to homosexual neighbors[29]				#	Homosexuality is never justified[30]				
	1990	1999	2008	2018		1981	1990	1999	2008	2018
Austria*	43	25	24	12	(35)		66	42	37	23
Czech R	51	20	23	23	(52)		52	41	46	29
Denmark*	12	8	6	2	(10)	45	44	27	18	8
Finland*	25	21	13	12	(33)		52	47	29	21
France	24	16	6	7	(27)	66	51	34	29	20
Germany*	34	13	17	8	(23)		54	35	36	15
Italy	39	29	23	12	(38)	78	61	44		26
Netherlands*	12	6	10	3	(10)	37	21	13	14	7
Norway*	19		6	3	(12)	64	75		21	9
Poland	70	55	53	30	(89)		89	72	75	59
Spain*	30	16	5	3	(23)	74	59	33	28	20
Sweden*	18	6	7	3	(12)	54	53	17	18	9
Switzerland			7	6	(18)		53		27	12

* Allowing lesbian couples
# Adding the two percentages of 2018

(23% and 29%, respectively). Acceptance[27] is the highest in Denmark, the Netherlands and Sweden, followed by Germany, Austria and Italy.

The acceptance of homosexuality mirrors regulation that allows for more or less access to ART for homosexual couples. The most permissive countries – Denmark, the Netherlands and Sweden – have opened ART to lesbian couples by law. The least permissive countries – the Czech Republic and Poland – have not. Neither has one of the countries in the middle group: Italy. The two other countries in the middle group – Austria and Germany – do allow lesbian couples access to ART.

Adding the five European countries mentioned before results in the same picture. Norway belongs to the most permissive group[28] and allows access to lesbian couples. The other added countries belong to the middle groups. Two of these countries have no legal barriers to this access (Finland and Spain), while the other two have (France and Switzerland).

To round up

In Europe, there is a trend towards the autonomy of children and the acceptance of homosexuality, although the pace differs considerably. Furthermore, there is a relation between values regarding child rearing and enacting laws lifting donor anonymity and between changed values regarding homosexuality and the existence of domestic laws regarding access for lesbian couples.

Therefore, based on the results of the EVS, one would not expect Italy and Poland to change their laws on donor anonymity in the near future. Furthermore, from this viewpoint, Denmark not lifting donor anonymity is not easy to understand. The results from the Czech Republic are too diverse to base a prediction on. With respect to access for lesbian couples by law, Italy, France and Switzerland would be candidates in the near future.

Rulings of the ECtHR as a driving force

McGleenan (1999) takes the position that the TFEU forces convergence upon the domestic laws of the countries of the European Union. Koffeman (2015), with one exception (outsourcing), takes the same position regarding the ECHR. In this section, I test the proposition that the rulings of the ECtHR lead to the convergence of domestic laws with respect to ART.

With regard to ART regulation, and in particular the right to know one's origins and the right to access to ART for lesbian couples, Article 8 of the ECHR (the right to respect for private and family life) proved important in the rulings of the ECtHR. Article 8 is an example of a provision with vaguely formulated rights and obligations, and therefore an article in which the "margin of appreciation" plays an important role.[31] The article reads:

1)   Everyone has the right to respect for his private and family life, his home and his correspondence.
2)   There shall be no interference by a public authority with the exercise of this right except such as is in accordance with the law and is

necessary in a democratic society in the interests of national security, public safety or the economic well-being of the country, for the prevention of disorder or crime, for the protection of health or morals, or for the protection of the rights and freedoms of others.

Besides Article 8, Article 14 (prohibition of discrimination) has proven important with respect to ART. The article reads:

The enjoyment of the rights and freedoms set forth in [the] Convention shall be secured without discrimination on any ground such as sex, race, color, language, religion, political or other opinion, national or social origin, association with a national minority, property, birth or other status.

The ECtHR and lifting of anonymous gamete donation

With respect to lifting donor anonymity in cases of assisted insemination with donor semen, there is one ruling of the court (*X,Y and Z v. the United Kingdom* 1997). At that time, the court took into account that:

there is no consensus amongst member states of the Council of Europe on the question whether the interest of a child conceived in such a way [assisted insemination with donor seed] are best served by preserving the anonymity of the donor of sperm or whether the child should have the right to know the donor's identity (para 44).

Therefore, the court granted the states a wide margin of appreciation and did not rule that the United Kingdom had violated Article 8 of the ECHR.

The legal question that plays an important role in the background of the lifting of anonymous gamete donation is – as we have seen in the country reports – whether children have the right to know their genetic origins. After the ruling in *X, Y and Z v. the United Kingdom*, the ECtHR has considered this question a number of times. In principle, the court has taken the position that children do have that right. The court justifies this with the statement:

In the Court's opinion, persons in the applicant's situation have a vital interest, protected by the Convention, in receiving the information necessary to uncover the truth about an important aspect of their personal identity (para 64 in *Mikulić v. Croatia* 2002).[32]

In later cases, the court specifies the idea of necessary information. For example, in *Odièvre v. France* (2003), the court stated:

Matters of relevance to personal development include details of a person's identity as a human being and the vital interest protected by the Convention in obtaining information necessary to discover the truth concerning important aspects of one's personal identity, such as the identity of one's parents (para 29) . . . people have a right to know their origins (para 44).[33]

And when a state objects that the applicant's personality has been developed even without such knowledge (*Jäggi v. Switzerland* 2006), the court ruled:

> Although it is true that . . . the applicant . . . has been able to develop his personality even in the absence of certainty as to the identity of his biological father, it must be admitted that an individual's interest in discovering his parentage does not disappear with age, quite the reverse. Moreover, the applicant has shown a genuine interest in ascertaining his father's identity, since he had tried throughout his life to obtain conclusive information on the subject. Such conduct implies mental and psychological suffering, even if this has not been medically attested (para 40).[34]

In the cases mentioned, the court not only examined whether the interests of the child had been violated but also whether there were other interests at stake that made a violation defensible. Two themes were discussed: regulations regarding the establishment of paternity (*Mikulić v. Croatia*) and regulations concerning anonymous birth giving (*Odièvre v. France* and *Godelli v. Italy*).

In *Mikulić v. Croatia*, the ECtHR[35] ruled that Article 8 of the ECHR was violated because the Croatian legal system did not provide procedural measures to provide "alternative means enabling an independent authority to determine the paternity claim speedily" (para 64).[36]

Odièvre v. France and *Godelli v. Italy* concern cases of children whose biological mother had opted for anonymous birth-giving, a legal option in their home countries. In *Odièvre v. France*, the court addressed the motivation of the possibility of anonymous birth: the protection of the health of mother and child during pregnancy and birth, the prevention of (illegal) abortion and of abandonment without proper procedure.[37] The right to respect for life,[38] a higher-ranking value guaranteed by the Convention, is one of the aims pursued by the French system (para 45). The ECtHR ruled that

> France has not overstepped the margin of appreciation which it must be afforded in view of the complex and sensitive nature of the issue of access to information about one's origins. . . . Consequently, there has been no violation of Article 8 of the Convention.[39]

The court's decision in *Odièvre* has been heavily criticized (Besson, 2007, p. 151). It is good to know that the court was divided. Seven judges – out of 17 – wrote a joint dissenting opinion, and 4 judges disagreed on parts. The dissenting judges stated that the majority of the court did not balance the rights at stake correctly and gave absolute priority to the rights of the mother. According to Besson, the court has taken this critique seriously (among others in *Jäggi v. Switzerland*) and "has demonstrated its intention to review very closely the weighing-up of the right to know at national level".[40]

Thereafter, in *Godelli v. Italy* (2012), the court's assessment differs from the former ruling:

> The Court notes that, unlike the French system examined in Odièvre, Italian law does not attempt to strike any balance between the competing rights and interests at stake. In the absence of any machinery enabling the applicants' right to find out her origins to be balanced against the mother's interests in remaining anonymous, blind preference is inevitably given to the latter (para 57) . . . the Court considers that the Italian authorities failed to strike a balance and achieve proportionality between the interests at stake and thus overstepped the margin of appreciation which it must be afforded (para 58).[41]

Thus, according to the reading of the ECtHR, children have the right to know their origins (even if they have become adults). This appears quite a strong right, because the court takes the position that states should have proper regulation to guarantee this right to offspring. Nevertheless, specific rules, namely to respect life and proper procedure, can overrule the interests of the child to know its origins. Currently two French cases on the right to information regarding the donor are pending: *Gauvin-Fournis v. France* and *Silliau v. France*.[42] We have to wait to see whether the court balances the right in the same way as it did in the 1997 ruling.

The ECtHR and access to ART for same-sex couples

Regarding the access of same-sex couples to ART, a decision of the ECtHR of February 2013 is important (*X and others*[43] *v. Austria* 2013).[44] The ruling is not so much about access to ART but the access of same-sex couples to second-parent adoption. In this case, Article 14 is important (in addition to Article 8).[45]

The applicants complained that they were being discriminated against the enjoyment of their family life on account of the first and third applicants' sexual orientation. They submitted that there was no reasonable and objective justification for allowing the adoption of one partner's child by the other partner where different-sex couples, whether married or unmarried, were concerned while prohibiting the adoption of one partner's child by the other partner in the case of same-sex couples.

The Austrian government argued that the Austrian Civil Code aimed to recreate the biological circumstances of the family unit, that the margin of appreciation should be wide in the case of adoption and that no formal consensus in Europe existed on the issue of second-parent adoptions (para 147).

The court disagreed. Its ruling does not so much give same-sex couples a specific right but regards the difference in treatment between unmarried different-sex couples and same-sex couples with respect to this type of adoption. The court did so by arguing that if an unmarried heterosexual couple has a right to adoption, an unmarried same-sex couple in the same circumstances is discriminated against if it does not have such a right. With respect to the consensus in Europe, the court argued that only member states which allow second-parent adoption by unmarried couples may be regarded as a basis of comparison and that this sample is too small. Furthermore, their regulations differ so much that a conclusion regarding the existence of a possible consensus among the member states cannot be drawn (para 149). The court noted that the Austrian government did not have to extend second-parent adoptions to unmarried heterosexual couples, and because it did, it was required to justify why it didn't extend it to unmarried same-sex couples as well (para 141 and 142).

> The distinction is therefore incompatible with the Convention (para 151). . . .
> In conclusion, the Court finds that there has been a violation of Article 14
> of the Convention taken in conjunction with Article 8 when the applicants'
> situation is compared with that of an unmarried different-sex couple in which
> one partner wishes to adopt the other partner's child (para 153).[46]

The same reasoning is most likely also valid regarding access of same-sex couples to ART. In any case, shortly after the ECtHR ruling (January 2014), the Austrian *Verfassungsgericht* ruled that it is unconstitutional to deny lesbian couples access to artificial insemination with donor gametes.

> The reason given for the decision is essentially that there are no "particularly
> convincing or serious grounds" for this regulation, which discriminates against
> women in same-sex relationships, as required by the case-law of the European
> Court of Human Rights. The reason put forward by the legislator, namely the
> avoidance of the risk of surrogacy, does not apply to sperm donation.[47]

Regarding access to ART, we have seen that lesbian couples, in countries where unmarried (heterosexual) couples have access to ART, can make a successful claim to access under the prohibition of discrimination. It also seems to be the case that a country that no longer holds to the traditional situation – a married heterosexual couple with fertility problems – should better motivate a limitation of access to ART than a country that does.

To round up

The question of whether the ECHR has a converging effect cannot be answered in general. It is clear that the margin of appreciation plays an important role. With regard to Article 8, the margin is quite wide, but this is less the case regarding the right to know one's origins. This right is acknowledged, but so are balancing rights (namely respect for life regarding anonymous birth giving). With regard to Article 14, the margin of appreciation is smaller, causing differences to be justified rather precisely.

Yet something can be said about the converging effect. With regard to pedigree information, the case law shows that the court attaches great importance to such information. The court seems to assume that such knowledge is necessary for the development of one's own identity.

Furthermore, it has become clear that if states do not have their procedures in order, that is, if the procedures are unclear, rigid, unreasonably motivated or non-proportional, little discretion is granted, and the right of the child prevails. And finally, it has become plain that the court does not want to go so far as to give all children the right to descent information. Where a country had a good reason (for example, the prevention of baby killing), the court did not conclude that a violation of Article 8 had occurred. The same could become true with respect to donor information if states provide good reasons to keep donor anonymity and their procedures are well developed. In such cases, it is safe to assume that the court will not conclude a violation of the ECHR has occurred, and the Czech, Danish, Italian and Polish laws don't have to be changed. Therefore, a convergence of domestic laws is not to be an expected result of ECtHR case law.

With respect to access for lesbian couples to ART, the margin of appreciation seems to be quite small if a country has a formal regulation regarding same-sex couples such as marriage or civil union. A country needs a sound motivation for making a difference between these couples and different-sex couples. Italy and the Czech Republic do have civil unions for same-sex couples and don't allow lesbian couples access to ART. Law cases have to show whether their motivation suffices to make this difference. Poland does not allow same-sex marriage or civil union and can therefore adhere more easily to its exclusion of lesbian couples to ART.

Conclusions and discussion

In this chapter, I tested two propositions regarding the convergence of domestic ART laws in Europe. The first concerned a converging effect based on a change in the values that people hold, the second a converging effect of the rulings of the ECtHR. The first proposition is confirmed; the conclusion regarding the second is less clear.

I concluded that in Europe, trends towards the autonomy of the child and acceptance of homosexuality exist. The expected relations were found. Most countries with populations that value obedience relatively low and independence relatively high lifted donor anonymity (and vice versa). The same conclusions can be drawn regarding the relation between values about homosexuality and domestic laws providing lesbian couples access to ART. Therefore, with respect to values as a driving force, in principle, we can expect a convergence of formal laws on the topics of this study.[48]

Besides that, it became clear that the ECtHR considers the child's interest to know its origins very important but not always outweighing the importance of the rights and interests of others. It is not clear yet whether the ECtHR will rule against donor anonymity. With respect to access to ART for lesbian couples, we have seen that the ECtHR estimates whether states differentiate between heterosexual and lesbian couples in an appropriate way. States must provide good reasons for discriminating between different-sex and same-sex couples. Therefore, the relation between rulings of the ECtHR and the convergence of domestic laws is more ambiguous.

Gravitating to the most liberal laws?

McGleenan not only formulated a proposition regarding convergence, he also proposed the direction of the convergence: towards the most liberal laws. Unfortunately, McGleenan does not define the word "liberal". His examples point in the direction of laws which permit more, that is, regarding ART, allowing all kinds of techniques and giving access for everyone. With regard to the latter, one of the topics of this chapter, McGleenan seems to be right. After first only allowing married couples access, then unmarried heterosexual couples, followed by lesbian couples, access is being discussed for singles and homosexual male couples.

Lifting donor anonymity, however, does not fit easily within the category of liberal. Is it more liberal to grant doctors, parents and donors the freedom of anonymity, or is it more liberal to give children the right to know their origins? The chapter makes clear that lifting donor anonymity is related to more permissive societies and at the same time to the emancipation of children. The least we can conclude is that McGleenan is not right in all respects.[49] There are regulations concerning ART which cannot simply be described as liberal.

Values and free movement of people

Kurzer (2001) argued that it is not so much the TFEU that led to the convergence of domestic laws but that national citizens are the agents of change. Their values have changed, and the removal of borders created an opportunity to act according to their preferences. Austria can serve as a good example in this respect. We do not know for sure whether the ruling of the ECtHR was the reason for the Austrian *Verfassungsgericht* to declare denial of access to lesbian couples to ART unconstitutional. We do know, however, that this ruling fits very well within the change in accepting homosexuality among the Austrian people.

But if, in the near future, the court would rule anonymous semen donation in France a violation of Article 8 of the EHCR and France would change its law on the topic accordingly, we can expect from the EVS that the majority of the French public would not support such a change. Therefore, Kurzer's idea that the convergence of laws in the European Union is built on changes in values probably needs to be nuanced. Court rulings can have an impact, too.

Outsourcing the law

According to Koffeman (2015), there is another way out for states than changing their domestic laws to make them accord with the values of the majority of their citizens: outsourcing. This comes down to not changing the law, knowing that their inhabitants will find what they seek abroad. According to Penasa (2012, p. 304), this has happened in the European Union with respect to ART "moving from a normative particularism to an interconnected, multilevel and multilayered regulatory system". However, none of the country reports mentioned something that could be described as outsourcing. One of the reasons for this is brought up by Koffeman: Outsourcing the law is always implicit. That outsourcing plays a role is indirectly shown in the Swedish report when the legislature named the cross-bordering of lesbian couples as a reason to allow them formal access and in the observation of the ECtHR in *A.H. and Others v. Austria* (2011). Besides, one can wonder whether outsourcing is a lasting solution. Patients prefer to receive their medical treatment in their home country, and crossing borders for treatment is not accessible for everyone. If the acceptance of homosexuality in Italy keeps growing, Italian lesbian couples forced to go abroad for ART will accept less and less that they cannot have treatment in their own country, and pressures to adapt the law to the new standards of the population will grow (Kurzer's approach).[50]

"Predicting is very difficult, especially about the future"[51]

I come to two conclusions. With respect to access for lesbian couples, I see both changes in values and decisions of the ECtHR pointing in the same direction: formally opening access for lesbian couples to ART. However, because objections to homosexuality are (still) widespread in Poland and the Czech Republic and these countries do not allow same-sex marriage and the like, it is not to be expected that Poland and the Czech Republic will enact a change in the law in this respect in the coming decades.

With respect to donor anonymity, it is less clear whether we should expect convergence of domestic laws. It is not clear yet whether value orientations and decisions of the ECtHR point in the same direction. If the ECtHR rules that Gauvin-Fournis and Silliau have the right to know their origins, it would.

Notes

1 I would like to thank Erich Griessler, Florian Winkler and Nicolle Zeegers for thoroughly reading the chapter and providing me with very useful comments.
2 Insofar as they allow heterologous donation.
3 In Germany and the Netherlands, lesbian couples formally have access to ART because of the prohibition of discrimination; this access is not recorded in a specific law (see the country reports).
4 The basic, rather elementary idea behind this is that in democracies, regulation mirrors public opinion.
5 ARTICLE 56 TFEU:
    Within the framework of the provisions set out below, restrictions on freedom to provide services within the Union shall be prohibited in respect of nationals of Member States who are established in a Member State other than that of the person for whom the services are intended.

ARTICLE 57 TFEU:
    Services shall be considered to be "services" within the meaning of the Treaties where they are normally provided for remuneration, in so far as they are not governed by the provisions relating to freedom of movement for goods, capital and persons.
"Services" shall in particular include:
(a) activities of an industrial character; (b) activities of a commercial character; (c) activities of craftsmen; (d) activities of the professions.

> Without prejudice to the provisions of the Chapter relating to the right of establishment, the person providing a service may, in order to do so, temporarily pursue his activity in the Member State where the service is provided, under the same conditions as are imposed by that State on its own nationals.

6 www.globalhealthrights.org/wp-content/uploads/2013/03/EWCA-1997-R-v.-Human-Fertilisation-and-Embryology-Authority-ex-parte-Blood.pdf

7 Margin of appreciation refers to a certain margin or latitude in determining whether a member state has violated the Convention.

8 An argument that is not elaborated on in this chapter is that states don't always follow up on the rulings of the ECtHR (www.coe.int/en/web/execution/statistics#{%2234782408%22:[0]}).

9 https://hudoc.echr.coe.int/eng#{%22itemid%22:[%22001-102332%22]} para 239.

10 https://hudoc.echr.coe.int/eng#{%22itemid%22:[%22001-107325%22]} para 114.

11 This is a very general statement. Political structure and culture and specific important events can prevent a change in legislation.

12 "The increasing emphasis on the realization of the individuals' rights in relation to other entities". More specific in the context of family history, individualization means "that individuals are less willing to take on the responsibilities and commitments that marriage and family entail" (Tomka, 2013, p. 90).

13 Secularization stands for the reduction of the influence of religious ideas and the control of the church of family life and thus a gradual diminishing of traditional dispositions (Tomka, 2013, p. 90).

14 With respect to the latter, the increase of female employment is considered an important factor in the changes to family values (Tomka, 2013, p. 59).

15 Astor and Dompnier (2017, pp. 16–17) use four scales: One relating to family liberalism, one to family duties, one to family happiness and one to women's commitment to the household.

16 That accept very varied forms of family life (Astor & Dompnier, 2017, p. 13).

17 "The coercive compulsory category . . . is characterized by a very weak level of liberalism. . . . It combines a very strong sentiment of duty with the absence of recognition of the family as an indispensable factor [in] generating happiness" (Astor & Dompnier, 2017, pp. 15–16).

18 That is, 35% of Czechs consider this an important quality.

19 In 2018, these countries have scores below the mean regarding obedience (17%) and above the mean regarding independence (63%).

20 In 2018, these three countries have scores above the mean regarding obedience and below the mean regarding independence. The expectation regarding the Czech Republic is not clear because of its unique combination of scores on the two topics.

21 Taken from Luijkx et al. (2016, p. 36).

22 Taken from Luijkx et al. (2016, p. 27).

23 Three countries which lifted donor anonymity – Finland, Norway, Switzerland – and two countries which did not – France and Spain. Adding these countries changes the mean a little: obedience, almost 19%; independence, 58%.

24 Because the mean regarding obedience is a little bit higher by adding countries, the Netherlands satisfies the condition of belonging to the countries with relatively low scores on obedience and relatively high scores on independence.

25 Finland, with a relatively high score on obedience (21%) and a relatively low score on independence (48%), did not.

26 Exceptions which we have already seen are the Czech Republic and Denmark.

27 Ranking by adding the two percentages of each country in 2018.

28 By adding the scores in 2018, I arrive at four categories: 0–15; 15–30; 30–45; above 45.

29 Taken from Luijkx et al. (2016, p. 84).

30 Taken from Luijkx et al. (2016, p. 285).

31 As previously indicated, the "margin of appreciation" stands for the discretion of national governments.

32 https://hudoc.echr.coe.int/eng#{%22itemid%22:[%22001-60035%22]}.

33 https://hudoc.echr.coe.int/eng-press#{%22itemid%22:[%22003-698999-70736 8%22]}.

34 https://hudoc.echr.coe.int/eng#{%22itemid%22:[%22001-76412%22]}, the same in *Godelli v. Italy* 2013 para 56 (https://hudoc.echr.coe.int/eng#{%22itemid%22: [%22001-113460%22]}).

35 The case is about a mother and a child who wanted to confirm paternity of a certain man. The man managed to avoid paternity tests.

36 In *Jäggi v. Switzerland*, the interests of the deceased (and his family) were weighed against those of Jäggi. The Court stated that the interests of the latter were more important.

37 There are several countries with such schemes. Blauwhoff (2008) indicates that anonymous birth is lawful in Italy, Luxembourg, the Czech Republic and Hungary, and it is condoned in Germany, Austria and Switzerland. In Poland, this option also exists (Besson, 2007, p. 153).

38 Part of the exception mentioned in Article 8.2.

39 https://hudoc.echr.coe.int/eng-press#{%22itemid%22:[%22003-698999-70736 8%22]}. The Court held that the French system of anonymous birth balanced the right of the mother and the child. The Court could do so because France, after a law reform in 2002, encourages leaving non-identifying information for the child and that the mother is entitled to change her mind at a later date and reveal her identity (para 49).

40 Besson takes the position that in *Jäggi v. Switzerland*, the Court made the dissenting judges' opinion in *Odièvre* its own.

41 https://hudoc.echr.coe.int/eng#{%22itemid%22:[%22001-113460%22]}.

42 https://eclj.org/family/echr/gauvin-fournis-and-silliau-v-france-n-21424/16–n45728/17

43 Two same-sex couples filed the complaint.

44 https://hudoc.echr.coe.int/eng#{%22itemid%22:[%22001-116735%22]}.

45 That LGBT couples can claim family life (protected under Article 8) has become clear in former cases such as *X, Y and Z v. the United Kingdom* 1997. X and Y are a transsexual couple; Z is Y's child conceived by using AID. They ask for recognition of X as Z's father, which is refused by the British courts. (https://hudoc.echr.coe.int/eng#{%22ite mid%22:[%22001-58032%22]}).

> The Court recalls that the notion of 'family life' in Article 8 is not confined solely to families based on marriage and may encompass other de facto relationships. . . . When deciding whether a relationship can be said amount to 'family life' a number of factors may be relevant, including whether the couple live together, the length of their relationship and whether they have demonstrated their commitment to each other by having children together or by any other means. (para 36)

46 In *E.B. v. France* (2008), the Court took a similar decision with respect to a homosexual single woman:

> The Court points out that French law allows single persons to adopt a child (see paragraph 49 above), thereby opening up the possibility of adoption by a single homosexual, which is not disputed. Against the background of the domestic legal provisions, it considers that the reasons put forward by the Government cannot be regarded as particularly convincing and weighty such as to justify refusing to grant the applicant authorization. (para 94)

47 www.vfgh.gv.at/downloads/samenspende_presseinformation.pdf. The legislature was given time until the end of the year to change the legal situation, and, as we saw in the country report, that happened.

48 As mentioned in endnote 11, political structure and culture and specific important events which can prevent a change in legislation are not taken into account in this chapter.
49 As the quote from Kurzer shows, she also found that convergence is not always in the more liberal direction.
50 This will certainly not guarantee a change of law; the proximity of the Vatican could be a reason to prevent this.
51 Attributed to Niels Bohr.

References

Ariès, P. (1965). *Centuries of childhood: A social history of family life*. Vintage.

Astor, S., & Dompnier, N. (2017). A geography of family values in Europe. In P. Bréchon & F. Gonthier (Eds.), *European values: Trends and divides over thirty years* (Vol. 17, pp. 9–28). Brill.

Besson, S. (2007). Enforcing the child's right to know her origins: Contrasting approaches under the Convention on the Rights of the Child and the European Convention on Human Rights. *International Journal of Law, Policy and the Family, 21*(2), 137–159. https://doi.org/10.1093/lawfam/ebm003.

Blauwhoff, R. J. (2008). Tracing down the historical development of the legal concept of the right to know one's origins – has to know or not to know ever been the legal question? *Utrecht Law Review, 4*, 99–116.

Halman, L., Sieben, I., & Zundert, M. van. (2012). *Atlas of European values. Trends and traditions at the turn of the century* (Vol. 14). Brill.

Koffeman, N. R. (2015). *Morally sensitive issues and cross-border movement in the EU: The cases of reproductive matters and legal recognition of same-sex relationships* (1st ed., Vol. 72). Intersentia.

Kurzer, P. (2001). *Markets and moral regulation: Cultural change in the European Union*. Cambridge University Press.

Luijkx, R., Halman, L., Sieben, I., Brislinger, E., & Quandt, M. (2016). *European values in numbers: Trends and traditions at the turn of the century* (Vol. 16). Brill.

McGleenan, T. (1999). Reproductive technology and the slippery slope argument: A message in blood. In E. Hildt & S. Graumann (Eds.), *Genetics in human reproduction* (pp. 273–283). Ashgate.

Penasa, S. (2012). Converging by procedures: Assisted reproductive technology regulation within the European Union. *Medical Law International, 12*(3–4), 300–327. https://doi.org/10.1177/0968533213485749

Tomka, B. (2013). *A social history of twentieth-century Europe*. Routledge.

11 What drives the politicization of ART in Western and Northern European countries?[1]

Nicolle Zeegers

Introduction

Not all of the dilemmas and problems connected to assisted reproductive technologies (ART) become political issues addressed by political parties and discussed in the parliamentary arena. As exemplified by some of the country chapters, there are jurisdictions in which ART rules are decided on in subsystems of experts, such as the medical profession, or in case law. Engeli et al. (2012) made a similar observation about how morality issues in the broader sense are defined and decided: Whereas in some countries, these are addressed in the arena of parliamentary politics and lead to passionate debates between political parties, in other countries, these are left to expert committees to decide on. In an effort to explain such a difference, the authors formulated the "two worlds of morality politics theory" (TWMP) that ascribes these different approaches to a difference in the countries' political party system revolving around the question of whether this represents a religious-secular cleavage. This theory is confirmed in the cases of morality policies in the countries addressed in their compilation.[2] However, does it also fit with cases of ART policy as addressed in our compilation? After elaborating on the TWMP theory in "The two worlds of morality politics" section and explaining the concepts of morality issues and politicization in "Central concepts and their operationalization", the subsequent section will answer this question for three European countries: Austria, the Netherlands and Sweden. The comparison between the process of politicization of ART in Austria and the Netherlands will lead to the identification of some shortcomings in the TWMP theory. "Closing the gap in the theory" section, will discuss Euchner's (2019) effort to repair these shortcomings by enriching the TWMP theory with insights into wedge issue politics. Section 6 is the conclusion.

The two worlds of morality politics theory

Engeli et al.'s (2012, 2013) theory regards the political party system and in particular the question of whether a strong religious-secular cleavage is reflected in this system as a driving force for the politicization of morality issues (including ART) (Euchner, 2019). Whether a strong religious-secular cleavage in the previous sense

DOI: 10.4324/9781003223726-11

is present in a countries' political system is visible through strong Christian Democratic parties, such as the German CDU and the Dutch CDA, or Conservative
parties, such as the Spanish Partido Popular (Bonafont & Roqué, 2012). On the
basis of this criterion, Engeli et al. (2012, 2013) consider, for example, Germany
and the Netherlands countries belonging to the religious world, whereas Portugal
and the United Kingdom exemplify countries belonging to the secular world.

Engeli et al. (2012) found that this typology in terms of countries belonging to
the religious or secular world better explains differences in attention patterns on
morality issues than the classic typologies of political systems, such as consensus
versus majority democracy (Banchoff, 2005; Fink, 2009; Rothmayr et al., 2004;
Stetson, 2001). The TWMP theory claims to explain, first, the variety in attention
patterns in different countries and, second, divergence and convergence in policy
choices concerning ART and other moral issues.

The TWMP theory has found a very specific policy dynamic behind morality
policy in the religious world, a dynamic that, rather paradoxically, often leads to
relatively permissive policies in the countries belonging to this world. An integral
part of this dynamic is the strategy that Christian Democratic parties followed
from the 1960s onwards. These parties transformed themselves from a largely confessional voter base to broad catch-all parties in order to cope with the growing
secularization in society (Engeli et al., 2013; Van Kersbergen, 1999). Part of this
transformation was an 'unsecular' strategy, existing in a focus on family values and
the welfare state and in not mentioning religion as such (Engeli et al., 2013; Kalyvas & Van Kersbergen, 2010). The latter means that Christian Democratic parties
from that moment on often tried to avoid rather than appropriate morality issues.
By addressing such issues, they would run the risk of mobilizing the more confessional voters and grass-roots activists in their constituency and thereby threaten
the broad appeal of the party (Engeli et al., 2013). This risk and effort of Christian
Democratic parties to avoid morality issues became an incentive for contesting
secular as well as orthodox religious parties to politicize morality issues. Liberal
parties define and promote issues concerning ART in terms of secular values such
as individual autonomy to stress the difference with political actors that define
them as religious values such as the sacredness of life or the importance of the
traditional family.

In the countries belonging to the secular world, much less of a general dynamic
is recognizable in the policy process concerning ART and other morality issues.
Each issue follows an issue-specific dynamic, often defined by the subsystem and
rather independent from parliamentary politics (Baumgartner & Jones, 1993).[3]
Whereas in the religious world, political parties have an angle they can hook onto
morality issues, this is not the case in the secular world. This is because no divide
between secular and confessional parties exists, and therefore the conflict that
would draw morality issues into the macro-political agenda is missing. In the countries belonging to the secular world, the question of whether ART and embryo
and stem cell research reaches the parliamentary arena at all depends on interest
groups and their ability to form alliances with individual members of Parliament
(MPs) who can raise the issue in the parliamentary arena (Engeli et al., 2013). In

general, in countries belonging to the secular world, political parties do not want to take a stance on or draw attention to ART and other morality issues.

The United Kingdom is the exemplary country belonging to the secular world with regard to morality issues. Although, in the mid-80s, it started out with Conservative backbenchers almost passing bills that would have banned nearly all IVF treatment and embryo research (Jackson, 2001), an alliance of scientists and MPs succeeded in preventing this (Jackson, 2001; Kirejczyk, 2000; Mulkay, 1997). Neither the governing conservative party's nor the opposition party's leadership were eager to have issues concerning ART and embryo research addressed in Parliament. Larsen et al. (2012) describe three phases of the Conservative leadership's avoidance strategy: First, it relegated questions concerning the issue to an expert commission, chaired by Mary Warnock (Department of Health & Social Security, 1984). Subsequently, after the publication of this commission's report, it kept the issue off the agenda by not allocating time for debate in Parliament; last, it only permitted fertilization treatment and embryo research to return to the agenda after the 1988 elections severely diminished the number of pro-life conservatives in the House of Commons. Larsen et al. (2012) and Engeli et al. (2013) point out how subsequently a lack of party conflict over ART issues as well as a focus on the economic growth potential of the new technologies involved have resulted in the most permissive regime concerning ART in Western Europe. The British subsystem of scientists and physicians has played an important role in pressing for such permissiveness.

In summary, the policy-making process concerning ART and other morality issues has shown a different pattern in the two types of countries distinguished by Engeli et al. (2012). In those belonging to the religious world, in contradiction to those belonging to the secular world, the regulation of ART issues is contested in the arena of parliamentary politics. The second expectation specifically regards the countries that belong to the religious world: Secular political parties and orthodox religious parties politicize ART issues, whereas Christian Democrats, as much as possible, avoid these issues.[4]

This chapter will answer the question of whether the way ART rules came into being in Austria, the Netherlands and Sweden fits with these expectations of the TWMP theory. In the next section, it will pay attention to the definition and operationalization of central concepts, for example, politicization.

Central concepts and their operationalization

Why can ART be regarded as belonging to the domain of morality issues? How to exactly delineate morality issues from other policy issues is a difficult question to answer, but political science scholars agree on the following common denominator: "conflicts about societal values rather than diverging material interests" (Euchner, 2019, p. 36). The issues concerned typically lead to debates and clashes concerning first principles as well as fights over what is right and wrong. The regulation of abortion, assisted dying and same-sex partnerships but also drugs and guns are policy examples of morality issues under this definition (Euchner, 2019).

However, the latter two subjects would be excluded in Engeli et al.'s (2012) definition, as these authors restrict morality issues to those that address questions relating to death, reproduction and marriage. ART clearly is included in this definition as well as in the broader one mentioned previously. From Engeli et al.'s (2012) more specific definition, it becomes clear that by studying morality issues, the authors want to focus attention on questions that historically belonged to spheres in which religion and the churches had a strong say (Euchner, 2019). What happens to such questions in times of secularization? What other spheres are expected to produce answers and rules: the medical, legal or political spheres?

This brings us to the second concept that needs explanation: politicization. Timmermans and Breeman (2012) define politicization as "a state of controversy in which political parties mobilize support by dramatizing an issue and increasing the stakes of policy decisions". Politicization concerns drawing attention to an issue by political parties, and by doing this, the issue is moved from the personal, medical or other sphere into the political. For example, although the regulation of in vitro fertilization (IVF) in Denmark, Germany and the Netherlands was initially left to the medical profession, the country reports show that at some point in recent history, the issue was put on the parliamentary agenda through questions by MPs, sometimes at the insistence of sections of the population. Thus, the regulation of in vitro fertilization in all three cases (Denmark, Germany and the Netherlands) seems to present examples of politicization.

However, from Timmermans and Breeman (2012) and Larsen et al. (2012), it can be inferred that two additional points have to be made about politicization as operationalized in Engeli et al.'s (2012) compilation. First, there are different degrees of politicization. There is a continuum of degrees of politicization, with intra-political party attention at the low end and government and parliamentary attention at the high end. If an issue leads to a government crisis, it is politicized to a higher degree than if it is only addressed briefly in a debate about another issue. Take, for example, political parties paying attention to an issue in their electoral program or in a report published by their scientific institute. Timmermans and Breeman (2012) do not regard these instances as such as clear signs of politicization. The authors explain how such attention by political parties to morality issues might merely serve a symbolic function, such as paying lip service to internal factions in the party. The authors only speak of politicization at the point when MPs raise an issue in the parliamentary arena, via bills, parliamentary questions, motions or urgent debates (Timmermans & Breeman, 2012). In other words, the institutional level at which ART is debated is an indication of the degree of politicization. In addressing the process of politicization of ART in Austria, the Netherlands and Sweden, attention will be paid to the different degrees of politicization in this sense.

Second, as becomes clear in Larsen et al.'s (2012) description of how IVF initially was addressed in the UK Parliament, it makes a difference whether a few isolated MPs ask questions or submit motions or bills in Parliament or these are MPs endorsed by the political party's leadership. Only if the party's leadership endorses this do the authors categorize this as politicization.

Therefore, this chapter will categorize instances of MPs dramatizing ART issues in the parliamentary and governmental arena as a high degree of politicization (provided that the MPs are not typical backbenchers). If ART is only discussed between political parties in the phases preceding parliamentary debate, this indicates a lower degree of politicization. Neither does the fact of a bill being tabled in Parliament – a formal requirement of law making – automatically lead to politicization of the issues involved. This is only the case if the issues are dramatized by MPs that call them into question.

The choice of country cases to investigate the expectations of the TWMP had different reasons. First, I needed cases for both categories of countries distinguished in the theory. The Netherlands, according to this typology, belongs to the religious world; the Christian Democrat party (CDA) – is historically a strong party. Therefore, in addition to the Netherlands, I needed a country that belongs to the secular world and therefore chose Sweden. Sweden belongs to the secular world, as the religious-secular cleavage historically has not been among the organizing principles of its party system.[5] This is because until the 1990s, there was no political party with a religious signature. In 1991, for the first time, a Christian Democratic party did enter the Swedish Parliament (Aylott et al., 2013). Although rather successful for a short while,[6] it never reached the powerful position of Christian Democratic parties in Western European countries such as Austria, Belgium, Germany and the Netherlands. Since the turn of the 19th to the 20th century, the religious-secular divide has been an organizing principle of the political party system in the latter countries, whereas in Sweden, the party system was organized solely along the labor-capital and the rural-urban cleavage lines (Sundberg, 1999).

Second, Austria, similarly to the Netherlands, belongs to the religious world.[7] However, there are striking differences between the ART regime in these two countries that call for closer investigation. For example, equal access for lesbian couples became the rule in the Netherlands in the year 2000 (in Sweden in 2004), whereas in Austria, lesbian couples had to wait for such access until 2015. A second striking difference might be connected to this; the countries followed different paths in the making of the rules. Whereas in the Netherlands, political debate from time to time revived, in Austria, politicians debated the issues before 1992 and for a short period of time preceding 2015, so ART for a long time had not been discussed in the general meetings of Austrian Parliament.

Austria, Netherlands and Sweden

In order to answer the previous question, in the following, I will address whether and to what extent IVF, mandatory donor registration and preimplantation genetic diagnosis (PGD) became a subject of real debate between political parties in the Parliament – a so called hot topic – in the three countries.[8] Table 11.1 addresses per technique whether and how issues became manifestly debated in the parliamentary arena.

Table 11.1 Did political parties debate the issue in a general Parliament meeting?

	Austria	The Netherlands	Sweden
IVF	The issues involved were only debated to a small extent, as FMedG 1992 was a precooked compromise between ÖVP and SPÖ. The issues were debated to some extent again in the preparation of FMedRag 2015.	Yes. The regulation through Planning Decrees is not conducive to such debate. However, the following issues were addressed: – Donation of egg cells debated in 1989. – Equal access for lesbian couples and single women in 2000.	No, the ban on egg donation was discussed between the medical profession and Insemination Committee but was not an issue of debate between political parties in the Parliament.
Mandatory donor registration	The issues involved were only debated to a small extent, as FMedG 1992 was a precooked compromise between ÖVP and SPÖ. The issue was debated to some extent again in the preparation of FMedRag 2015.	Yes, this issue was raised in the early 90s and agreed on at the end of the 1990s.	No, the ban on donor anonymity was discussed between the medical profession and Insemination Committee but was not an issue of debate between political parties in the Parliament.
PGD	Yes, this issue was raised in the early 90s but only later settled in *Gentechnikgesetz*. The issue was debated again in the preparation of FMedRag 2015.	Yes, in 2008, a proposal to widen access was fiercely discussed and accepted.	No information.

Source: (Country chapters in this book and Hadolt, 2007)

Austria

The first ART law in Austria, *Fortpflanzungsmedizingesetz* (FMedG), was debated between interest groups and political parties for ten years before – after extensive consultation – being accepted in 1992. As in other Western European countries, AID and IVF were increasingly practiced, leading to questions concerning the status of children in family law as well as concerns about abuse of the IVF technique. In the early 1980s, Catholic conservatives were first in urging for regulations. Groups of law scholars, theologians, medical professionals and religious and feminist activists followed suit, together with big political parties such as ÖVP and Austrian Social Democrats (SPÖ), as well as smaller political parties such as FPÖ and Grünen (Hadolt, 2007).[9] Hadolt describes the political process preceding the acceptance of the bill in 1992 by all parties participating in Parliament in four phases (2007).[10] There was a wide consensus about the bill in the Parliament; Griessler and Hager (2016) ascribe this consensus at the moment of acceptance in the Parliament to the precooking that had been done by the governing parties in the years before: The conservative ÖVP and the social-democratic SPÖ each had different core values. However, an intersection existed, for example, between the former's norm of traditionally structured family (ÖVP) and the latter's protection of women from exploitation (SPÖ), and years of consultation and negotiation led to them formulating a compromise. The compromise between them existed of a rather restrictive law that limited access to IVF to married or cohabiting heterosexual couples.

Despite the fact that physicians and other stakeholders repeatedly asked to amend the law, foremost because the law excluded some groups from access to ART, it was more than 20 years before a new law was passed by Parliament. Griessler and Winkler (2022) explain why the Austrian ART regime had been in gridlock for such a long period and why things changed in the period preceding the passing of the FMedRag on 5 February 2015. The cultural process of individualization is pivotal in the explanation of the latter, as it led to pressures for law change through two channels. The first channel was the judiciary, because the ECtHR as well as Austrian's Constitutional Court ruled about access to ART. In *S.H. and others v. Austria* (GC), no 57813/00 (European Court of Human Rights, 2011), the applicants were two married couples who wished to use medically assisted reproductive techniques banned under Austrian law at the time.[11] The ECtHR considered in this case "that the right to conceive a child and to make use of medically assisted procreation for that purpose is also protected by Article 8 ECHR". (Van Beers, 2014, p. 119).[12] The case submitted to the Austrian Supreme Court and the Austrian Constitutional Court concerned a lesbian couple demanding access to egg donation.[13] The Austrian Constitutional Court judged that several clauses of the FMedG were unconstitutional and demanded rectification (10 December 2013).

The second channel was the arena of political parties, as liberal wings had developed in the ÖVP and in the SPÖ that also wanted to make the ART law less restrictive (Hadolt, 2007). The feminists within the SPÖ moved from emphasizing protection of women from exploitation to self-determination. A less religious fraction in the ÖVP became dominant which was tired of the battles fought over abortion and IVF.

In addition to these developments, the background of these changes within the traditional political parties was the breakdown of the dual polar political system – existing in a conservative and a social democratic camp. In 2013, the two parties together only gained 51% of the votes, illustrating how, in the last three decades, voting has become unpredictable and volatile (Plasser & Ulram, 2006). Since the upsurge of the FPÖ in the mid-80s, it has become clear to both traditional parties that they have to compete with other political parties for their share of power in Parliament, henceforth making them try to listen more to the preferences of the voters, at least as far as expressed in the polls. This also played out in renewed attention to demands regarding the FMedG. Added to the fact that the Constitutional Court had not left much room for maneuver, the new attention led to the appearance of the issues concerning ART on Austria's parliamentary agenda. Griessler and Winkler (2022), describe how the populist political parties FPÖ and Team Stronach countered allowing egg donation – which would widen access to IVF – as well as opposing making PGD available, whereas the majority of parliamentarians from SPÖ, ÖVP, the Greens and the NEOS were in favor of more permissive regulations.

We must conclude about the decision making concerning ART rules in Austria that this only confirms the first expectation formulated in the TWMP. The issues involved and the proposals to resolve these are indeed addressed in the political-parliamentary arena, as can be expected from a country belonging to the religious world. However, until the end of the last century, the larger part of contestation and debate was done in the early phases of the political process, making it possible for the political elites of ÖVP and SPÖ to formulate compromises and to precook the decisions preceding the plenary debate in Parliament. This prevented a high degree of politicization of ART as defined and operationalized in this chapter. In addition, after the acceptance of the FMedG, the two traditional parties kept the ranks closed and for decades avoided addressing calls for change. A strategy of depoliticization, or at least avoidance of political conflict, is recognizable here, but, different from what the theory expects, both the conservative ÖVP and the social-democratic SPÖ applied this strategy.

A second deviation from the theory is that the – long-existing – pact between these parties was not cracked by secular or orthodox Christian political parties. Nor did the FPÖ or the Greens politicize access to ART. Instead, subgroups of individuals within the ÖVP and SPÖ did this, encouraged by citizens claiming access to ART in court as well as the fact that ART physicians helped patients in getting treatment abroad (Griessler & Winkler, 2022). The courts urged a review of the restrictive law, and this created momentum for these subgroups to enforce amendments. Notable is how populist parties such as FPÖ and Team Stronach – that have been important in breaching the dual polar political system – in discussing the FMedRag have rather defended the existing restrictive ART regime than contributed to its liberalization.

The Netherlands

Planning decrees regulate the quantity of IVF treatments and stipulate the quality requirements concerning these treatments as well as access to PGD, whereas Parliament accepted a law in order to make donor registration mandatory. In the process preceding the formulation of these regulations, the Christian Democrats in the Netherlands were the first to convey a clear opinion concerning IVF and mandatory donor registration (Weyers & Zeegers, 2022). The party paid attention to these subjects in its electoral program in 1986 (Timmermans & Breeman, 2012). In addition, its Scientific Institute published the report *Zinvol Leven*, among others, claiming that IVF should only be allowed if there was a biological reason for childlessness. Following Timmermans and Breeman's (2012) definition of politicization, as explained in section 3, this is only a low degree of politicization. This allows the conclusion that IVF initially was not politicized to a noticeable degree. The Dutch government used planning decrees as an instrument to prescribe the boundaries within which the number of IVF treatments would be allowed to develop, as well as other requirements. In general, governing through decrees prevents debate from occurring in Parliament. As a matter of fact, it can be regarded as a strategy of governmental parties to evade debate, and it has been applied successfully quite often. However, in this case, after two CDA ministers agreed on a Planning Decree (1989) that in fact put a ban on IVF treatments with donated egg cells, there was a public outcry in the media, as banning treatments with donated egg cells would discriminate against women, especially those without egg cells of their own (Kirejczyk, 1996). After two MPs of D66, a left-liberal party, asked questions in Parliament, the ministers felt forced to amend the Planning Decree before the end of 1989.[14] After this, subsequent governments left issues such as whether to allow using donated egg cells and who had access to IVF to hospitals to decide. This led to diverse treatment in hospitals, some giving lesbian couples and single women access to IVF treatment, whereas others refused such access. In 2000, on the instigation of the Equal Treatment Commission, the minister asked hospitals not to categorically exclude these groups from treatment anymore.

With respect to mandatory donor registration, the Lubbers II government, a coalition of the Christian democrat CDA and the right-wing liberal VVD, proposed a bill on the initiative of the CDA. The bill was briefly discussed in Parliament in the early 90s, with the secular parties showing reluctance to agree with mandatory donor registration and asking for more research into whether persons need to know their origins. At the end of the 90s, the bill returned to Parliament after the Dutch Supreme Court issued the Valkenhorst I Ruling that concerned a woman who had been born in a single mother's home and was refused information about her biological father. With this ruling, the case was settled and the court confirmed the right to know one's parents, referring to the right to personality (Weyers & Zeegers, 2022). Subsequently, the political parties in Parliament developed a consensus about this right, and the bill was almost unanimously accepted in Parliament in 2002.

In 2008, PGD had been heavily discussed in the parliamentary arena after a Social Democratic secretary of state proposed widening its availability by making a wider category of hereditary diseases indicative. Parliament accepted this proposal after fierce opposition by the more orthodox religious Christian Union, under the condition of strict oversight by a committee of medical professionals.

Having addressed rulemaking concerning these three subjects, we can safely conclude that political parties to a considerable extent have addressed issues concerning ART in the parliamentary arena, confirming this part of the TWMP theory about countries belonging to the religious world. The second expectation can be confirmed for how IVF and PGD came to be politicized. Here, secular political parties such as the social democratic PvdA and left liberal D66 initiated parliamentary debate, whereas the CDA kept the issues as much as possible off the parliamentary agenda, among other things by using planning decrees to formulate rules and conditions. However, with regard to mandatory donor registration, the Christian Democratic CDA took the initiative by proposing a bill. This might be regarded as contradicting the TWMP theory somewhat. However, the issue of mandatory donor registration concerns family values; the CDA stressing these values rather than more fundamental religious principles is in line with the unsecular strategy that the TWMP theory expects this party to follow (Engeli et al., 2013; Kalyvas & Van Kersbergen, 2010).

Sweden

The Swedish legislature permitted the use of donor sperm for insemination in the 1984 Insemination Act and in the same act stipulated that donor registration was mandatory. This act had been carefully prepared by the Insemination Committee formed by the government in 1981 with Tor Sverne as special examiner. The issue of mandatory donor registration met with resistance from the medical professionals involved in ART (Singer, 2022). In the preparatory phase of the 1988 IVF Act, the proposal to ban egg donation – while permitting IVF under certain conditions – appeared to be another issue for this group of medical professionals. However, as Singer explains, neither mandatory donor registration nor the ban on egg donation was politicized in the sense of the definition used in this chapter, as the issues were not debated between political parties in the parliamentary arena. With its cautious approach to ART, the Insemination Committee precooked the 1984 Insemination Act, and it did this again with the 1988 IVF Act. Through this process of precooking, it made sure that these bills were widely accepted by political parties and did not lead to fierce discussions between them in the general meetings of Parliament (Singer, 2022; Swedish Government Official Report, 1985).[15] In addition, when the question of banning egg donation appeared to keep simmering in the subsystem of medical professionals (Nordic Council of Ministers, 2006), the political parties did not take the issues up to bring them into the arena of parliamentary debate. Instead, the government assigned the Swedish National Council on Medical Ethics (*Statens medicinsk-etiska råd*), to review the issues mentioned, in addition to a number of other questions about fertilization outside the body.[16] In 1995, this council advised permitting egg donation; in light of sex equality, it argued that infertile women should not be denied the opportunity of becoming mothers via donated eggs (Nordic Council of Ministers, 2006).[17] The Swedish government followed this advice, although the ban on egg donation lasted until 2003.[18] The next relevant step taken by the legislature was to allow lesbian couples access to assisted reproduction.[19] Again, as Singer observes, no real resistance to the proposal had arisen in Parliament. This time, the preparatory investigations by the parliamentary Committee on Children in Homosexual Families had done the appeasement work. This committee investigated legal differences between homosexual and heterosexual couples as well as the facts about children living in homosexual families.[20] In addition, Singer describes the wide consensus that had existed for a long time about the entitlement of children to two parents, which barricaded the access of single women to donor insemination and IVF (Singer, 2022). This barricade is an issue that politicians did address in Parliament: In 2005, a left-wing MP submitted a motion asking the government to allow single women such access.[21] This motion as well as subsequent motions of MPs from five out of six parties in 2006 and six out of seven parties in 2008 were denied. However, in 2008, the Committee on Health and Welfare started an investigation into the matter, and in 2013, the government appointed the Committee on Increased Possibilities to Address Involuntary Childlessness to resolve the issue.[22] In 2016, Parliament accepted legislation enabling single women to access assisted fertilization to the same extent as married and cohabiting couples.[23] Singer (2022) observes that this legislation was widely supported in Parliament, with the exception of the Swedish Christian Democrats.

Does the account of developments in the Swedish rules concerning ART confirm the TWMP theory and the idea that Sweden belongs to the secular world? In the secular world, each morality issue would follow an issue-specific dynamic, often defined by the subsystem and rather independent from parliamentary politics.

With the exception of allowing single women access, ART issues indeed hardly seem to have led to debate in general meetings of Parliament; instead, the issues were resolved by committees predominantly consisting of experts. Two subsystems have been paramount for finding solutions and anticipating possible differences of opinion, as they played a big role in conducting investigations and formulating and discussing the Swedish rules for ART. First, the subsystem of medical professionals specialized in ART and second, the subsystem of experts dedicated to what is "the best interest of the child". When there were potential conflicts because of differences of opinion between the children's rights experts and the medical experts, for example, with respect to the ban on donor anonymity, the former experts won because of the compelling character of arguing in the child's best interests. In any case, things were almost completely settled without much parliamentary debate and without political parties taking much interest in the issues concerned. Issues, such as access to ART for homosexual couples, could be resolved in the course of time, because together with the newly generated evidence, the insights about what is in the best interests of the child changed. In addition, equal treatment (gender; sexual orientation) grew in importance. Although through these cultural changes, most issues could be resolved quite smoothly, this was different for allowing access for single women, as the idea that a child needs two parents appeared to be persistent. The government used the fact that "many women go abroad to have donor insemination" as an inducement to convince Parliament (Singer, 2022).[24]

The only political party that really aligned itself with the issue of ART was the Swedish Christian Democratic party. The 2001 program of this party mentions human dignity as a guiding principle, "each and every person's absolute, unique, and inalienable dignity shall inform the rules and practices of medical ethics" (Kristdemokraterna, 2001). The party has – unsuccessfully – sought to promote this principle through parliamentary motions to amend the Swedish law with a constitutionally guaranteed right to life. This conveys how this party has a more orthodox Christian ideology than the Christian Democratic parties referred to in the TWMP theory.

The absence of conflict and divided debate between political parties about the issues involved in ART seems to confirm the TWMP in the Swedish case. However, precooking things in committees, sometimes involving experts exclusively, sometimes including MPs, seems to be a general characteristic of the Swedish political system. Therefore, the extent to which the absence of politicization of ART (as defined in the TWMP) is convincing evidence for the theory remains to be seen. We have come across a general pattern in Swedish politics that also occurs when ART or other morality issues are at stake.

Conclusion about the TWMP theory

The process of formulating rules concerning ART in Austria, the Netherlands and Sweden to some extent does fit with the TWMP theory about politicization processes. Close comparison of the country cases, however, begs for some reflection on how politicization is defined in this theory and is rather about moving issues to a higher level of contestation than about where politics takes place.

When we look at where politics with regard to ART takes place, both in Austria and Sweden, this is often done in the early – preparatory – phases of law making, more often than in the Netherlands.[25] However, as described in section 3, politicization is about whether political parties mobilize the activity of resolving conflicts to higher levels of visibility and political contestation. In the Austrian case, there is clear evidence that ÖVP and SPÖ actively prevented such mobilization from happening, among other things by forming a pact in the preparation phase of the FMedG and subsequently keeping the ranks closed. Here we see forces at work that counteract and even block (potential) politicization forces, and we might label the former depoliticization. The resulting rather low level of politicization of ART is in fact the sum of these two contradictory forces. This is different for the low to negligible level of politicization of ART observed in Sweden: Here MPs were often grouped together with experts involved in the decision making concerning ART. However, there is no sign that they tried to mobilize the issues to a higher level of contestation or had to prevent other MPs from doing so.

Comparing Austria and the Netherlands might provide deeper insight into the degrees of politicization and the underlying forces. The process of decision making about ART in the Netherlands has known a much higher degree, as on different occasions, issues led to debates in general parliamentary meetings, in the case of PGD even leading to a small government crisis. Secular political parties, such as D66 and the Social Democratic party PvdA, as well as orthodox Christian parties, are the drivers of this process of politicization in the Dutch case. D66 and PvdA sided in challenging rules that restricted access to techniques and in calling for more equality for homosexuals. The orthodox Christian party, Christian Union, opposed the proposal of a Social Democratic secretary of state to widen the availability of PGD in government and in Parliament. No analogy can be found in the role that secular political parties played in the Austrian case. Notwithstanding the presence of secular parties in the opposition, the call for liberalization of the ART rules and more equality in access mostly came from concerned couples who wanted to have access to ART and physicians who wanted to broaden its applications. In the end, only after the courts demanded a law review was this call taken up by subgroups of politicians that had formed within the Social Democratic and the Christian Democratic party, and the bill to liberalize ART rules was submitted to Parliament. Although politicization of ART issues occurred in both countries belonging to the religious world, in the Austrian case, depoliticization seems to have been more successful, resulting in a degree of politicization that was relatively low.

The TWMP theory does not go into how processes of politicization and depoliticization interact. A difference in degree of politicization will result from the interaction between political parties trying to politicize and political parties trying to depoliticize ART issues, as exemplified by the comparison between Austria and the Netherlands. The next section will try to deepen insights into these processes and interactions and supplement the theoretical framework.

Closing the gap in the theory?

In order to explain why ART in the Netherlands has been politicized to a higher degree than in Austria, although both countries belong to the religious world, differences in their political (party) system might be relevant. Euchner (2019) offers a clue for finding a relevant difference in this respect by proposing to enrich theory about morality politics by acknowledging the mechanism of "wedge issue politics". She introduces this mechanism in her work on morality politics in four countries belonging to the religious world: Austria, Germany, the Netherlands and Spain. While endorsing the TWMP theory for explaining how these countries differ from those belonging to the secular world, she criticizes it for not explaining, first, differences in morality issue politicization across these countries and, second, differences in morality attention patterns in such a country over time. This criticism fits with the conclusion of the former section, and therefore the mechanism of "wedge issue politics" might offer a missing link in the explanation.

Euchner describes "wedge issue politics" as political parties politicizing a topic in order to drive a wedge between the supporters of the opponent in order to electorally gain from the division sown (2019). Pointing at this mechanism, she argues that political parties may use morality issues to challenge opponents and that they will do this only when conditions are favorable. The conditions for the political parties to do this are favorable when they are in the position of an opposition party and able to challenge a governing party that is more powerful but also vulnerable to wedge issue politics. Powerful opponents are vulnerable to such politics in the case of intra-party conflict or – in situations of coalition government – inter-party conflict (Euchner, 2019; Riker, 1986; van de Wardt et al., 2014). In the religious world, this is not only the case for Christian Democratic parties but also for the political parties that participate in government coalitions with them. Euchner finds confirmation of this theory in her analysis of how parliamentary attention to homosexuals' rights and prostitution developed in her case studies.

By acknowledging the mechanism of wedge issue politics, the situation of the governing parties comes into play as a variable that scholars should take into account in explaining differences in the degree of politicization of morality issues between countries. With respect to the difference in the politicization of ART between Austria and the Netherlands, we should look into the differences in the composition of subsequent government coalitions in the two countries. Similar in the two countries – more or less – is the frequency of government coalitions that are a mix of a secular party and a Christian Democratic party. In the period of time relevant for ART rules, such mixes existed in the Netherlands from 1986 to 1994 and again from 2002 to 2012 and from 2017 to the moment of this writing and in Austria from 1986 to 2000 and again from 2007 to 2016. However, in the Netherlands, the secular party in the coalition was either a liberal or a social democratic party; the VVD and the PvdA more or less took turns in being the coalition partner of the Christian Democratic party. The Austrian political system is different because the third party that was strong enough to gain governance power was the FPÖ, as the Greens for a long time were still too weak. However, after Jörg Haider and his far-right populists came into power in the FPÖ, this party lost all its liberal elements. This resulted in a strategic position for the strong secular party in Austria that was different from the strong secular parties in the Netherlands: The secular parties in the Netherlands each had the other secular party as a coalition partner alternative to the Christian Democratic party, whereas the SPÖ in Austria did not have such an alternative, as entering government with the FPÖ was out of the question given its Nazi heritage. The ÖVP was the only choice for the SPÖ. Therefore, the incentive to compete with the governing Christian Democrats by driving wedges was much stronger in Dutch politics than in Austrian politics because both secular parties in the former had an alternative to forming government coalitions. In Austria, both the ÖVP and SPÖ were better off by keeping the ranks as closed as possible in order to continue in government. The SPÖ driving wedges between the voters of the ÖVP by politicizing ART was not an option because there was a risk of losing the ÖVP's willingness to govern with them.

As the examples of Austria and the Netherlands show, the mechanism of "wedge issue politics" can help to explain the differences in morality issue politicization between countries belonging to the religious world and through time. In Austria, the depoliticization of ART was a joint strategy of ÖVP and SPÖ and probably therefore more successful. The wedge issue mechanism indeed seems to offer an enrichment of the TWMP theory as it explicitly theorizes the situation of the governing parties. As long as the TWMP theory paid attention to governing parties, it one-sidedly focused on the Christian Democratic parties in this position. By addressing the situation of governing parties as a variable more broadly, the theoretical framework can be improved in two ways. First, it can be acknowledged how depoliticization of ART or other morality issues might also be part of the governing strategy of parties other than Christian Democratic ones. Second, more attention can be paid to the processes of depoliticization of ART issues that occur in addition and reaction to (potential) processes of politicization, how these two processes interact and under what conditions the one prevails over the other.

Conclusion

Engeli et al.'s (2012, 2013) theory that a religious-secular cleavage in the party system is a driver of the politicization of morality issues is more or less confirmed in the Dutch and the Swedish case of rulemaking about ART; in the Austrian case, this seemed to be less so. The latter case offered a puzzle, as in comparison to the Dutch case, it showed a much lower degree of politicization of ART issues, whereas, according to the TWMP, both countries belong to the religious world. This puzzle could be solved by following the insights about wedge issue politics and looking into the situation of the governing parties of the three decades preceding 2016. The situation of the governing parties in the Dutch situation offered better incentives for "driving wedges" in support of the Christian Democratic parties than in Austria, where the Social Democrats also had an interest in the depoliticization of ART.

The assessment of the fit of TWMP theory with the processes of ART politicization in the three countries also delivered insights into some tensions and seeming contradictions in applying the concept of politicization and depoliticization. First, this chapter reflected on how the concept of politicization is concerned with the movement of an issue to a higher level of contestation. However, this higher level refers to the institutional level at which the issue is debated – general parliamentary meetings are, for example, higher than parliamentary committee meetings – as well as a higher level of expressed disagreement between political parties. These different aspects of politicization and the manner in which they are or can be operationalized in research need further specification and explanation. The concept of depoliticization is even more puzzling. First, it cannot simply be seen as a counter-movement – from higher to lower levels of contestation. It is much more concerned with preventing issues from moving to higher levels of contestation. Second, such efforts to prevent others from dramatizing issues and putting these on the political agenda are often less visible than efforts to politicize and at the same time prevent politicization from happening. This chapter noted how the low level of politicization of ART in Austria in fact is the sum of politicizing and depoliticizing forces contradicting each other, the latter mainly blocking the former. The understanding of the political processes involved in ART regulation would be served by a fuller detection of these forces, and clearer definitions and operationalizations of politicization would help to accomplish this task.

Notes

1 I want to thank Erich Griessler and Florian Winkler for thoroughly reading the chapter and providing me with very useful comments and Heleen Weyers for, in addition to this, also motivating me at a crucial moment to continue writing the chapter.
2 These are Denmark, Netherlands, Spain, Switzerland and United Kingdom.
3 Engeli et al. (2013) call for future research that would provide a more detailed understanding of the subsystem politics structuring morality issues in the secular world.

4 Engeli et al. (2012) formulate a third expectation, not addressed in this chapter: The change of government coalitions is decisive for the laws and rules that result from contestation about the proper scope of ART.
5 Sundberg (1999) describes how the labor-capital and rural-urban cleavages instead are the organizing principles of the Swedish party system.
6 In 1998, the party peaked by gaining 11% of the votes.
7 Krouwel, A. (2012) describes how the ÖVP (Austrian Peoples Party) is a Conservative and also Christian Democratic party. The ÖVP originated in the *Christlich Soziale Partei* founded in 1889 and was itself founded in 1945, following attempts to unite Christian Democracy beginning as early as 1870.
8 Since 2017, this technique has been called pre-implantation genetic testing (PGT).
9 The FPÖ is the result of a merger in 1956 of the *Verband der Unabhangigen* and the *Freiheitspartei*.
10 Although FPÖ and Grünen accepted with a proviso (Hadolt, 2007).
11 One couple needed the use of sperm from a donor and the other couple ova that had been donated.
12 *S.H. and others v. Austria* (GC), para 114.
13 The court asked the Austrian Bioethics Commission for advice. In 2012, this commission advised reforming the FMedG and permitting egg and sperm donation and PGD as well as widening access to ART more generally.
14 See electoral program.
15 This committee with Tor Sverne as special examiner was formed in 1981 in order to prepare legislation on donor insemination (Singer, 2022).
16 Regeringsbeslut 1994–06–23 nr 34.
17 In addition, the Council argued against the idea that confusion concerning maternity would arise, as the woman who gives birth to the child is the mother, irrespective of the existence of a genetic link. See Singer (2022) on the amendment to the Children and Parents Code that was necessary to solve the case of a non-genetically related birth mother.
18 Government Bill, Prop. 2001/02:89 Treatment of involuntary childlessness (*Behandling av ofrivillig barnlöshet*).
19 Government Bill, Prop 2004/05:137 pp. 41–42; Parliamentary Committee Report, Bet. 2004/05:LU25 Assisted fertilization and parenthood (*Assisterad befruktning och föräldraskap*).
   In order to give all prospective children two parents, the rules concerning the establishment of parenthood were also amended.
20 Swedish Government Official Report, SOU 2001:10 Children in Homosexual Families. (*Barn i homosexuella familjer*) p. 18.
21 Parliamentary motion, Motion 2005/06:L262 Assisted fertilization and egg donation. (*Assisterad befrukting och äggdonation*)
22 *Utredningen om utökade möjligheter till behandling av ofrivillig barnlöshet.*
23 Government Bill, Prop. 2014/15:127.
24 Government Bill, Prop 2014/15: 127 p. 12.
25 Departing from Dahl's (1961) definition of politics as resolving inevitable conflicts in a peaceful manner.

References

Aylott, N., Blomgren, M., & Bergman, T. (2013). *Political parties in multi-level polities. The Nordic countries compared* (1st ed.). Palgrave Macmillan.
Banchoff, T. (2005). Path dependence and value-driven issues: The comparative politics of stem cell research. *World Politics, 57*(2), 200–230.

Baumgartner, F. R., & Jones, B. D. (1993). *Agendas and instability in American politics* (1st ed.). The University of Chicago Press.

Bonafont, L. C., & Roqué, A. M. P. (2012). From prohibition to permissiveness: A two-wave change on morality issues in Spain. In I. Engeli, C. Green-Pedersen, & L. T. Larsen (Eds.), *Morality politics in Western Europe: Parties, agendas and policy choices* (pp. 62–87). Palgrave Macmillan. https://doi.org/10.1057/9781137016690_5

Dahl, R. A. (1961). *Who governs? Democracy and power in an American city.* Yale University Press.

Department of Health & Social Security. (1984). *Report of the Committee of Inquiry into Human Fertilisation and Embryology.* www.bioeticacs.org/iceb/documentos/Warnock_Report_of_the_Committee_of_Inquiry_into_Human_Fertilisation_and_Embryology_1984.pdf

Engeli, I., Green-Pedersen, C., & Larsen, L. T. (2012). Theoretical perspectives on morality issues. In I. Engeli, C. Green-Pedersen, & L. T. Larsen (Eds.), *Morality politics in Western Europe: Parties, agendas and policy choices* (pp. 5–26). Palgrave Macmillan. https://doi.org/10.1057/9781137016690_2

Engeli, I., Green-Pedersen, C., & Larsen, L. T. (2013). The puzzle of permissiveness: Understanding policy processes concerning morality issues. *Journal of European Public Policy, 20*(3), 335–352. https://doi.org/10.1080/13501763.2013.761500

Euchner, E.-M. (2019). Morality politics in a secular age: Strategic parties and divided governments in Europe. In E.-M. Euchner (Ed.), *Morality politics in a secular age: Strategic parties and divided governments in Europe.* Springer. https://doi.org/10.1007/978-3-030-10537-2_9

European Court of Human Rights. (2011). *Case of S.H. And others v. Austria* [Case Report]. http://hudoc.echr.coe.int/eng?i=001-107325

Fink, S. (2009). Churches as societal veto players: Religious influence in actor-centred theories of policy-making. *West European Politics, 32*(1), 77–96. https://doi.org/10.1080/01402380802509826

Griessler, E., & Hager, M. (2016). Changing direction: The struggle of regulating assisted reproductive technology in Austria. *Reproductive Biomedicine & Society Online, 3,* 68–76. https://doi.org/10.1016/j.rbms.2016.12.005

Griessler, E., & Winkler, F. (2022). Emerging from standstill: Austria's transition from restrictive to intermediate ART policies. In *This book.*

Hadolt, B. (2007). Die Genese der Reproduktionstechnologiepolitik in Österreich: Überlegungen zum Politiklernen in neuen Politikfeldern. *Österreichische Zeitschrift für Politikwissenschaft, 36*(3), 285–302.

Jackson, E. (2001). *Regulating reproduction. law, technology and autonomy.* Hart Publishing.

Kalyvas, S. N., & Van Kersbergen, K. (2010). Christian democracy. *Annual Review of Political Science, 13,* 183–209. https://doi.org/10.1146/annurev.polisci.11.021406.172506

Kirejczyk, M. (1996). *Met technologie gezegend? Gender en de omstreden invoering van in vitro fertilisatie in de Nederlandse gezondheidszorg.* Uitgeverij Jan van Arkel.

Kirejczyk, M. (2000). Beleidsculturen en menselijke embryo's: Een vergelijking van beleidsontwikkeling in Nederland en het Verenigd Koninkrijk. *Beleidswetenschap, 14*(3), 203–228.

Kristdemokraterna. (2001). *Principprogram.* https://snd.gu.se/sv/vivill/party/kd/p/2001

Krouwel, A. (2012). *Party transformations in European democracies.* SUNY Press.

Larsen, L. T., Studlar, D. T., & Green-Pedersen, C. (2012). Morality politics in the United Kingdom: Trapped between left and right. In I. Engeli, C. Green-Pedersen, & L. T. Larsen (Eds.), *Morality politics in Western Europe: Parties, agendas and policy choices* (pp. 114–136). Palgrave Macmillan. https://doi.org/10.1057/9781137016690_7

Mulkay, M. (1997). *The embryo research debate: Science and the politics of reproduction.* Cambridge University Press.

Nordic Council of Ministers. (2006). *Assisted reproduction in the Nordic countries: A comparative study of policies and regulation*. Nordic Council of Ministers.

Planningsbsluit IVF. (1989, juli 20). *Staatscourant*.

Plasser, F., & Ulram, P. (2006). Wahlverhalten. In H. Dachs, P. Gerlich, H. Gottweis, H. Kramer, V. Lauber, W. C. Müller, & E. Tálos (Eds.), *Politik in Österreich: Das Handbuch*. Manz.

Riker, W. H. (1986). *The art of political manipulation*. Yale University Press.

Rothmayr, C., Varone, F., Serdült, U., Timmermans, A., & Bleiklie, I. (2004). Comparing policy design across countries: What accounts for variation in art policy? In I. Bleiklie, M. L. Goggin, & C. Rothmayr (Eds.), *Comparative biomedical policy: Governing assisted reproductive technologies* (pp. 228–253). Routledge.

Singer, A. (2022). From safeguarding the best interest of the child to equal treatment. Legislating assisted reproductive techniques in Sweden. In *This book*.

Stetson, D. M. (2001). *Abortion politics, women's movements, and the democratic state: A comparative study of state feminism*. Oxford University Press.

Sundberg, J. (1999). The enduring Scandinavian party system. *Scandinavian Political Studies*, *22*(3), 221–241. https://doi.org/10.1111/1467-9477.00014

Swedish Government Official Report. (1985). *Befruktning utanför kroppen*.

Timmermans, A., & Breeman, G. (2012). Morality issues in the Netherlands: Coalition politics under pressure. In I. Engeli, C. Green-Pedersen, & L. T. Larsen (Eds.), *Morality politics in Western Europe: Parties, agendas and policy choices* (pp. 35–61). Palgrave Macmillan. https://doi.org/10.1057/9781137016690_4

Van Beers, B. C. (2014). Is Europe 'giving in to baby markets?' Reproductive tourism in Europe and the gradual erosion of existing legal limits to reproductive markets. *Medical Law Review*, *23*(1), 103–134. https://doi.org/10.1093/medlaw/fwu016

van de Wardt, M., De Vries, C. E., & Hobolt, S. B. (2014). Exploiting the cracks: Wedge issues in multiparty competition. *The Journal of Politics*, *76*(4), 986–999. https://doi.org/10.1017/S0022381614000565

Van Kersbergen, K. (1999). Contemporary Christian democracy and the demise of the politics of mediation. In G. Marks, H. Kitschelt, J. D. Stephens, & P. Lange (Eds.), *Continuity and change in contemporary capitalism* (pp. 346–370). Cambridge University Press and Cambridge Core. https://doi.org/10.1017/CBO9781139175050.014

Weyers, H., & Zeegers, N. (2022). Avoiding ideological debate. Assisted reproduction regulation in Netherlands. In *This book*.

12 Regulating change in human procreation

Value changes and imaginaries of assisted reproductive technologies in eight European countries[1]

Erich Griessler

Introduction

More than 40 years after the first child ever conceived by in vitro fertilization (IVF) was born, survey data indicate that Europe is still divided in its assessment of assisted reproductive technologies (ART). An online poll carried out in France, Germany, Italy, Spain, Sweden and the United Kingdom that surveyed more than 6,000 people concluded that, taken together, a majority of 54% of the respondents was positive about IVF (Fauser et al., 2019). However, this relative majority in favour faces a strong minority of sceptics. All together, 46% of the respondents agreed that they "never had, nor would . . . ever consider IVF treatment" (Fauser et al., 2019). Public attitudes also vary between European countries. In France and Germany, sceptics were in majority (62% and 57%, respectively); in the United Kingdom, opponents are a strong minority (46%); in Sweden, Italy and Spain, they were more than a third (Sweden, 39%, Italy and Spain 38%). Another consideration is the diversity of regulations in Europe, as a recent overview again showed (Calhaz-Jorge et al., 2020).

Given the diversity of attitudes towards ART in Europe and the variation amongst relevant legal regulations, this chapter addresses two questions: What can the comparison of the country cases of this volume tell us about differences and similarities of ART policies in Europe, and what long-term changes and trends of ART policies can we observe?

To address these questions, the first section of this chapter will give an overview on ART regulation in our country sample. The second part will explore the country cases for meanings of ART in order to detect similarities and differences and to analyze their development over time. For that, I will take a theoretical position that is inspired by cultural (Douglas, 1993; Elias, 1991; Geertz, 1995; Knorr-Cetina, 1991) and radical constructivism (von Foerster, 1985) and constructivist strands of science and technology studies literature (Pinch & Bijker, 1984), which postulate that technology is not fixed and bound to influence society

DOI: 10.4324/9781003223726-12

in a particular way. In contrast to such a perspective of "technological determinism" (Wyatt, 2008), ART and its regulation need to be understood, as any other technology, as culturally dependent, socially constructed, contingent and subject to change; ART in this perspective has no fixed and universal meaning – it only carries specific meaning in specific discursive and historic contexts.

In the second part of this chapter, I will look into the case studies for such specific meanings in specific contexts and for similarities and differences between the countries. I will also look for shifts and continuities in the meanings of ART and related themes such as attitudes towards the basic availability of human procreation for medical intervention, changes in the significance of marital status, changes of family values and the meaning of parenthood, kinship and relatedness, same-sex relations, surrogacy and preimplantation genetic diagnostics (PGD). Following the aforementioned position of constructivism, I will try to apply in my analysis as much as possible "agnostic lenses" (Metzler & Pichelstorfer, 2020, p. 76), which means to avoid a normative understanding of what ART policies should look like and rather attempt to understand their actual shape, development and patterns.

In the third part of this chapter, I will utilize the concept of "socio-technical imaginaries" developed by Jasanoff and Kim (2009) and will synthesize from the empirical material of the country cases and literature four contesting socio-technical imaginaries of ART. Socio-technical imaginaries express and promote a vision of how science, technology and society are related and determine the path of technological development. They "encode . . . visions of what is attainable through science and technology" as well as "how life ought, or ought not, to be lived; in this respect they express a society's shared understanding of good and evil" (Jasanoff, 2015, p. 5). From the case studies I identify four contesting imaginaries of ART, that is, the imaginaries of unavailability, cure, equality and optimization.

In the last part of this chapter, I will finally summarize my results, put ART and its regulation in a broader historical and societal perspective and draw conclusions for the discussion of ART regulations.

Using the country cases as an empirical basis for addressing the question of similarities, differences and changes has its limitations. Although all chapters address the same questions, each of them does it in its own way, highlights particular aspects, develops a specific story and, as a result, covers the shared topics in varying depth and detail. As a consequence, this chapter is limited to providing a panoramic and granular comparison. More detailed studies of the meaning of ART in Europe and differences and similarities of regulatory approaches, as well as related socio-technical imaginaries, will necessitate further research.

ART regulation in different European countries

Engeli and Rothmayr-Allison (2016) suggest distinguishing between permissive, restrictive and intermediate ART policies and propose categorizing them along "(1) the autonomy granted to the medical community to practice ARTs; (2) the constraints imposed upon access to treatment; and (3) the availability of health-care coverage for fertility-related treatment" (Engeli & Rothmayr Allison, 2016,

p. 89).[2] Whereas restrictive and permissive ART regulations lean one way or the other, intermediate policies combine characteristics of both dimensions. The category of intermediate policies recognizes that "states are not systematically restrictive or permissive in their regulations regarding ART access and parenthood" (Leibetseder & Griffin, 2019, p. 4). In addition, ART policies are not fixed but "change over time" (Engeli & Rothmayr Allison, 2016, p. 90; Leibetseder & Griffin, 2019, p. 9).

Table 12.1 builds upon the typology and data of Engeli and Rothmayr-Allison (2016). They coded permissive ART policies as "broad patients' access, AND broad medical autonomy, AND full/quasi full reimbursement"; intermediate as "patients' access under conditions, OR limited medical autonomy, OR low or no reimbursement" and restrictive as "patients' access under conditions, AND limited medical autonomy, AND/OR no or low reimbursement" (Engeli & Rothmayr Allison, 2016, p. 90). The following table adds the Czech Republic and Poland to their initial comparison of 2017 and updates their data to current ART policies in 2020.[3]

Our sample includes three permissive, two intermediate and three restrictive countries. The group of permissive countries consists of Denmark, the Netherlands and Sweden, which, over the years, moved gradually from restrictive to permissive policies (Herrmann, 2022; Singer, 2022; Weyers & Zeegers, 2022).

Austria and the Czech Republic are examples of intermediate ART policies. Austria's regulation shifted in 2015 from restrictive to intermediate after permissive reforms had been blocked for a long time (Griessler & Winkler, 2022; Leibetseder & Griffin, 2019). Czech regulation combines permissive elements in allowed procedures with restrictive access criteria (Slepičková, 2022).[4]

Germany, Italy and Poland are restrictive. In Germany, the restrictive federal law remains unchanged since the 1990s (Geyken, 2022). Italy did not have a specific law on ART for many years, which led to the development of a "wild west" of ART (Corti, 2022). The situation completely reversed in 2004, when Parliament enacted a restrictive law. Yet, in the following years, the Constitutional Court

Table 12.1 Classification of ART policies in Western Europe.

	Permissive	*Intermediate*	*Restrictive*
Austria		x	
Czech Republic		x	
Denmark	x		
Germany			x
Italy			x
Netherlands	x		
Poland			x
Sweden	x		

Source: (Engeli and Rothmayr, 2016, p. 90; adapted and updated by the author)

rewrote large parts by repealing some of its restrictive statutory provisions (Corti, 2022). Poland did not have a specific law on ART for a very long time and passed restrictive regulations in 2015 (Krawczak & Radkowska-Walkowicz, 2022).

The variable meaning of ART

After this introduction into the variation of ART policies in our sample, I will look into the development of the diverse European landscape of ART regulation. I will probe the country cases for meaning attributed to ART, values affiliated with ART and potential value shifts.

From "unavailability of procreation" to "ART as accepted intervention" – country specifics in the developing meaning of ART

The current political debate in Poland shows that strong rejection of ART exists and impacts today's ART policies (Krawczak & Radkowska-Walkowicz, 2022). The ruling Polish conservatives and the influential Catholic Church perceive ART as transgression of nature. The Catholic Church rejects ART in any form, arguing that "the child has the right to be conceived, carried in the womb, brought into the world and brought up within marriage which unequivocally means that IVF and most forms of heterologous fertilization are considered wrong" (Krawczak & Radkowska-Walkowicz, 2022). This radical position exemplifies a standpoint which considers intervention in human procreation in principle illegitimate and unavailable.

Reservations about ART

Opposition towards ART is, and was, not idiosyncratic to Poland but existed[5] and still exists in many countries and global regions.[6] Comparison shows that all countries collected in this volume experienced in the last decades a value shift from basic scepticism about ART towards increased acceptance. This development manifested in more permissive ART regulation. Yet, countries differ, *when*, on *what topic*, and *in what context* this change happened. The next section will illustrate the basic value shift with examples from our country cases.

In Denmark, government was rather reluctant about ART in the 1980s and 1990s as several examples in this country case show. In its guidelines for physicians, the National Board of Health considered IVF only one of several options for treatment a physician should inform a couple about. In 1996, the spokesperson of the Danish Social Party, for example, described ART as "monstrous research". The name of the respective law, Artificial Fertilization Act, expresses reservation towards ART and implies that the technology is "inherently unnatural" (Herrmann, 2022).

In the Netherlands, Protestant and Catholic Churches opposed assisted insemination (AI) in the 1950s, and only a few physicians were willing to do it. This attitude was in line with Dutch culture at the time, "a traditional religious country with rather strict views on family and morals" (Weyers & Zeegers, 2022).[7] This scepticism decreased in the decades to follow; homologous AI and even artificial insemination by donor (AID) became acceptable. Yet, with IVF, things were different again. In the mid-1980s, many Dutch churches had reservations about IVF. The feminist movement was split; one part was in favour, but others were critical because of the medical risks ART created for women and the embryo and the increased medicalization of reproduction. It was thought this might further increase female repression by men as well as carrying the threat of embryo selection and enhancement. In contrast to sceptical voices, the Health Council, a highly influential, semi-public advisory body to the government, compared IVF with the already accepted technique of AI and did not raise ethical concerns as long as access to IVF was limited to stable heterosexual relationships, which I will return to later in the context of access to ART. Thus, the shift towards acceptance of ART as legitimate intervention into human procreation had already happened in the Netherlands long before IVF was practiced in the context of AI.

In contrast to their Dutch colleagues of the 1950s, Swedish physicians were in general more lenient towards AI, which they had already practiced since the 1920s. In 1947, a government report considered homologous and donor insemination for married couples acceptable. However, with IVF, there was a sentiment of potential limits of progress. It was felt that ART was causing change and raised problems "of legal, ethical and psychological nature" (Singer, 2022). A government committee that looked into AI and AID in 1985 mentioned "a limit (to) be set how far to go regarding manipulations to remedy childlessness". It declared that it "can never be a human right to have children" and used a concept of increasing grades of technology and an idea of "naturalness" to evaluate ART methods. Whereas it considered AI and AID acceptable because of similarities to sexual intercourse, the committee perceived IVF as increasing the degree of manipulation. It recommended permitting the use of the sperm and egg of a married or cohabiting couple for IVF but thought that egg donation was "completely against the natural life process . . . having so many features of technical construction for solving the problem of childlessness that the method is ethically indefensible" (Singer, 2022).

In Germany, the debate on ART was also occupied with the question of whether intervention in human reproduction is in principle justifiable, and, in the beginning, there were enormous reservations. In the late 1950s, the German Medical Assembly dealt for the first time with the question of AI. It considered AI acceptable only in exceptional cases and objected to AID for medical, legal and psychological reasons (Geyken, 2022). In Italy, the attitude towards ART was unreceptive as well. In the 1950s and 1960s, several parliamentary bills tried to ban AID because it would contradict the basic value that family is based on marriage (Corti, 2022).

These examples show that in the beginning, there were fundamental reservations against ART in many countries. The Czech Republic is an outlier in our sample. ART was accepted in this country from the very beginning, and "infertility is perceived . . . primarily as a medical problem requiring high technology treatment" (Slepičková, 2022). Slepičková connects this attitude to the "very low level of religiosity" in the Czech Republic (2022).

From the concept of procreation as "act of love" to ART as high-technology intervention

A key argument in the controversy about the basic justification of ART, besides the previously mentioned recourse to nature, is the claim that ART would change procreation from an intimate act of love into a technological procedure. However, the idea that procreation always happened in an "act of love" is in itself an idealizing myth of the past. Ideals and practices of love and sexuality are culturally diverse, change over time and can differ in one and the same culture between social strata (e.g., farmers, burghers, nobility, even particular professions). In Europe, for example, sexuality has only become increasingly important as an expression of one's self and one's autonomy since the 18th century (Shorter, 1971). The bourgeois ideal of marital intimacy gained importance in Europe only starting in the 19th century, and intimacy between spouses varies between social strata and historical periods (Mitterauer & Sieder, 1991).

Today, the Catholic Church maintains that procreation must remain within the act of loving union between man and woman (Krawczak & Radkowska-Walkowicz, 2022). This argument is not only used in Poland as of today; in the past, it was also used in other countries of our sample. In Germany, a draft bill in the 1960s planned to penalize heterologous insemination by arguing that an "artificial" child did not result from love between a couple, and such practices might affect "the roots of moral order and the human culture" (Geyken, 2022). Similarly, in 1984, an Italian Ministerial Commission considered it in principle also preferable that children should be born "from an act of love of their parents" (Corti, 2022). Although it seems that these attitudes carry little weight in today's political debate, they nevertheless might be important for individual patients and their partners and children (Lebersorger, 2019), as well as for the acceptance of ART in society and everyday life. I will return to this argument later in the context of ART and kinship and donor anonymity.

Change towards acceptance

Negative sentiments towards ART changed over time. In Denmark, a clear indication of the completion of this transformation was substituting the term "artificial" in the naming of the relevant law with "assisted" in 2011. In Sweden, the turning point was giving same-sex female couples access to ART. Then, equal treatment was considered more important than the previously held argument of ART not being in accord with the "natural life process" (Singer, 2022). The German Medical Association, which rejected AI and AID in the 1950s, changed its position in the 1970s as well. By then, it considered these techniques reasonable, though not recommendable because of the legal problems they created. Only in the mid-1980s did the Association accept "extracorporeal insemination and embryo transfer as a therapy to treat infertility" (Geyken, 2022) and work out relevant directives which were implemented by the responsible state chambers of physicians. Italy also experienced a basic value shift. In 1984, a Ministerial Commission advised the government to permit homologous and heterologous insemination in vivo and in vitro in cases of infertility as a medical last resort. In 1995, a second Ministerial Commission recommended allowing homologous insemination but was, however, split regarding access to heterologous insemination. In 2014, Law Nr. 40 prohibited heterologous donations, but the Constitutional Court lifted this ban in 2015 and permitted heterologous insemination both for sperm and egg donation (Corti, 2022). Processes and changes such as these clearly show how values towards ART in the many countries were not set in stone but slowly changed at different paces towards a more accepting attitude.

From ART as infertility treatment to ART as means to create new family forms

When ART was accepted as an, in principle, legitimate and accepted intervention, the question of entitlement to treatment became pertinent. Therefore, the next important value shifts concern family values and the piecemeal transformation of ART from a medical intervention to treat infertility in heterosexual couples into a technology that enables people to have children independently of marital status and sexual orientation. Table 12.2 provides an overview of whether and when this shift occurred in our country sample. The table indicates the year in which access to ART was provided to a particular group. If the year is not provided in the country cases, then it indicates only whether access of a particular group is or is not permitted in the year 2020.

As Table 12.2 shows, the sample is again divided into permissive, intermediate and restrictive countries. Denmark, Sweden and the Netherlands allow ART for married and cohabiting heterosexual and same-sex female couples as well as single women. Austria takes a middle position by including same-sex female couples but excluding single women. Germany, the Czech Republic, Italy and Poland ban both

Table 12.2 Access to ART by country and year.

Access for	AT	CZ	DK	GER	I	NL	PL	SE
Heterosexual married couples	1992	Yes	1997	Yes	2004	1984	2015	1984
Heterosexual cohabiting couples	1992	2006	1997	Yes	2004	1984	2015	1984
Same-sex female couples	2015	No	2006	No[8]	No	2000	No	2005
Single women	No	No	2006	No[9]	No	2000	No	2016
Parental skills	No	No	Yes	No	No	No	No	Yes

Source: (Own compilation from country cases)

same-sex female couples and single women from ART treatment. Table 12.2 also shows temporal changes. Countries with permissive and intermediate ART policies began as restrictive and gradually broadened access. This process of change consists of several steps.

First, all countries in our sample abandoned marriage as obligation for ART treatment and accepted stable heterosexual relationships. That cohabitation became more accepted in Europe starting in the 1970s can be seen from the growing number of children born outside marriage (Figure 12.1). Second, access to ART for same-sex female couples was put on the table. Again, countries in the sample are divided. Whereas Austria, Denmark, the Netherlands and Sweden moved towards opening, the Czech Republic, Germany, Italy and Poland limited access to ART to heterosexual couples living in marriage or in stable relationships. Third, the Netherlands, Sweden and Denmark opened ART for single women, while Austria, Germany, the Czech Republic, Italy and Poland retain exclusion. The following section describes the last two value shifts in more detail.

Children born outside wedlock as example of historical and cultural contingency of family and procreation

Sexuality and procreation have been heavily regulated in the past and are regulated in the present.[10] Attitudes towards, and regulation of, procreation are not uniform; they vary between countries, regions and social strata. In addition, they change continually. The number of children born outside wedlock is an example of the cultural variation of patterns of procreation from an historical, regional and social perspective. Prior to the 18th century, the number of children born outside marriage, then often heavily discriminated against socially and economically and considered "illegitimate", was rather small. After the Napoleonic wars, the numbers increased across Europe, though with differences between countries and regions (Lee, 1977). They declined sharply again at the turn of the 20th century (Sumnall, 2020, p. 365). As Figure 12.1 indicates, in the 1960s, the "golden age of marriage", children born outside marriage were rather uncommon in Europe (Klüsener et al., 2012, p. 149). Still, countries and regions were very diverse. In 1960, the Netherlands had the lowest share of children born outside marriage in our sample, followed by Italy, the Czech Republic and Germany. In Sweden and Austria, the share was above 10%. Thereafter, numbers of birth outside marriage increased dramatically in all selected countries. However, again, countries differ in their pattern. In 2019, 54.5% of all living children in Sweden were born outside marriage; in Denmark, the share was 54.1%, and in the Netherlands 52.4%. However, in Poland, Germany and Italy, the share is lower (25.4%, 33.3% and 35.4%, respectively).

This short excursus on the development of the numbers of children born outside wedlock illustrates the historical and cultural diversity and malleability of the social process of procreation. It also highlights that we should critically question our own assumptions about family and procreation and put them into a wider societal and historical context. I will return to this point later in the conclusion.

Departure from an intermediate station: the "golden age of marriage"

Access criteria to ART have to be perceived against the background of the afore-mentioned trend of declining importance of marriage for procreation and the cultural diversity in Europe in this matter.

In the late 1980s, the Danish Council of Ethics pondered the questions of what constitutes a family and – as a consequence – who was entitled to ART. The committee was divided about whether access should be given to single women. In 1993, the Danish National Board of Health, an agency under the Ministry for Health, limited ART in its guidelines to "treatment for infertile heterosexual couples". Subsequently, the law of 1997 restricted access to married couples or couples living in marriage-like relations (Herrmann, 2022).

In the Netherlands, same-sex female couples and single women did AI and AID starting in the late 1970s. However, access to IVF was a different story. Although the Dutch Health Council, as already said, considered AI and IVF in 1984 comparable and acceptable, it stated that IVF should be reserved for "infertile women in a stable heterosexual relationship" (Weyers & Zeegers, 2022). Likewise, a draft bill in the late 1980s showed a reluctance to treat same-sex female couples and single women.

Sweden also started with limiting ART treatment to heterosexual couples. As early as 1947, a special committee thought that AI should be restricted to married women with consent of their husband. Decades later, in 1984, the Swedish Insemination Act permitted access to AID only for married or cohabiting

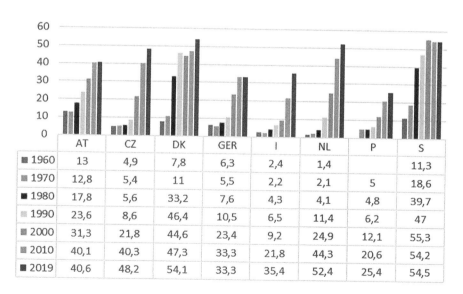

	AT	CZ	DK	GER	I	NL	P	S
■ 1960	13	4,9	7,8	6,3	2,4	1,4		11,3
■ 1970	12,8	5,4	11	5,5	2,2	2,1	5	18,6
■ 1980	17,8	5,6	33,2	7,6	4,3	4,1	4,8	39,7
▨ 1990	23,6	8,6	46,4	10,5	6,5	11,4	6,2	47
■ 2000	31,3	21,8	44,6	23,4	9,2	24,9	12,1	55,3
■ 2010	40,1	40,3	47,3	33,3	21,8	44,3	20,6	54,2
■ 2019	40,6	48,2	54,1	33,3	35,4	52,4	25,4	54,5

Figure 12.1 Live births outside marriage, selected years, 1960–2019 (share of total life births %).

Source: (Eurostat, 2021)

couples. AID was perceived as medical treatment and not as an alternative to sexual intercourse. The law in 1984 stressed that the child should have two parents and therefore excluded single woman. The explanatory to the law stated that this expresses the traditional family, which would be the prevailing view in society (Singer, 2022). Also, Austrian legislators restricted ART in 1995 to heterosexual married or cohabiting couples (Griessler & Winkler, 2022).

These examples illustrate that most countries in our sample started out from a traditional family model: heterosexual couples, living in a stable relationship, which in most countries in the 1980s meant being married (see Figure 12.1).

Disparate change towards broader access

However, all these countries changed their access criteria in the 2000s and 2010s. A development that is particularly noteworthy in this context is the one in the Netherlands. Because of the emphasis on professional self-regulation, it was actually always the medical profession and individual hospitals that decided whether same-sex female couples and single women were treated. This resulted in inconsistent practices across the country. Some hospitals accepted single women and same-sex female couples; others did not. In the year 2000, the Equal Treatment Commission considered exclusion of these groups in some hospitals discriminatory, and – as a consequence – the minister of health instructed hospitals to stop this practice (Weyers & Zeegers, 2022).

In Sweden, opening ART to same-sex female couples and single women took a long time as well. In 1988, the IVF Act limited treatment to married and cohabiting couples. Governmental reports in the 1980s and 1990s concluded that the adoption of children by same-sex couples should remain prohibited because it was "assumed to most likely be in contradiction with the current values of society" (Singer, 2022). This changed in the early 2000s, when a parliamentary committee no longer found justification for this position. Married same-sex female couples were given the right to apply for adoption in 2003, and in 2005, same-sex female couples were permitted access to ART.

Concerning access of single women to ART in Sweden, from 2005 to 2011, a number of parliamentary motions demanded widening access with increasing support. However, the Committee on Health and Welfare rejected all of them, arguing that the child would have the right to two parents, that Swedish authorities were obliged by law to ascertain paternity for all children and that the UN convention would stipulate the child's right to know its parents and be cared for. In 2014, a government-appointed committee concluded that the ban of single women from ART was not justified. In 2016, this position became law. It explained that family norms had changed, single parenthood was more accepted and research showed no indication that upbringing of children with one parent would be unfavourable.

In Denmark, access for single women and same-sex female couples was permitted in the early 2000s. In 2006, Parliament considered ART "no longer . . . as a cure of infertility, but also as a means to make families for people who could not have a child for other reasons than infertility" (Herrmann, 2022). Austria took the decision to open ART to same-sex female couples as the last of these countries. Dissatisfied citizens and the Constitutional Court were the instigators for change. In 2013, the Constitutional Court ruled in favour of a claimant that the exclusion of same-sex female couples was unconstitutional and required legislative change. Today, same-sex female couples are permitted to receive ART treatment, but single women are still excluded (Griessler & Winkler, 2022).

In summary, whereas marriage as obligatory prerequisite for ART was abandoned rather swiftly in all countries of our sample, providing same-sex female couples and single women access to ART took much longer in permissive and intermediate countries and did not happen at all in restrictive countries. However, access criteria do not always include marital status and sexual orientation only. As our country cases show, Denmark and Sweden, for example, also link access to parents' competence to raise a child.[11]

Complex, multiparty arrangements to enable "procreation projects"

ART transforms procreation in many ways: it turns it from an experience in private into a medical intervention and, in many instances, takes it from privacy into the technical ambiance of a semi-public treatment room. It transforms procreation into what Weyers and Zeegers (2022) and Corti (2022) call a "project". Procreation includes an increasing number of "meaningful others" (Lebersorger, 2019, p. 153) such as physicians; nurses; lab technicians; medical assistants; donors of egg, sperm and embryo; surrogates; hospital administrations; intermediaries; brokers; and lawyers. The roles, rights and obligations of these meaningful others in the "procreative process" (Leibetseder & Griffin, 2019, p. 12) have to be negotiated and clarified, and legal and contractual arrangements have to be made. Donor information is one of the examples of contractual definitions which become necessary. In the Netherlands, for example, such registers have to include "medical data, physical features, education, occupation, data regarding personal characteristics, family name, surnames, date and place of birth address" (Weyers & Zeegers, 2022). Similar regulations exist in other countries of our sample.

Not only did ART transform the procreation process in the sense that additional actors are enrolled into it, but ART also annulled two ancient assumptions. The donation of eggs, embryos and mitochondria and/or surrogacy changed the certainty of who the mother is ("mater semper certa"), and sperm donation undoes the supposition – because "pater semper incertus" – that the father of a child is the man who is married to the woman giving birth.[12] Thus, ART necessitates a re-definition of maternal and paternal status, rights and obligations. This change has several elements:

1. Abandoning donor anonymity in favour of the child's "right to know";
2. Breaking up the assumption of unity of biological and social fatherhood and privileging the social father as (irrevocable) legal father/parent;[13]

3. Breaking up the assumption of a unity of biological, legal and social parenthood, which necessitates the definition of complex, multiparty, contractual relations;
4. Breaking up the unity of genetic mother, surrogate and social mother and privileging the latter as legal mother.

In the following section, I will look into some of these changes in more detail.

Moving from donor anonymity to "the right to know"

An important shift in the context of ART concerns donor anonymity and the increasing importance attributed to children's right to know their biological parents.

The country cases are difficult to read when it comes to arguments in favour of *donor anonymity*,[14] because the sources used in reports often remain very vague in their arguments. Weyers and Zeegers (2022), for example, report that prior to the 1990s, it was perceived in the Netherlands as "obvious that children should not be told about them being donor offspring. Informing them was supposed to raise many problems in education and family".[15] Questioning their genetic ties, they continue, might negatively affect the parent-child relation and strain family relations. Not to touch on this sensitive issue was considered the preferential choice. But the nature of these "many problems" remains unexplained in the country report. In the Czech Republic, supporters of donor anonymity argued in 2017 that donor anonymity was important because parents and donors need to be protected "from violation of their privacy" (Slepičková, 2022). Again, it remains unclear what exactly these issues of "privacy" are.

Corti (2022) reports that the use of donation was considered problematic in Italy. In 1995, one faction within the National Bioethics Committee held "that participation of an outsider in the procreative process is seen to have negative effects on the couple's relationship and on that between parents and children" (Corti, 2022). In Sweden, the Insemination Committee "considered it problematic (that) these methods made it possible to create relationships between children and parents not based on genetics" (Singer, 2022). In both country cases, Italy and Sweden, the "negative effects" and "problems" they allude to are not mentioned. In Poland, physicians claim that donor anonymity would be in the best interest of the entire family. Donor anonymity, in combination with the stipulation that physicians should pick donors based on physical resemblance, works as "social neutralization of donation" to blur "the traces of the 'other blood' and physical differences between parents and children" (Krawczak & Radkowska-Walkowicz, 2022). The reasons "neutralization" is necessary remain implicit in the country case.

In summary, the case studies indicate that revealing the donor (1) could create problems in education and family, (2) could call into question established ties between a couple and (3) parents and children and (4) could violate the privacy of a family. Donation could be problematic because it (5) involves a third person in the procreative act and (6) creates relations between parents and children that are not based on genetics. Finally, (7) donor anonymity would enable parents to neutralize and conceal donation.

All these issues are difficult to grasp because they have many conscious and sub-conscious psychological elements[16] and are embedded in complex social relations. They involve questions of identity and identity building (Lebersorger, 2019) and concepts of origin of oneself and of relatedness to partners, parents and children. In an attempt to get a grip on these complex and elusive questions, the concept of *family secrets* is helpful. Carol Smart ranks "reproductive secrets" prominently among such family secrets. They include stories about "illegitimacy, informal adoptions, premarital conceptions and secrets surrounding illicit conceptions and assisted conceptions" (2009, p. 557). She perceives family secrets not as a question of individual integrity but puts them in their social, legal and cultural context. It might be necessary for someone to keep a family secret to avoid shaming; punishment; violence; and the disruption, or even destruction, of important social relations (Turney, 2005). We have to remember that adultery was a criminal offence in many European countries until well in the middle of the 20th century (Corti, 2022) and still is in some countries. Thus, reproductive secrets are not bygones of a less liberal past; they continue and change as legal and social norms change. Smart suggests that "contemporary secrecy over assisted reproduction has its precursor in secrecy over illegitimacy, adoption and paternity" (2009, p. 557).

However, what kind of family secrets are connected with donor anonymity? Jeanett Martin studied the recent German controversy about so-called "cuckoo children" and "ostensible fathers" (2017), which is about men who suspect that they are not the biological father of their child and secretly use paternity tests to reach certainty of their *genetic link*. Martin reports "hate speeches of cheated men" (2017, p. 12) when the German Federal Court decided that secret paternity tests cannot be admitted in paternity suits. The terms "hate" and "cheated" indicate strong emotions. In similarly strong language, observers of the debate liken genetic testing to "bioweapons in the battle of sexes" (Martin, 2017, p. 10). Yet what is the battle about, and how? What are these men cheated about? Why these strong emotions? Martin reports that "ostensible fathers" assert a "claim on certainty"; they "doubt" (2017, p. 10) that a child procreated by a different man has been "deliberately foisted" onto them (p. 12). They feel betrayed by their partners, deceived about fatherhood and taken advantage of, because they raised a child they are not biologically connected to. Their negative emotions are primarily directed towards their partner. Admittedly, sperm donation is not about infidelity and unfaithful partners. But it includes similar themes, like the involvement of another man in conception and the absence of a biological tie between father and child. Yet is this a problem in our "modern" European context?

According to Martin, the increasing public attention paid to "cuckoo children" indicates the growing biologization and naturalization of fatherhood in the context of increased genetic testing. She argues that fatherhood was considered in Europe for a long time a more social and legal, rather than a biological, category. She provides non-European anthropological examples that fatherhood is not always attributed via the concept of sexual intercourse. However, she also mentions that "the topos of uncertain fatherhood is a red thread running through Europe's history and literature from the antique to the present" (Martin, 2017, p. 14) and that there was a "historically consistent worry about cuckoo children" (p. 15). She recounts procedures for how physicians and courts since antiquity have tried to ascertain biological fatherhood, ranging from ordeal, oracle, sworn declaration, physical similarities, blood tests and genetic testing. The significance attributed to transgenerational biological connection is not restricted to Europe. Hörbst reports from her anthropological field work in Mali and Uganda that men are reluctant to use donor sperm because they "would have no corporeal bond with the child" (2016, p. 113). Consequently, it is believed that "neither a man's lineage would be perpetuated nor the spiritual relationship to the ancestry could be granted – both aspects important for many Christians and Muslims in Mali and Uganda" (Hörbst, 2016, p. 113). Similarly, Inhorn and Tremayne (2016) report that it is considered a "moral imperative" for Sunni Muslims to preserve the genealogical "origin" of each child, that is, the knowledge of biological father and mother. Therefore, both egg and sperm donation are banned by Sunni Islam.

The consistent worry of men about fatherhood throughout European history – including the recent phenomenon of clandestine genetic testing – indicates the importance attributed to biological fatherhood in Europe.[17] This has repercussions on the question of donation in ART and *donor anonymity*. Reasoning from the hints provided in the country cases, advocates of donor anonymity argue that it would give recipients the chance to conceal donation and allow the family to keep "reproductive secrets". Anonymity helps to avoid questioning and straining of established emotional ties between parents and children, which partly rest on the concept of biological kinship. It helps to protect the relationship between partners from possible conflicts. It protects recipients and children from unwelcomed interference into their families. Moreover, it saves donors from inquiries by their biological children and potential alimony claims (Geyken, 2022). A more businesslike argument and very different from the previous ones is provided by ART physicians, who argued in several countries against the "right to know" because they were afraid it might decrease the number of donors (Griessler & Winkler, 2022; Singer, 2022; Slepičková, 2022).

When it comes to policies towards donor anonymity, a majority of five countries in our sample, that is, Austria, Germany, Italy, the Netherlands and Sweden, gives children conceived by ART the right to know their biological parents. In Denmark, women and couples can decide between anonymous donation and a known donor. The "right to know" was a constant in the ART regulation in Austria, Germany and Sweden, but Italy and the Netherlands changed their laws towards banning donor anonymity. Poland and the Czech Republic decided for obligatory donor anonymity. In Denmark, it was thought important to keep the option of donor anonymity. Denmark therefore moved from mandatory anonymity to the choice between known and anonymous donor. Thus, there is no right to know in Denmark.

The Dutch case illustrates very well the radical shift from the preference of "not knowing" to the "right to know". The argument in favour most often used was the best interest of the child. However, the interpretation of what's in the best interest of the child reversed completely. As already mentioned, the dominant assumption in the first years of AID in the Netherlands was that donor anonymity was desirable. In the late 1980s, Dutch Christian Democrats questioned this postulation and demanded a mandatory donor registry. They claimed that it would be in the best interest of the child to know his or her father and mother. The knowledge of genetic origin would be important to know oneself. Non-religious parties challenged this assumption. However, the perceived importance of genetic origin took roots in Dutch society. In 1994, the Constitutional Court ruled in favour of a claimant that she has a right to know her genetic father, despite her mother's objection. In 2004, anonymous donation was legally banned, and, as already mentioned, a mandatory register was required that includes the donor's medical and personal data. The explanation of the law elaborates on the right to know

> Not knowing and not be able to know who is your father and mother, affects many heavily, especially those who don't and aren't. Knowledge of genetic origins offer human beings a footing. Without this footing, human beings lack materials which can offer a deeper insight in oneself.
>
> (Weyers & Zeegers, 2022)

Defining new roles

Leibetseder and Griffin suggest to make the "procreative process" transparent by adding every "pro-creator" on a birth certificate. This would include the "sperm donor, the egg donor, the surrogate, the social parent/s" (2019, p. 12). Also, obligations in surrogacy have to be clarified: "the duty of the surrogate mother to be fertilized, the duty of the surrogate mother to cede the child after birth, the duty of the prospective parents to take the child after birth, and their duty to pay the agreed expenses" (Weyers & Zeegers, 2022). Surrogacy contracts include many more obligations which the surrogate has to follow in order to safeguard a healthy child. Additional contractual obligations to be laid down in order to practice ART include, for example, the definition of legal parenthood, regulation of adoption, professional obligations of IVF clinics or contracts for semen donation laying down documentation, traceability, reporting obligation and data protection (Geyken, 2022).

Further significant developments

In this section, I will briefly discuss two other important developments in the use of ART important to understanding overall patterns of use of ART, which I will discuss in a later section of this chapter in the context of socio-technical imaginaries of ART. These developments concern the critical stance of ART policies in our country sample towards surrogacy, which contrasts, for example, the practice in the United States as well as the cautious use of pre-implantation genetic diagnostics, which is limited to severe hereditary diseases.

Surrogacy

AID has been controversially discussed in the countries of our sample. Surrogacy is even more controversial. All countries in our sample discourage surrogacy; however, they do this with different intensity. Austria, Germany, Italy, Poland and Sweden[18] ban surrogacy directly or indirectly, and the Netherlands and Denmark ban commercial surrogacy. In the Czech Republic, surrogacy is neither allowed nor forbidden and practiced unofficially.

PGD

All countries in our sample allow PGD for medical reasons. Denmark allows the creation of saviour siblings.[19] Austria, Denmark, Italy and Germany changed their policies and allowed PGD.

The Austrian FMedG 1992 did not allow PGD. Some Austrian physicians circumvented the ban by offering polar body analysis, which provides similar information like blastocyst analysis but without directly testing the fertilized egg. After many years of controversial discussions, the Parliament passed an amendment in 2015. Today, PGD is limited to strictly defined severe hereditary diseases. Supporters of PGD in Austria argued that it would help to avoid severe hereditary diseases and suffering through miscarriage and stillbirth. In addition, it would avoid "pregnancy on trial" in which carriers of hereditary diseases would be forced to conceive a child, have it tested by prenatal genetic diagnostics and, if found positive, have an abortion. Opponents of PGD stated that PGD would imply discrimination of physical and mental disabilities and hereditary diseases, involve the destruction of fertilized egg cells and select between worthy and unworthy, respectively perfect and imperfect, life (Griessler & Winkler, 2022).[20]

Germany changed its law regarding PGD after long and intense discussion. Although the Embryo Protection Law prohibits PGD in principle, it can be carried out under strict conditions if there is a high risk because of the genetic disposition of the parents for severe hereditary diseases of the child or stillbirth or miscarriage. An ethics committee at the authorized PGD centre checks whether these requirements are fulfilled (Geyken, 2022).

In Italy, Law No. 40 banned all forms of selection of embryos or gametes for eugenics, modification of the genetic heritage or to "predetermine genetic characteristics". PGD should only be allowed for diagnostics and therapeutic purposes which are necessary to safeguard the health and development of the embryo. However, the Constitutional Court ruled against the general prohibition of PGD (Corti, 2022).

Already in 1984, a working group installed by the Danish Minister of Health considered the issue of selecting "certain lives" and emphasized the consideration of the nature and severity of a disease in these decisions. In 1989, the newly established Danish Council of Ethics dealt with the question "selection of lives (as) a pressing and important ethical issue", and PGD was at the centre of parliamentary debate of the report. Whereas Socialists and the Conservatives were strongly opposed to PGD, the Red-Green alliance was more positive. In contrast, PGD was little discussed in 1997 when passing the Act on Artificial Fertilization, and PGD was permitted for fertile and infertile women "in case of a known risk of the child being born with severe genetic disorders or to diagnose or rule out chromosomal disorders". The rationale was that PGD was preferable to abortion in a later stage of pregnancy. This regulation has remained unchanged ever since. The reform of the act in 2006 allowed PGD to create saviour siblings. This was discussed controversially as well. Whereas Socialists and Red-Greens were critical, Liberals supported the amendment, which was backed by the University Hospital in Copenhagen but refused by the Council of Ethics, arguing that "children were no 'spare parts'". The Act on Assisted Reproduction stipulates that ovum and sperm must be genetically unmodified. Sex selection is prohibited with the exception of avoiding serious gender-related diseases in the child (Herrmann, 2022).

In summary, all countries in our sample implemented policies which are critical of surrogacy and which limited PGD to strictly restricted medical reasons.

Sociotechnical imaginaries of ART

After having dealt with diversity of the European ART policies as well as significant shifts of values and practices connected with ART in our country sample, I will systematize in this section my observations by using Jasanoff's and Kim's (2009) concept of sociotechnical imaginaries. Socio-technical imaginaries are "collectively imagined forms of social life and social order reflected in the design and fulfilment of nation-specific scientific and/or technological projects" (Jasanoff & Kim, 2009, p. 120). Socio-technical imaginaries are not limited to nation states, as Jasanoff concedes in a later paper (2015, p. 5) but

> can be articulated and propagated by other organized groups, such as corporations, social movements, and professional societies. Though collectively held, sociotechnical imaginaries can originate in the visions of single individuals, gaining traction through blatant exercises of power or sustained acts of coalition building. Only when the originator's vision comes to be commonly adopted, however, does it rise to the status of an imaginary.
>
> (2015, p. 4)

Moreover, Jasanoff acknowledges that

> multiple imaginaries can coexist within a society in tension or in a productive dialytic relationship. It often falls to legislatures, courts, the media, or other institutions of power to elevate some imagined futures above others, according them a dominant position for policy purposes.
>
> (2015, p. 5)

ART can be conceptualized as scientific/technological project including different imaginaries.

The multiplicity and co-existence of different socio-technical imaginaries is apparent in the case of ART in Europe. From the country cases, I synthesize four different, ideal-typical imaginaries of ART: the imaginaries of (1) unavailability, (2) cure, (3) equality and (4) optimization. They combine different visions of the individual, society and technology and answer the following questions differently:

- Is intervention in human procreation, as done in ART, basically permissible? Why or why not? Who is the dominant actor in answering this question? How strong is the reference to nature?
- What is a legitimate objective of ART?
- Who should have access to ART? What is the meaning of marital status, family and sexual orientation of parents in the context of ART?
- What ART intervention is legitimate (donation, surrogacy, PGD, embryo research, genetic modification)?
- What is the right time for parenthood (age limits and limits of storage)?
- What is the meaning of identity and kinship (donor anonymity, donation)?

Although the four ideal typical imaginaries are on a spectrum of increasing permissiveness, this by no means implies a natural progress over time from restrictive to permissive regulation; neither is there any claim of quasi-natural progression from one imaginary to another.

Unavailability

The imaginary of unavailability is the antitheses to ART. Based on a religious worldview or a concept of original and unavailable nature, it completely rejects this intervention. Instead, it advocates alternative medical strategies to IVF or adoption and the acceptance of involuntary childlessness. The imaginary is based on the belief that human procreation and life are unavailable for human intervention. Churches and affiliated political parties are dominant actors. Having children is perceived as based on an act of love between a heterosexual couple without interference of a donor, either sperm or egg. Therefore, only homologous AI is acceptable. Marriage and, at the most, cohabitation, are the only legitimate spaces of procreation. Traditional family is the only legitimate family form. PGD is perceived as leading to negative eugenics and discriminating against people who are physically or mentally challenged. Surrogacy violates human dignity.

Cure

The cure imaginary considers ART a legitimate medical treatment of infertility. It is based on the idea of helping failing nature and restoring a natural state by healing a disease. As a consequence, only heterosexual, married or cohabiting couples who, for medical reasons, cannot conceive children by sexual intercourse should have access. Parents should be within an age range of "natural" fertility. Same-sex couples and single women are excluded from treatment. The imaginary supports many technical possibilities of ART but maintains the traditional family model. Sperm and egg donation are considered legitimate. There are age limits for women donating to collect eggs with the best chances to develop and receiving egg cells to avoid very late maternity. Storage of gametes is allowed for medical reasons, and there are time limits, again to avoid late maternity. Commercial donation is banned, but in some countries, financial compensation of actual and strictly confined expenses is possible. In most cases, the right for children to know their biological parents prevails, but donor anonymity exists in some countries. PGD is restricted to cases where severe hereditary diseases should be avoided. Genetic modification and surrogacy are banned. Embryo research is only allowed for limited medical purposes.

Equality

The gist of the equality imaginary is captured by an Austrian policy maker, who stated in an interview "in principle, whoever wants children should have them" (Griessler, 2012, p. 54) The objective of this imaginary is to enable all people to fulfil their wish to have children, independent of their sexual orientation and marital status. While human rights are driving this imaginary, in particular the right to non-discrimination, family and private life, it also insists on non-commercialization of the body. Therefore, heterosexual and same-sex female couples, as well as single women, have access to ART. Male gay couples are excluded because surrogacy is banned in most countries. Donation of egg and sperm is permitted, either altruistically or with limited financial compensation. Age limits for access to ART and donation exist; there are time limits for storage of egg and sperm; post-mortem ART is possible. In most of our cases, the right for children to know the donor prevails. PGD is more permissive than in the cure imaginary but still limited to medical indication. Embryo research is allowed for a broader set of purposes than in the cure imaginary. Genetic modification is banned. Surrogacy is not banned but also not encouraged. Altruistic surrogacy is possible, but commercial surrogacy is banned.

Optimization

The optimization imaginary offers all ART technologies that are available today and is open to new ones. It is based on the idea of fulfilling the desire to have children for everybody regardless of gender, sexual orientation and age (by ART, gamete donation, surrogacy, storage of gametes); to have healthy children (by PGD, PND) of the desired gender (by sex selection); to have optimized children with traits the future parents/mother desire (by PGD, selection of gametes and embryos, genetic modification). Claims of ART physicians illustrate the imaginary.

For example, the Austrian Society of Reproductive Medicine and Endocrinology and the Austrian IVF Society argue their demands for a more permissive law with changed family images, self-determination of women and scientific progress. They demand to provide single woman access to ART up to an age limit of 50 years, social egg freezing for non-medical reasons, raising the age limit for egg donation to 50 years for the recipient, giving choice in donor anonymity, abolishing the limitation of compensation for expenses, egg and embryo sharing, using spare eggs and embryo from routine treatment cycles and allowing meditation. Repeatedly, they warn about reproductive tourism if their demands are not fulfilled (Griessler & Winkler, 2022).[21]

Table 12.3 provides an overview of the four ideal typical imaginaries of ART.

The imaginaries express contesting worldviews and differ along questions of access to ART, availability of the human body and temporal flexibility. While access to ART relates to the question of who, according to marital status and sexual orientation, should be entitled to ART treatment, the questions regarding availability of the human body include several issues: Is the human body available for IVF in principle? Is donation of egg, sperm and embryo acceptable? Is surrogacy permissible? Should donation be limited to altruistic donation, or is compensation or payment acceptable? Should sex selection and PGD be allowed? Can embryos which were not used for IVF be used for research instead? Should genetic modification of the embryo be permissible? The four imaginaries take different positions regarding these questions.

ART, by cryo-conserving eggs, sperm and embryos, but also by egg and embryo donation, can be used to extend the span in which a recipient can become pregnant, even when the donor is deceased (post-mortem donation). This increased temporal flexibility of pregnancy allows recipients to adapt their wish for children to their individual biography. To what extent legal regulations allow for technological possible temporal flexibility is connected to societal concepts about right mother- and fatherhood and issues such as: Do age limits for recipients and their partners exist to receive ART, and what are these limits? Do time limits exist for the storage of eggs, sperm and embryos, and what are these limits? Is egg or embryo donation allowed for women above a certain age limit with lower chances to become pregnant because of increased age? Is post-mortem ART allowed? Again, the four imaginaries provide different answers to these questions.

Imaginaries in international perspective

How do the four socio-technical imaginaries of ART distribute in our country sample? In order to answer this question, I categorized their manifestation in the different countries of our sample using the criteria dominant (+++), medium (++), weak (+) and no (-). A dominant imaginary is an imaginary that is the basis for the current ART regulation. A medium imaginary co-exists with the dominant imaginary and is supported by important actors within society. A weak imaginary also co-exists with the current dominant imaginary but has little support from important actors in society. Table 12.4 provides an overview of the strength of different imaginaries in our country sample.

Table 12.3 Imaginaries of ART.

	Unavailability	Cure	Equality	Optimization
Is ART ethically permissible?	No	Yes	Yes	Yes
Objective of ART	ART is in principle illegitimate	Treat infertility	Enable people to have children	Optimize children
Why is ART permissible or not?	Religious belief, cultural customs and nature	Right to medical treatment; cure disease, reinstating natural state	Human rights (non-discrimination, family and private life)	Pursuit of individual happiness
Dominant actors	Churches	Health sector	Courts; individual citizens claiming fundamental rights	Autonomous individual in markets
Access to ART?	Married couples	Heterosexual couples, married or in stable relationships	Heterosexual, same-sex female couples and single women	Heterosexual and same-sex male and female couples, single women
Donation of egg, sperm, embryo	No	Yes, but only altruistic	Yes, altruistic or with compensation of expenses	Yes, payment and commercial mediation
Donor anonymity	n/a	Obligatory donor anonymity or right to know	Right to know	Choice between donor anonymity and right to know
PGD	No	Yes, but limited to severe hereditary diseases	Yes, with a broader set of medical indications	Yes, for broad medical and non-medical objectives
Embryo research	No	Yes, for limited research objectives	Yes, for broader research objectives	Yes, for medical and non-medical purposes
Genetic modification	No	No	No	Yes
Surrogacy	No	No	Yes, altruistic	Yes, with payment and commercial mediation
Age limits for ART treatment for patients and partners?	Yes	Yes (low)	Yes (high)	No (self-regulation of physicians)
Time limits for storage?	n/a	Yes	Yes	No

Source: (Own compilation)

Table 12.4 Imaginaries of ART across country cases as of 2020.

	AT	CZ	DK	GER	I	NL	P	S
Unavailability	+	-	-	+	+	+	+ +	-
Cure	+ +	+ + +	+	+ + +	+ + +	+	+ + +	+
Equality	+ + +	+ +	+ + +	+ +	+ +	+ + +	+	+ + +
Optimization	+	-	+ +	-	-	+	-	+ +

Source: (Own compilation)

Table 12.4 shows that in our sample, all imaginaries of ART are present. However, cure and equality are the most frequent ones. The cure imaginary is dominant in the Czech Republic, Germany, Italy and Poland, whereas the equality imaginary is dominant in Austria, Denmark, the Netherlands and Sweden. The imaginaries of unavailability and optimization are dominant in none of our countries. However, unavailability has medium strength in Poland and is weak in Austria, Germany, Italy and the Netherlands. The optimization imaginary has medium strength in Denmark and Sweden.

Summary and discussion

In the last section, I will return to the questions I posed at the beginning of this paper: What can the comparison of the country cases tell us about similarities and differences of ART policies in European countries and about long-term changes, trends and continuities of ART policies? I will also try to put ART into a historical as well as broader societal perspective and will end with a discussion of what this means for the assessment of ART policies.

A heterogeneous and changing landscape of European ART policies

The case studies show a multifaceted landscape of European ART regulation. In 2020, Denmark, the Netherlands and Sweden had permissive; Germany, Italy and Poland restrictive; and Austria and the Czech Republic intermediate ART policies.

Shifts in value and policies

To make the picture even more complex, the European landscape of ART is in constant flux: ART policies and underlying values change. In broad strokes, these changes comprise several interconnected shifts that I will summarize in this section.

ART was initially received with mixed reactions in all countries of our sample. Positions ranged from complete rejection to unquestioning embracing. However, over the years, all countries departed from the idea that human reproduction is in principle unavailable for medical intervention. Today, ART is a legitimate and established medical treatment in Europe. It is widely accepted that procreation does not necessarily happen in privacy and in an act of love but can be turned into a high-technology medical intervention that happens in the semi-public of a surgery. It is also widely accepted that procreation does not necessarily happen in a dyadic relationship but can involve, with increasing complexity, an increasing number of "meaningful others" (Lebersorger, 2019), such as physicians; nurses; medical technical assistants; donors of eggs, sperm and embryos; surrogate mothers; brokers; and lawyers. The formal arrangement, rights and obligations of these meaningful others are negotiated and (re-)defined. Patients, their partners, donors and surrogates have to cope individually with the consequences of this transformation.

In addition to this basic acceptance, countries of our sample widened their access criteria for ART. However, how and to what extent they did this varied.

As a first step, all countries in our sample changed one access criterion for ART, marital status, from marriage to stable heterosexual relationships. Marriage, which in the middle of the 20th century was a heavily protected social norm, is no longer perceived as the only legitimate family status entitled to parenthood.

Second, access has also been broadened with regard to sexual orientation of ART patients and their partner. Austria, Denmark, the Netherlands and Sweden departed from limiting ART to heterosexuals and provide access to ART to same-sex female couples. Lawmakers in the Czech Republic, Germany, Italy and Poland did not make this shift.[22]

Third, Sweden, Denmark and the Netherlands also shifted towards allowing assisted pro-creation outside dyadic relationships and gave single women access to ART. In these countries, two parents are no longer perceived as a prerequisite to create a family. Austria, the Czech Republic, Germany, Italy and Poland maintain the concept of a two-parent family and deny single women access to ART.

Another shift relates to donation of egg and sperm and the question of whether the involvement of a third or fourth person in procreation as a donor would harm the couple's relationship and the relationship between parent and child. This question also concerns the significance attributed to genetic links between parents and children. Over time, all countries in our sample shifted towards allowing heterologous insemination, and all countries but Germany allow heterologous egg donation.

The donation of gametes and surrogacy breaks up the assumption of a unity of biological, social and legal parenthood. Thus, the definitions of fatherhood, motherhood and parenthood are renegotiated. This brought several changes: All countries of the sample shifted towards privileging social fatherhood. Austria, Germany, Sweden, the Netherlands and Italy shifted from donor anonymity towards "the right to know". They privilege the child's right to know his/her biological origins against privacy considerations that protect ART patients, their partners and donors. Denmark gives prospective parents the right to choose between anonymous and non-anonymous donation. Poland and the Czech Republic decided for obligatory donor anonymity.

All countries of our European sample started to allow PGD in cases of severe hereditary diseases. In some countries, this happened earlier than in others. It also generated more discussion in some than in others. Most countries in our sample allow PGD and sex selection to avoid severe hereditary diseases. The definition of indications for PGD is often left to the medical profession.

In summary, all countries shifted from strongly binding, religiously based and socially sanctioned morals towards a stronger emphasis on individual autonomy, self-determination, equality and non-discrimination. In many countries, the state is no longer perceived as legitimate decision maker in these matters. Still, this shift is slower and more contested in some countries than in others.

Positions maintained

Apart from changes, the countries also maintain certain axioms, such as:

- The legal mother of the child is the woman who gives birth.[23]
- All countries reject the commodification of the body. In many countries, commercialization of egg, sperm and embryo donation is banned, but allowance of expense is often accepted.
- Many countries ban surrogacy completely – in particular commercial surrogacy. The concept prevails that motherhood should be solely built on love. Some countries allow altruistic surrogacy. In many countries, the recognition of parenthood in cases of reproductive tourism for commercial surrogacy generates legal dilemmas.
- In all countries of our sample, positive eugenics for non-medical reasons, including sex selection, is illegitimate.
- Genetic modification of the embryo is not accepted in the countries of our sample.

The practice of procreation as continuously changing construction in a wider fabric of society

At the outset of this chapter, I stated my intention to apply a broad constructivist approach and use an agnostic lens to analyze ART policies. This approach showed similarities and differences between European countries in ART policies as well as several historical changes in the understanding and regulation of ART.

However, literature from anthropology, demography, historical science and sociology shows that these changes are by far not the first and only ones in the history of the social practice of procreation. On the contrary, almost everything that we might consider fixed in this context proves culturally and historically flexible. Our own concepts and assumptions about procreation are often difficult to see, address and understand because we take them for granted. Cross-cultural and historical comparison helps in noticing our ethnocentric perspectives.

In this chapter, I touched upon many culturally and temporally contingent themes in the context of ART, such as the idea of unavailability of life, concepts and practices of sexuality and procreation (Foucault, 1983; Shorter, 1971), the concept and role of children (Aries, 1978), parents and family (Mitterauer & Sieder, 1991), attitudes towards children born outside marriage (Klüsener et al., 2012; Lee, 1977; Shorter, 1971; Sumnall, 2020), sentiments like motherly (Badinter, 1988) and parental affection (Mitterauer & Sieder, 1991), kinship and relatedness (Hörbst, 2016; Martin, 2017) and the process of individuation (Lebersorger, 2019), as well as the importance and ambivalence of family secrets (Smart, 2009). The previously mentioned shifts in ART policies are elements in this constant line of historical transformation.

ART, which dawned in the 1950s and picked up speed after 1978 when the first IVF baby was born, proves to be one in a continuous succession of historical changes in the practice of human procreation. However, ART brings particularly far-reaching changes because it is an "enabling technology", which means a technology that, in combination with others, creates radical and often unexpected change. ART, in combination with cryo-conservation, genetic testing, genome editing, cloning and embryo research, generated and keeps generating a "veritable explosion" (Inhorn & Tremayne, 2016) of new possibilities in human reproduction (Metzl, 2019). Already in 1982, the U.S. American ART pioneer Howard J. Jones discussed a potential "domino effect" of IVF, leading to procedures such as "genetic manipulation, i.e. embryo modification, surrogate motherhood, cloning, and such" (p. 148).[24]

How can we explain the shifts in values and attitudes towards ART, procreation, sexuality and family values identified in this volume? They cannot solely and simply be attributed to a vague process of "modernization" (Sumnall, 2020, p. 365), "liberalization" or "sexual revolution", which is understood as departing from strict morals propagated by churches and a growing understanding of sexuality as a way of hedonistic self-expression and autonomy (Shorter, 1971). Churches and state often lost a grip on people's sexuality and lamented their immorality (Lee, 1977; Mitterauer & Sieder, 1991).

Historians repeatedly point out that changes in procreation are embedded in broader transformation of the "wider fabric of society" (Sumnall, 2020, p. 365). This wider fabric includes, for example, available natural and financial resources; social organization of work; demand for human labour; marriage restrictions; courting patterns; and family, marriage and inheritance laws (Mitterauer & Sieder, 1991; Sumnall, 2020). The values shift identified in this chapter and the increasing as well as diversifying practice of ART must be understood against the backdrop of such changes in the wider fabric of society. However, what is today's wider fabric of society? I suggest positioning the rise of ART within the wider fabric of a neo-liberal economy and social organization of work, which prioritizes paid labour, limits the function of the family to social placement and emotional functions and outsources important parts of childcare to semiprofessionals and professionals. In an ideal typical form, a neo-liberal regime of ART includes:[25]

- The idea that the human body is available in procreation for medical intervention. This includes the acceptability of donation of sperm, eggs and embryos.[26]

- Body products and parts of the body as well as reproductive services are available and tradable in a free globalized "reproductive market" (Van Beers, 2014, p. 105) which takes advantage of legal differences and economic inequality.
- Full temporal flexibility of procreation by storage of eggs, sperm and embryos without age restrictions for donors and recipients.
- Full spatial flexibility of procreation by mobility of donors, donations, recipients and surrogate mothers in a free global reproductive market.
- Individual self-determination primarily interpreted as consumer power and economic freedom of recipients to buy and of donors to sell bodily products, parts and reproductive services.

The rise and diversification of ART, the transformation of values and attitudes connected with ART and a neo-liberal economy are intertwined developments; ART both results from and fuels a neo-liberal economic regime.

The process of normalization of ART

As already described, many countries of our sample experienced within 40 years a massive, and in some countries at times heavily contested, transformation of values concerning the legitimacy of intervention into human life, different forms of sexuality, gender issues and family values, kinship and autonomy. This value change is closely interrelated with but not limited to the growing technological possibilities of ART in combination with other life science technologies.

The change of reproductive practices and the accompanying shift of value and policies from restrictive to permissive can be described as a process of normalization of ART. Once normalization is accomplished, ART seems rational, indisputable and normal. Normalization has a dual nature; it carries an element of liberalization, but it also has emotional and economic costs on collective and individual level (e.g., Lebersorger, 2019). Previous reproductive practices appear outdated, at odds and irrational, even irresponsible, and people who stick to them might experience pressure to justify their decision (Maasen, 2008).[27]

The case studies provide several examples of accomplished normalization of ART, for example, the already mentioned renaming of the Danish Act on Artificial Reproduction to the Act on Assisted Reproduction. To give another example, in the Netherlands, it is now "acceptable to procreate in other ways than via sexual intercourse and in addition to the traditional family other ways of living with children are acknowledged and accepted" (Weyers & Zeegers, 2022). Since 2003, Sweden has a "more open view towards assisted reproduction" which allows an increased pace in the development of ART regulation (Singer, 2022).

Discussion

What can we learn from an international and historical comparison of the development of ART policies?

First, historic comparison indicates that concepts and practices of procreation, family and kinship are neither universal nor fixed. They are culturally diverse, constructed and in constant flux. We cannot base our judgement on an ethnocentric idea of original states of procreation and family that need to be preserved and which justify restrictions and lead to banning permissive ART policies.

Second, international comparison also shows that there is no quasi-natural progress towards permissiveness. In contrast, several competing socio-technical imaginaries of ART, which are based on very different worldviews, co-exist in Europe. Certain values are stronger in one country than in others; certain shifts did not occur in some countries and maybe will never happen at all. History plays a role in the regulation of ART. Comparison shows that changes in ART regulation are not predestined, linear, uniform or irreversible. Thus, neither can we use the idea of quasi-natural technological progress to legitimate permissive ART policies.

Third, historical comparison also shows that understandings and practices of family, procreation and sexuality are always connected to a wider economic and social fabric which might not become apparent to contemporary members of the respective society. Thus, what people desire, aspire to and yearn for and how they perceive themselves, their family and children are strongly connected to the economic and social make-up of the society they live in. This also applies to us and the society we live in. Thus, our own desires and wishes are not unquestionable, independent and an absolute reference point. Current western society ideals, including the idea of an independent individual, emerge within the wider fabric of a neo-liberal economy. Individual and society, and the very idea that there is something like an individual, are inseparably intertwined (Elias, 1991). Therefore, we must also reflect our own wishes and aspirations and cannot use them as the sole basis to legitimate particular ART policies.

The changes triggered by ART as enabling technology are vast and far reaching, and they will further grow with further technological development. Societies must cope with these changes and make choices. Historical and cross-cultural comparison shows that the number and complexity of ethical, legal, social and psychological aspects connected with ART is abundant. ART even cuts to the very questions of self-formation. Comparison also shows that there are no simple answers on how to regulate ART. It throws us back to the conclusion that we can make choices and must make well-reasoned decisions. It also shows that we can no longer justify our decisions with readymade concepts from religion, nature, ideas of a quasi-natural progress or our own desires. Comparison proves none of them are stable and unquestionable reference points. One way out of this dilemma could be to weigh our individual and collective decisions using the principles of bioethics and assess what the use of ART concretely means for all involved actors in terms of their autonomy, in terms of beneficence and non-maleficence and in terms of justice.

Notes

1   I want to thank Anna Krawczak, Doris Leibetseder, Janne Rothmar-Herrmann, Anna Singer, Lenka Slepičková, Florian Winkler, Heleen Weyers and Nicolle Zeegers for their encouragement and their valuable comments on earlier versions of this chapter. I also want to thank Shauna Stack for language editing.

2 These are not the only possible criteria to categorize ART policies. Leibetseder and Griffin (2019, p. 3), for example, suggest additional criteria to reflect the situation of trans and queer people.

3 Engel and Rothmayr-Allison covered of our country sample: Austria, Denmark, Germany, Italy, the Netherlands, Sweden.

4 Despite its in many ways permissive ART policies, treatment of single women and same-sex female couples is controversial and prohibited in the Czech Republic. Until 2006, ministerial guidelines restricted access to medical conditions and married couples. Then, non-married heterosexual couples living in stable relationships were included. In 2008 and 2017, attempts to open ART failed in Parliament because of opposition from conservative parties and the Church. Church representatives argued that this would eliminate fatherhood and contradict the ideal type of family with biological parents. In 2017, government was split on this issue. In daily life, however, restrictions are side-stepped by presenting "fake" partners to physicians. They are not obliged to verify the nature of the relationship between partners (Slepičková, 2022).

5 For personal recollections of physicians who developed ART in the 1970s and 1980s about early protests, see Cohen et al. (2005); for ART physicians' rejection of such criticism, see Jones (1982).

6 Scepticism towards ART is not limited to Europe and the United States. For the diversity of perspectives on ART in Islam, see Inhorn and Tremayne (2016). For different attitudes towards ART in Africa, see Hörbst (2016).

7 The low numbers of children born outside marriage in the Netherlands of the 1960s illustrate these "strict morals" (see Figure 12.1).

8 In Germany, ART is only available for heterosexual couples who are either married or live in a stable relationship. Professional self-regulation of the German Medical Association, which was adopted by most of the 17 State Chambers of Physicians, excludes single women and same-sex female couples from treatment (Geyken, 2022).

9 See endnote 8.

10 One of the most prominent scholars who showed this is Michel Foucault (1983).

11 Danish law stipulates that "intended parents must not give rise to doubts in terms of their ability to care for the child after birth". Regional authorities decide on access (Herrmann, 2022). The Swedish law stipulated that physicians should assess whether the would-be parents' medical, social and psychological circumstances would allow the child to grow up under good conditions (Singer, 2022).

12 On the other hand, today, genetic testing provides the means to ascertain fatherhood, which generates new problems (see below).

13 In many countries, such as, Austria, Germany and Sweden, the potential impact of ART, in particular egg and sperm donation, on family law sparked regulatory efforts. The Italian and Swedish cases demonstrate the consequences of this question for children. In the 1950s and 1990, Italian courts permitted disavowal of fatherhood after AID in several cases (Corti, 2022). In Sweden, the Supreme Court decided in 1983 in favour of a claimant who wanted to revoke fatherhood after his divorce of a child which was conceived by anonymous AID. This decision left the child without a biological father and indicated that new regulation was necessary (Singer, 2022).

14 For aspects of the discussion whether to tell children about ART and donation, see, for example, Martin (2017), Lebersorger (2019) or Smart (2009).

15 This perception was also held in the United Kingdom. For a short discussion on "the right to know", see Smart (2009).

16 Conscious and unconscious elements of ART might impact the conjugal and parent-child relationship but also have psychological consequences for the child's development. For a short discussion of these issues from a psychoanalytical perspective, see Lebersorger (2019).

17 This section focused on donor anonymity in sperm donation. Literature suggests that attitudes of intending mothers towards egg donation are different, because they are in constant connection with their child during pregnancy (Hörbst, 2016). ART adjusts to the importance ascribed to bonding with the unborn child during pregnancy. A newspaper reported in 2018 on ART for a U.S. American same-sex female couple in which both parents carried the baby for some time during pregnancy (Steussy, 2018).

18 There is no explicit ban on surrogacy in Sweden, but Swedish law does not enable it. There is no explicit ban on commercial surrogacy; no form of surrogacy is legally recognized (Singer, 2022).

19 A saviour sibling is "a child who is born with particular genes that have been chosen in order to treat an older brother or sister who has a disease" (Cambridge Dictionary, 2021)

20 Polish conservative groups who oppose PGD refer to PGD as "Nazi eugenics" (Krawczak & Radkowska-Walkowicz, 2022).

21 For an illustrative example of the optimization imaginary, see Metzl (2019).

22 However, we also have to bear in mind that legal regulation and practice of ART do not always coincide (see, for example, endnote 4).

23 Adoption is an exception to this rule.

24 However, he refused to discuss these far-reaching consequences of IVF and insisted instead on limiting the assessment of IVF to IVF itself and excluding the already dawning future possibilities from discussion. "These should only be discussed when they arise" (Jones, 1982, p. 148). These, as I would call it, salami tactics of technology assessment are pervasive and not limited to ART. This eases the introduction of enabling technologies by systematically underplaying their impact. By focusing on one single technology at a time and refusing to take a systemic and future-oriented view, the vast societal impact of IVF in combination with other technologies remains outside perspective and thus always unaddressed. Therefore, technology assessment of an enabling technology is often not comprehensive but remains a sequence of single and fragmented assessments of individual technologies that have to accept previous fait accompli.

25 For a critique of this neo-liberal regime in general, and circumventive tourism in particular, see van Beers (2014).

26 An example for this position is again Howard H. Jones, who refers to the U.S. Bill of Rights and states: "No one is required to seek such benefits as may be available from abortion or from in vitro fertilization. . . . It is fundamental to our freedom that the rights of those who wish to participate in these programs not be compromised" (1982, p. 149).

27 Metzl (2019) is a good example to illustrate how a justification imperative develops in ART and exercises power on individual level.

References

Aries, P. (1978). *Geschichte der Kindheit* (1st ed.). Deutscher Taschenbuch Verlag.

Badinter, E. (1988). *Die Mutterliebe. Geschichte eines Gefühls vom 17. Jahrhundert bis heute.* Piper Verlag GmbH.

Calhaz-Jorge, C., De Geyter, C. h, Kupka, M. S., Wyns, C., Mocanu, E., Motrenko, T., Scaravelli, G., Smeenk, J., Vidakovic, S., & Goossens, V. (2020). Survey on ART and IUI: Legislation, regulation, funding and registries in European countries: The European IVF-monitoring consortium (EIM) for the European society of human reproduction and embryology (ESHRE). *Human Reproduction Open*, 2020(1), 1–15. https://doi.org/10.1093/hropen/hoz044

Cambridge Dictionary. (2021). *Savior sibling.* https://dictionary.cambridge.org/dictionary/english/saviour-sibling

Cohen, J., Trounson, A., Dawson, K., Jones, H., Hazekamp, J., Nygren, K.-G., & Hamberger, L. (2005). The early days of IVF outside the UK. *Human Reproduction Update, 11*(5), 439–459. https://doi.org/10.1093/humupd/dmi016

Corti, I. (2022). Assisted procreation in Italy: A long and winding road. In *This Book.*

Douglas, M. (1993). *Ritual, Tabu und Körpersymbolik. Sozialanthropologische Studien in Industriegesellschaft und Stammeskultur.* Suhrkamp.

Elias, N. (1991). *Die Gesellschaft der Individuen.* Suhrkamp.

Engeli, I., & Rothmayr Allison, C. (2016). Governing new reproductive technologies across Western Europe: The gender dimension. In M. Lie & N. Lykke (Eds.), *Assisted reproduction across borders: Feminist perspectives on normalizations, disruptions and transmissions* (1st ed., pp. 87–99). Routledge.

Eurostat. (2021). *Live birth outside marriage, selected years, 1960–2019 (share of total life births, %).* Retrieved October 10, 2021, from https://ec.europa.eu/eurostat/statistics-explained/images/4/42/Live_births_outside_marriage%2C_selected_years%2C_1960-2019_%28share_of_total_live_births%2C_%25%29_May_2021.png

Fauser, B. C. J. M., Boivin, J., Barri, P. N., Tarlatzis, B. C., Schmidt, L., & Levy-Toledano, R. (2019). Beliefs, attitudes and funding of assisted reproductive technology: Public perception of over 6,000 respondents from 6 European countries. *PLoS One, 14*(1), e0211150. https://doi.org/10.1371/journal.pone.0211150

Foucault, M. (1983). *Der Wille zum Wissen. Sexualität und Wahrheit 1* (1st ed.). Suhrkamp Taschenbuch Wissenschaft.

Geertz, C. (1995). *Dichte Beschreibung. Beiträge zum Verstehen kultureller Systeme.* Suhrkamp.

Geyken, S. (2022). A regulatory jungle: The law on assisted reproduction in Germany. In *This book.*

Griessler, E. (2012). *'Selbstbestimmung' versus 'Kind als Schaden' und 'Familie': Die politische Debatte um Pränataldiagnostik und Eizellspende in Österreich anhand der Beispiele des Entwurfs zum Schadenersatzänderungsgesetz und des Urteils des Europäischen Gerichtshofs für Menschenrechte* (Sociological Series). IHS. https://irihs.ihs.ac.at/id/eprint/2123/

Griessler, E., & Winkler, F. (2022). Emerging from standstill: Austria's transition from restrictive to intermediate ART policies. In *This book.*

Herrmann, J. R. (2022). Taming technology: Assisted reproduction in Denmark. In *This book.*

Hörbst, V. (2016). 'You cannot do IVF in Africa as in Europe': The making of IVF in Mali and Uganda. *Reproductive Biomedicine & Society Online, 2,* 108–115. https://doi.org/10.1016/j.rbms.2016.07.003

Inhorn, M. C., & Tremayne, S. (2016). Islam, assisted reproduction, and the bioethical aftermath. *Journal of Religion and Health, 55*(2), 422–430. https://doi.org/10.1007/s10943-015-0151-1

Jasanoff, S. (2015). Future imperfect: Science, technology and the imaginations of modernity. In S. Jasanoff & S.-H. Kim (Eds.), *Dreamscapes of modernity: Sociotechnical imaginaries and the fabrication of power* (pp. 1–33). The University of Chicago Press.

Jasanoff, S., & Kim, S.-H. (2009). Containing the atom: Sociotechnical imaginaries and nuclear power in the United States and South Korea. *Minerva, 47,* 119–146. https://doi.org/10.1007/s11024-009-9124-4

Jones, H. W. (1982). The ethics of in vitro fertilization – 1982. *Fertility and Sterility, 37*(2), 146–149. https://doi.org/10.1016/S0015-0282(16)46030-9

Klüsener, S., Perelli-Harris, B., & Sánchez Gassen, N. (2012). Spatial aspects of the rise of nonmarital fertility across Europe since 1960: The role of states and regions in shaping patterns of change. *European Journal of Population/Revue Européenne de Démographie*, 29(2), 137–165. https://doi.org/10.1007/s10680-012-9278-x

Knorr-Cetina, K. (1991). *Die Fabrikation von Erkenntnis. Zur Anthropologie der Naturwissenschaft*. Suhrkamp.

Krawczak, A., & Radkowska-Walkowicz, M. (2022). IVF in Poland: From political debates to biomedical practices. In *This book*.

Lebersorger, K. (2019). "Als das Wünschen nicht geholfen hat" – Urszene, Ödipuskomplex und Familienroman in Zeiten assistierter Reproduktion. In U. Kadi, S. Schlüter, & E. Skale (Eds.), *Mutter, Vater und andere Genealogien* (pp. 148–161). Eigenverlag der Wiener Psychoanalytischen Akademie.

Lee, W. R. (1977). Bastardy and the socioeconomic structure of South Germany. *The Journal of Interdisciplinary History*, 7(3), 403–425. https://doi.org/10.2307/202573

Leibetseder, D., & Griffin, G. (2019). States of reproduction: The co-production of queer and trans parenthood in three European countries. *Journal of Gender Studies*, 29(3), 310–324. https://doi.org/10.1080/09589236.2019.1636773

Maasen, S. (2008). Bio-ästhetische Gouvernementalität – Schönheitschirurgie als Biopolitik. In P.-I. Villa (Ed.), *Schön normal: Manipulationen am Körper als Technologien des Selbst* (pp. 99–118). Transcript Verlag.

Martin, J. (2017). Auf der Suche nach dem ›richtigen‹ Vater: Aktuelle Debatten um ›Kuckuckskinder‹ in Deutschland. *ZIF-Mitteilungen*, 2, 11–20.

Metzl, J. (2019). *Hacking Darwin: Genetic engineering and the future of humanity*. Sourcebooks, Inc.

Metzler, I., & Pichelstorfer, A. (2020). Embryonic silences: Human life between biomedicine, religion, and state authorities in Austria. In M. Weiberg-Salzmann & U. Willems (Eds.), *Religion and biopolitics* (pp. 73–96). Springer International Publishing. https://doi.org/10.1007/978-3-030-14580-4_4

Mitterauer, M., & Sieder, R. (1991). *Vom Patriarchat zur Partnerschaft. Zum Strukturwandel der Familie* (5th ed.). Beck'sche Reihe.

Pinch, T. J., & Bijker, W. E. (1984). The social construction of facts and artefacts: Or how the sociology of science and the sociology of technology might benefit each other. *Social Studies of Science*, 14(3), 399–441. JSTOR.

Shorter, E. (1971). Illegitimacy, sexual revolution, and social change in modern Europe. *The Journal of Interdisciplinary History*, 2(2), 237–272. https://doi.org/10.2307/202844

Singer, A. (2022). From safeguarding the best interest of the child to equal treatment. Legislating assisted reproductive techniques in Sweden. In *This book*.

Slepičková, L. (2022). Assisted reproduction in the Czech Republic. In *This book*.

Smart, C. (2009). Family secrets: Law and understandings of openness in everyday relationships. *Journal of Social Policy*, 38(4), 551–567. https://doi.org/10.1017/S0047279409003237

Steussy, L. (2018, October 29). Same-sex couple makes history by carrying same baby. *New York Post*. https://nypost.com/2018/10/29/same-sex-couple-makes-history-by-carrying-same-baby/

Sumnall, C. (2020). The social and legal reception of illegitimate births in the Gurk Valley, Austria, 1868–1945. *Studies in Church History*, 56, 362–382. https://doi.org/10.1017/stc.2019.20

Turney, L. (2005). Paternity secrets: Why women don't tell. *Journal of Family Studies*, 11(2), 227–248. https://doi.org/10.5172/jfs.327.11.2.227

Van Beers, B. C. (2014). Is Europe 'giving in to baby markets?' Reproductive tourism in Europe and the gradual erosion of existing legal limits to reproductive markets. *Medical Law Review*, 23(1), 103–134. https://doi.org/10.1093/medlaw/fwu016

von Foerster, H. (1985). *Sicht und Einsicht. Versuche zu einer operativen Erkenntnistheorie.* Springer.

Weyers, H., & Zeegers, N. E. H. M. (2022). Avoiding ideological debate. Assisted reproduction regulation in Netherlands. In *This book*.

Wyatt, S. (2008). Technological determinism is dead; Long live technological determinism. In E. J. Hackett, O. Amsterdamska, M. E. Lynch, & J. Wajcman (Eds.), *The handbook of science and technology studies* (3rd ed., pp. 165–180). MIT Press.

Index

Note: Page numbers in **bold** indicate a table on the corresponding page. Page numbers followed by "n" indicate a note.

For Product Safety Concerns and Information please contact our EU representative GPSR@taylorandfrancis.com Taylor & Francis Verlag GmbH, Kaufingerstraße 24, 80331 München, Germany

Printed and bound by CPI Group (UK) Ltd, Croydon, CR0 4YY

08/06/2025

01897008-0012